# Neurological and Developmental Outcomes of High-Risk Neonates

*Editors*

NATHALIE L. MAITRE
ANDREA F. DUNCAN

# CLINICS IN PERINATOLOGY

www.perinatology.theclinics.com

*Consulting Editor*
LUCKY JAIN

March 2023 • Volume 50 • Number 1

**ELSEVIER**

1600 John F. Kennedy Boulevard • Suite 1800 • Philadelphia, Pennsylvania, 19103-2899

http://www.theclinics.com

**CLINICS IN PERINATOLOGY Volume 50, Number 1**
**March 2023 ISSN 0095-5108, ISBN-13: 978-0-323-96191-2**

Editor: Kerry Holland
Developmental Editor: Karen Justine S. Dino

Clinics in Perinatology (ISSN 0095-5108) is published quarterly by Elsevier Inc., 360 Park Avenue South, New York, NY 10010-1710. Months of issue are March, June, September, and December. Business and Editorial Offices: 1600 John F. Kennedy Blvd., Ste. 1800, Philadelphia, PA 19103-2899. Customer Service Office: 3251 Riverport Lane, Maryland Heights, MO 63043. Periodicals postage paid at New York, NY and additional mailing offices. Subscription prices are $341.00 per year (US individuals), $713.00 per year (US institutions), $387.00 per year (Canadian individuals), $872.00 per year (Canadian institutions), $461.00 per year (international individuals), $872.00 per year (international institutions), $100.00 per year (US and Canadian students), and $195.00 per year (International students). International air speed delivery is included in all Clinics subscription prices. All prices are subject to change without notice. **POSTMASTER:** Send address changes to Clinics in Perinatology, Elsevier Health Sciences Division, Subscription Customer Service, 3251 Riverport Lane, Maryland Heights, MO 63043. **Customer Service: Telephone: 1-800-654-2452** (U.S. and Canada); **1-314-447-8871** (outside U.S. and Canada). **Fax: 1-314-447-8029. E-mail: journalscustomerservice-usa@elsevier.com** (for print support); **journalsonlinesupport-usa@elsevier.com** (for online support).

Reprints. For copies of 100 or more, of articles in this publication, please contact the Commercial Reprints Department, Elsevier Inc., 360 Park Avenue South, New York, NY 10010-1710. Tel. 212-633-3874; Fax: 212-633-3820; E-mail: reprints@elsevier.com.

Clinics in Perinatology is also published in Spanish by McGraw-Hill Interamericana Editores S.A., P.O. Box 5-237, 06500 Mexico D.F., Mexico.

Clinics in Perinatology is covered in MEDLINE/PubMed (Index Medicus) Current Contents, Excepta Medica, BIOSIS and ISI/BIOMED.

# Contributors

## CONSULTING EDITOR

**LUCKY JAIN, MD, MBA**
George W. Brumley Jr Professor and Chairman, Emory University School of Medicine, Department of Pediatrics; Chief Academic Officer, Children's Healthcare of Atlanta; Executive Director, Emory + Children's Pediatric Institute, Atlanta, Georgia, USA

## EDITORS

**NATHALIE L. MAITRE, MD, PhD**
Professor, Department of Pediatrics, Emory University School of Medicine, Children's Healthcare of Atlanta, Atlanta, Georgia, USA

**ANDREA F. DUNCAN, MD, MSClinRes**
Associate Professor of Pediatrics, University of Pennsylvania Perelman School of Medicine, Distinguished Endowed Chair in the Department of Pediatrics, Associate Chair, Diversity and Equity, Department of Pediatrics, Medical Director, Neonatal Follow-up Program, Children's Hospital of Philadelphia, Philadelphia, Pennsylvania, USA

## AUTHORS

**ELAINE ATTRIDGE, MLS**
Quality and Performance Improvement Librarian, Claude Moore Health Sciences Library, University of Virginia, Charlottesville, Virginia, USA

**SARAH L. BAUER HUANG, MD, PhD**
Department of Pediatric and Developmental Neurology, Department of Neurology, Washington University School of Medicine in St. Louis, St Louis, Missouri, USA

**KRISTEN L. BENNINGER, MD, MSc**
Center for Perinatal Research, The Abigail Wexner Research Institute, Nationwide Children's Hospital, Columbus, Ohio, USA

**SAMUDRAGUPTA BORA, PhD**
Mothers, Babies and Women's Health Program, Mater Research Institute, The University of Queensland, South Brisbane, Queensland, Australia

**RACHEL BYRNE, PT**
Cerebral Palsy Foundation, New York, New York, USA

**DEBORAH E. CAMPBELL, MD**
Division of Neonatology, Children's Hospital at Montefiore, Professor, Department of Pediatrics, Albert Einstein College of Medicine, The Bronx, New York, USA

**LINA F. CHALAK, MD, MSCS**
Professor of Pediatrics and Psychiatry, Director of Neuro-NICU Program, The University of Texas Southwestern Medical Center, Dallas, Texas, USA

**SHIVAANG CHAWLA, BS**
Marcus Autism Center, Department of Pediatrics, Emory University School of Medicine, Children's Healthcare of Atlanta, Atlanta, Georgia, USA

**DIANE DAMIANO, PhD, PT**
Rehabilitation Medicine Department, National Institutes of Health, Bethesda, Maryland, USA

**RAYE-ANN DEREGNIER, MD**
Ann & Robert H. Lurie Children's Hospital of Chicago, Northwestern University, Feinberg School of Medicine, Chicago, Illinois, USA

**ANDREA F. DUNCAN, MD, MSClinRes**
Associate Professor of Pediatrics, University of Pennsylvania Perelman School of Medicine, Distinguished Endowed Chair in the Department of Pediatrics, Associate Chair, Diversity and Equity, Department of Pediatrics, Medical Director, Neonatal Follow-up Program, Children's Hospital of Philadelphia, Philadelphia, Pennsylvania, USA

**STACEY C. DUSING, PT, PhD, FAPTA**
Certified Specialist in Pediatric Physical Therapy, Sykes Family Chair of Pediatric Physical Therapy, Health and Development, Associate Professor, Director of Pediatric Research, Division of Biokinesiology and Physical Therapy, University of Southern California, Los Angeles, California, USA

**CHARLETA GUILLORY, MD, MPH**
Professor of Pediatrics, Baylor College of Medicine, Neonatologist, Texas Children's Hospital, Director, Neonatal-Perinatal Public Health Program, Houston, Texas, USA

**DARRAH N. HAFFNER, MD, MHS**
Division of Pediatric Neurology, Department of Pediatrics, Nationwide Children's Hospital and the Ohio State University, Columbus, Ohio, USA

**SUSAN R. HINTZ, MD, MS**
Division of Neonatal and Developmental Medicine, Department of Pediatrics, Stanford University School of Medicine, Palo Alto, California, USA

**DAWN ILARDI, PhD**
Emory University School of Medicine, Children's Healthcare of Atlanta, Atlanta, Georgia, USA

**SONIA IMAIZUMI, MD**
Neonatologist, Senior Medical Director, MultiPlan.com, Newtown Square, Pennsylvania, USA

**YVETTE R. JOHNSON, MD, MPH**
Associate Professor of Pediatrics, Texas Christian University, Burnett School of Medicine, Neonatologist, Cook Children's Medical Center, Medical Director, N.E.S.T. Developmental Follow-up Clinic, Fort Worth, Texas, USA

**CHERYL KLAIMAN, PhD**
Marcus Autism Center, Department of Pediatrics, Emory University School of Medicine, Children's Healthcare of Atlanta, Atlanta, Georgia, USA

**AMI KLIN, PhD**
Marcus Autism Center, Department of Pediatrics, Emory University School of Medicine, Children's Healthcare of Atlanta, Atlanta, Georgia, USA

**LAZAROS KOCHILAS, MD, MSCR**
Emory University School of Medicine, Children's Healthcare of Atlanta, Atlanta, Georgia, USA

**LISA LETZKUS, PhD, RN, CPNP-AC**
Assistant Professor of Pediatrics, Division of Neurodevelopmental and Behavioral Pediatrics, Department of Pediatrics, University of Virginia, Charlottesville, Virginia, USA

**JONATHAN S. LITT, MD, MPH, SCD**
Department of Neonatology, Beth Israel Deaconess Medical Center, Assistant Professor, Department of Pediatrics, Harvard Medical School, Department of Social and Behavioral Sciences, Harvard TH Chan School of Public Health, Boston, Massachusetts, USA

**NATHALIE L. MAITRE, MD, PhD**
Professor, Department of Pediatrics, Emory University School of Medicine, Children's Healthcare of Atlanta, Atlanta, Georgia, USA

**JENNIFER M. McALLISTER, MD**
Cincinnati Children's Hospital Perinatal Institute, University of Cincinnati College of Medicine, Cincinnati, Ohio, USA

**DANA B. McCARTY, PT, DPT**
Board Certified Specialist in Pediatric Physical Therapy, Assistant Professor of Physical Therapy, Division of Physical Therapy, Department of Health Sciences, The University of North Carolina at Chapel Hill, Chapel Hill, North Carolina, USA

**LYNDA MCNAMARA, BPhty (HONS)**
The Children's Hospital Westmead Clinical School, The University of Sydney, Sydney, New South Wales, Australia

**EMMA McQUEEN, BS**
Marcus Autism Center, Department of Pediatrics, Emory University School of Medicine, Children's Healthcare of Atlanta, Atlanta, Georgia, USA

**ADRIANA I. MENDEZ, MA**
Department of Psychology, Emory University, Marcus Autism Center, Department of Pediatrics, Emory University School of Medicine, Children's Healthcare of Atlanta, Atlanta, Georgia, USA

**STEPHANIE L. MERHAR, MD, MS**
Cincinnati Children's Hospital Perinatal Institute, University of Cincinnati College of Medicine, Cincinnati, Ohio, USA

**GINA MILANO, MD**
The University of Texas Southwestern Medical Center, Dallas, Texas, USA

**CATHERINE MORGAN, PhD, BAPPSC (PHTY)**
Cerebral Palsy Alliance Research Institute, Specialty of Child and Adolescent Health, Sydney Medical School, Faculty of Medicine and Health, The University of Sydney, Forestville, Sydney, New South Wales, Australia

**MARY LAUREN NEEL, MD, MSCI**
Division of Neonatology, Emory University School of Medicine, Children's Healthcare of Atlanta, Atlanta, Georgia, USA

**IONA NOVAK, PhD, MSC (HONS), BAPPSC OT**
Cerebral Palsy Alliance Chair of Allied Health, Cerebral Palsy Alliance Research Institute, Specialty of Child and Adolescent Health, Sydney Medical School, Faculty of Medicine and Health, The University of Sydney, Forestville, Sydney, New South Wales, Australia

**ATHINA PAPPAS, MD**
Wayne Medical School, Detroit, Michigan, USA

**TRISHA PATEL, MD**
Emory University School of Medicine, Children's Healthcare of Atlanta, Atlanta, Georgia, USA

**WILLIAM G. SHARP, PhD**
Associate Professor, Department of Pediatrics, Emory University School of Medicine, Director, Multidisciplinary Feeding Program, Center for Advanced Pediatrics, Children's Healthcare of Atlanta, Atlanta, Georgia, USA

**HANNAH TOKISH, BA**
Marcus Autism Center, Department of Pediatrics, Emory University School of Medicine, Children's Healthcare of Atlanta, Atlanta, Georgia, USA

**BETTY R. VOHR, MD**
Division of Neonatology, Department of Pediatrics, Women & Infants Hospital, The Warren Alpert Medical School of Brown University, Providence, Rhode Island, USA

# Contents

Advances in perinatal care have led to remarkable long-term survival for infants who are born preterm. This article reviews the broader context of follow-up care, highlighting the need to reenvision some areas, such as improving parental support by embedding parental involvement in the neonatal intensive care unit, incorporating parental perspectives about outcomes into follow-up care models and research, supporting their mental health, addressing social determinants of health and disparities, and advocating for change. Multicenter quality improvement networks allow identification and implementation of best practices for follow-up care.

Infants and children with prenatal opioid exposure generally have development within the normal range; however, they seem to be at risk for behavioral problems and for lower scores on cognitive, language, and motor assessments than children without prenatal opioid exposure. It is as of yet unclear whether prenatal opioid exposure itself causes issues with development and behavior or whether it is simply correlated, due to other confounding factors.

Neonatal hypoxic-ischemic encephalopathy (HIE) is a leading cause of death and neurodevelopmental impairment in neonates. Therapeutic hypothermia (TH) is the only established effective therapy, and randomized trials affirm that TH reduces death and disability in moderate to severe HIE. Traditionally, infants with mild HIE were excluded from these trials due to the perceived low risk for impairment. Recently, multiple studies suggest that infants with untreated mild HIE may be at significant risk of abnormal neurodevelopmental outcomes. This review will focus on the changing landscape of TH, the spectrum of HIE presentations, and their neurodevelopmental outcomes.

Even before birth, children with congenital heart disease (CHD) are at risk for neurodevelopmental concerns, with additional insults occurring as part of their treatment course and from subsequent exposures to socioeconomic stressors. With multiple affected neurodevelopmental domains, individuals with CHD face lifelong cognitive, academic, psychological, and quality-of-life difficulties. Early and repeated neurodevelopmental evaluation is key to receiving appropriate services. However, obstacles at the level of the environment, provider, patient, and family can make the completion of these evaluations difficult. Future neurodevelopmental endeavors should aim to evaluate CHD-specific programs, their effectiveness, and barriers to access.

Long-standing health disparities in maternal reproductive health, infant morbidity and mortality, and long-term developmental outcomes are rooted in a foundation of structural racism. Social determinants of health profoundly affect reproductive health outcomes of black and Hispanic women disproportionately; they have higher rates of death during pregnancy and preterm birth. Their infants are also more likely to be cared for in poorer-quality neonatal intensive care units (NICUs), receive poorer quality of NICU care, and are less likely to be referred to an appropriate high-risk NICU follow-up program. Interventions that mitigate the impact of racism will help to eliminate health disparities.

Premature infants and infants later diagnosed with autism spectrum disorder (ASD) share many commonalities in clinical presentations. However, prematurity and ASD also have differences in clinical presentation. These overlapping phenotypes can lead to misdiagnoses of ASD or missing a diagnosis of ASD in preterm infants. We document these commonalities and differences in various developmental domains with the hope of aiding in the accurate early detection of ASD and timely intervention implementation in children born premature. Given the degree of similarities in presentation, evidence-based interventions designed specifically for preterm toddlers or toddlers with ASD may ultimately aid both populations.

This review summarizes the current state of evidence regarding interventions for executive function in high-risk infants and toddlers. Currently, there is a paucity of data in this area, with the interventions that have been studied highly variable in their content, dosage, target, and results. Self-regulation is the executive function construct targeted the most, with mixed results. The few studies that report later child outcomes in

accelerate progress, current priorities are to generate more high-quality data; engage with diverse local stakeholders including families of infants born preterm to identify neurodevelopmental outcomes meaningful to them within their contexts; and develop sustainable, scalable, high-quality models of neonatal follow-up, codesigned with local stakeholders, addressing the unique needs of low- and middle-income countries. Advocacy is critical to recognize optimal neurodevelopment as an "outcome of priority" along with the reduction in mortality.

Preterm infants are at heightened risk for chronic health problems and developmental delays compared with term-born peers. High-risk infant follow-up programs provide surveillance and support for problems that may emerge during infancy and early childhood. Although considered standard of care, program structure, content, and timing are highly variable. Families face challenges accessing recommended follow-up services. Here, the authors review common models of high-risk infant follow-up, describe novel approaches, and outline considerations for improving the quality, value, and equity of follow-up care.

Infants born prematurely or with other medical complexities are at high risk for developing long-term feeding problems that extend beyond infancy. Intensive multidisciplinary feeding intervention (IMFI) represents the standard of care for children with chronic and severe feeding issues, with a professional team that should involve, at a minimum, psychology, medicine, nutrition, and feeding skill expertise. IMFI seems to hold benefit for preterm infants and those with medical complexities; however, there remains a need to develop and investigate new therapeutic pathways to reduce the number of patients who likely require this level of care.

Dedicated neonatal intensive care unit (NICU) follow-up programs are recommended for ongoing surveillance for infants at high-risk for future neurodevelopmental impairment (NDI). Systemic, socioeconomic, and psychosocial barriers remain for referrals and the continued neurodevelopmental follow-up of high-risk infants. Telemedicine can help overcome these barriers. Telemedicine allows standardization of evaluations, increased referral rates, and reduced time to follow-up as well as increased therapy engagement. Telemedicine can expand neurodevelopmental surveillance and support all NICU graduates, facilitating the early identification of NDI. However, with the recent expansion of telemedicine during the COVID-19 pandemic, new barriers related to access and technological support have arisen.

Nathalie L. Maitre, Diane Damiano, and Rachel Byrne

Early detection and intervention for CP is best practice for all high-risk infants according to international guidelines, consensus statements and research. It allows family support and optimization of developmental trajectories into adulthood. Implementation of CP early detection in high-risk infant follow-up programs across the world has proven feasible. The largest clinical implementation network in the world sustained for >5 years an average CP diagnosis age of <12 months. As high-risk infant follow programs decrease the age of CP detection, Targeted referrals and interventions for CP can then be offered during optimal periods of neuroplasticity, and new therapies researched.

Nathalie L. Maitre and Andrea F. Duncan

As this issue of *Clinics in Perinatology* illustrates, a profound shift has occurred in the driving purpose of high-risk infant follow-up (HRIF) over the past 5 years. As a result, HRIF has evolved from primarily providing an ethical compass, concerned surveillance, and documentation of outcomes to developing novel models of care; considering new high-risk populations, settings, and psychosocial factors; and incorporating active, targeted interventions to improve outcomes.

## PROGRAM OBJECTIVE
The goal of *Clinics in Perinatology* is to keep practicing perinatologists, neonatologists, obstetricians, practicing physicians and residents up to date with current clinical practice in perinatology by providing timely articles reviewing the state of the art in patient care.

## TARGET AUDIENCE
Perinatologists, neonatologists, obstetricians, practicing physicians, residents and healthcare professionals who provide patient care utilizing findings from *Clinics in Perinatology.*

## LEARNING OBJECTIVES
Upon completion of this activity, participants will be able to:
1. Recognize the effect of health disparities on maternal and neonatal health outcomes, especially among Black and Hispanic populations leading to poor health outcomes of high-risk born neonates and children.
2. Discuss the necessity for research and development of novel interventions and practice guidelines to reduce the impact of social determinants and health disparities on child development and to improve health outcomes.
3. Review interventions that are supported by evidence-based practices for multidisciplinary care, shared decision-making, parental and community participation, equitable care, and screening for adverse social determinants of health.

## ACCREDITATION
The Elsevier Office of Continuing Medical Education (EOCME) is accredited by the Accreditation Council for Continuing Medical Education (ACCME) to provide continuing medical education for physicians.

The EOCME designates this journal-based CME activity for a maximum of 16 *AMA PRA Category 1 Credit*(s)™. Physicians should claim only the credit commensurate with the extent of their participation in the activity.

All other health care professionals requesting continuing education credit for this enduring material will be issued a certificate of participation.

## DISCLOSURE OF CONFLICTS OF INTEREST
The EOCME assesses conflict of interest with its instructors, faculty, planners, and other individuals who are in a position to control the content of CME activities. All relevant conflicts of interest that are identified are thoroughly vetted by EOCME for fair balance, scientific objectivity, and patient care recommendations. EOCME is committed to providing its learners with CME activities that promote improvements or quality in healthcare and not a specific proprietary business or a commercial interest.

**The planning committee, staff, authors, and editors listed below have identified no financial relationships or relationships to products or devices they or their spouse/life partner have with commercial interest related to the content of this CME activity:**
Elaine Attridge, MLS; Sarah L. Bauer Huang, MD, PhD; Kristen L. Benninger, MD, MSc; Samudragupta Bora, PhD; Rachel Byrne; Deborah E. Campbell, MD; Lina F. Chalak, MD, MSCS; Shivaang Chawla; Diane Damiano, PhD; Raye-Ann deRegnier, MD; Andrea F. Duncan, MD, MSClinRes; Stacey C. Dusing, PT, PhD, FAPTA; Charleta Guillory, MD, MPH; Darrah N. Haffner, MD, MHS; Susan R. Hintz, MD, MS; Dawn Ilardi, PhD; Sonia Imaizumi, MD; Yvette R. Johnson, MD, MPH; Cheryl Klaiman, PhD; Ami Klin; Lazaros Kochilas, MD, MSCR; Lisa Letzkus, PhD, RN, CPNP-AC; Jonathan S. Litt, MD, MPH, ScD; Nathalie L. Maitre, MD, PhD; Jennifer M. McAllister, MD; Dana McCarty, PT, DPT; Lynda McNamara; Emma McQueen; Adriana I. Mendez, MA; Stephanie L. Merhar, MD, MS; Gina Milano, MD; Catherine Morgan, PhD; Mary Lauren Neel, MD, MSCI; Iona Novak, PhD, MSc; Athina Pappas, MD; Trisha Patel, MD; William G. Sharp, PhD; Jeyanthi Surendrakumar; Doreen Thomas-Payne, MSN, BSN, RN, PMHNP-BC; Hannah Tokish, ; Betty R. Vohr, MD

## UNAPPROVED / OFF-LABEL USE DISCLOSURE
The EOCME requires CME faculty to disclose to the participants:
1. When products or procedures being discussed are off-label, unlabelled, experimental, and/or investigational (not US Food and Drug Administration [FDA] approved); and
2. Any limitations on the information presented, such as data that are preliminary or that represent ongoing research, interim analyses, and/or unsupported opinions. Faculty may discuss information about pharmaceutical agents that is outside of FDA-approved labelling. This information is intended solely for CME

and is not intended to promote off-label use of these medications. If you have any questions, contact the medical affairs department of the manufacturer for the most recent prescribing information.

## TO ENROLL
To enroll in the *Clinics in Perinatology* Continuing Medical Education program, call customer service at 1-800-654-2452 or sign up online at https://www.theclinics.com/cme. The CME program is available to subscribers for an additional annual fee of USD 254.00.

## METHOD OF PARTICIPATION
In order to claim credit, participants must complete the following:
1. Complete enrolment as indicated above.
2. Read the activity.
3. Complete the CME Test and Evaluation. Participants must achieve a score of 70% on the test. All CME Tests and Evaluations must be completed online.

## CME INQUIRIES/SPECIAL NEEDS
For all CME inquiries or special needs, please contact elsevierCME@elsevier.com.

# CLINICS IN PERINATOLOGY

---

**SERIES OF RELATED INTEREST**

*Obstetrics and Gynecology Clinics of North America*
https://www.obgyn.theclinics.com

---

**THE CLINICS ARE AVAILABLE ONLINE!**
Access your subscription at:
www.theclinics.com

# Dedication

This issue is dedicated to two leaders in High-Risk Infant Follow-Up.

We dedicate this issue to Dr Ricki Goldstein: Ricki, you are an inspiration. Thank you for getting so many of the most obstinate and passionate people together to create guidelines and recommendations for High-Risk Infant Follow-Up. Thank you also for being the first person to take a chance on mentoring me (Dr Nathalie L. Maitre) in this field, and the person who gave my son the greatest gift he could ever receive. You helped his mother find hope that he could have a healthy and happy future. Your legacy will endure.

We also dedicate this to the memory of Dr Ira Adams-Chapman, dedicated physician to infants and children most vulnerable to developmental concerns, and passionate advocate for families of those at the highest risk for injustice. She lived as a shining role model of compassion, kindness, and service to all of us who follow in her footsteps. Ira was the first person to welcome this newbie into the national follow-up research world (Dr Andrea F. Duncan). For me, she exemplified grace, giving, and making room at the table. She adored her work with these vulnerable children, and she was an inspiration and friend to me. We miss you, Ira.

Nathalie L. Maitre, MD, PhD
Pediatrics
Emory University School of Medicine
Children's Healthcare of Atlanta
1123 Zonolite Road, Suite 22
Atlanta, GA 30306, USA

Andrea F. Duncan, MD, MSClinRes
Children's Hospital of Philadelphia
3401 Civic Center Boulevard
2nd Floor main, Division of Neonatology
Philadelphia, PA 19104, USA

*E-mail addresses:*
n.maitre@emory.edu (N.L. Maitre)
duncana2@chop.edu (A.F. Duncan)

# Foreword

# Nothing Matters More Than the Long-Term Outcomes of High-Risk Newborns

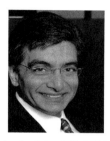

Lucky Jain, MD, MBA
*Consulting Editor*

It has been 5 years since the last issue of the *Clinics in Perinatology* devoted to long-term follow-up of high-risk newborns was published. In that issue edited by Drs Adams-Chapman and DeMauro, we discussed how predicting long-term outcomes of high-risk newborns is singularly challenging.[1] In fact, no other area of medicine faces a prognostic challenge of this magnitude, where developmental and neurologic indicators in the first year or two of life are expected to shed light on potential outcomes decades later. Doing so when the brain is highly plastic and developing is hard enough, add to it the uncertainty of environmental factors and nurturing (**Fig. 1**).[2] It is no surprise that real-life outcomes are often quite different from assessments based on neurodevelopmental studies done early on in infancy or even in preschool years. Clinicians and scientists, therefore, were mostly content with using developmental assessments to validate short-term safety of new interventions used in the neonatal period. There was little emphasis on using such information to navigate models of care.[3]

As the editors of this new issue of *Clinics in Perinatology* Drs Maitre and Duncan point out, a significant shift has occurred in the overarching goal of high-risk infant follow-up over the past 5 years. Rather than limit themselves to static documentation of developmental findings, programs are expanding to include new high-risk populations and developing novel models of care. This bodes well for the field of neonatal-perinatal medicine given the opportunity to proactively change care delivery and modify factors with detrimental impact on outcomes.

This remarkable issue of *Clinics in Perinatology* has not only expanded the scope and purpose of the discipline of developmental follow-up but also provides hope that the field is shifting from a passive focus to one that aims to actively develop new models of care delivery that will improve outcomes. Drs Maitre and Duncan are

Clin Perinatol 50 (2023) xix–xx
https://doi.org/10.1016/j.clp.2022.12.001
0095-5108/23/© 2022 Published by Elsevier Inc.

**perinatology.theclinics.com**

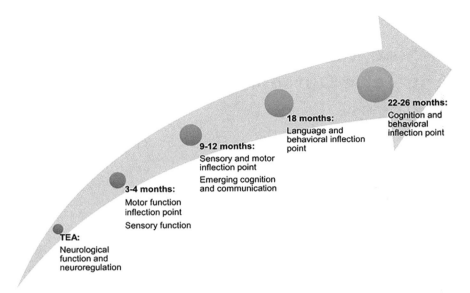

**Fig. 1.** A true neurodevelopmental trajectory. An ideal early neurodevelopmental trajectory includes a variety of time points, each of which represents a specific developmental domain inflection point with targeted assessments from TEA to 2 years. TEA, term-equivalent age. (*From* Benninger KL, Inder TE, Goodman AM, Cotton MC, Nordli DR, Shah TA, Slaughter JC, Maitre NL. Perspectives from the Society for Pediatric Research-Neonatal Encephalopathy Clinical Trials: Developing the Future. Pediatr Res. 2021;89:74-84.)

to be congratulated for engaging top experts in the field to assemble a true state-of-the-art offering. As always, I am grateful to the authors for their valuable contributions and to my publishing partners at Elsevier (Kerry Holland and Karen Solomon) for their help in bringing this valuable resource to you.

Lucky Jain, MD, MBA
Department of Pediatrics
Emory University School of Medicine
Children's Healthcare of Atlanta
1760 Haygood drive, W409
Atlanta, GA 30322, USA

*E-mail address:*
ljain@emory.edu

### REFERENCES

1. Jain L. The business of predicting long-term neonatal outcomes. Clin Perinatol 2018;45:xv–xvi.
2. Benninger KL, Inder TE, Goodman AM, et al. Perspectives from the Society for Pediatric Research-Neonatal Encephalopathy clinical trials: developing the future. Pediatr Res 2021;89:74–84.
3. Adams-Chapman I, Heyne RJ, DeMauro SB, et al. Follow-up study of the Eunice Kennedy Shriver National Institute of Child Health and Human Development Neonatal Research Network. Pediatrics 2018.

# Preface

# Neurologic and Developmental Outcomes of High-Risk Neonates

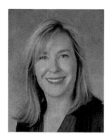 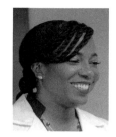

Nathalie L. Maitre, MD, PhD     Andrea F. Duncan, MD, MSClinRes
*Editors*

For too long, neonatal follow-up was seen as a necessary means to the end of completing developmental assessments, as endpoints for clinical trials conducted in the neonatal intensive care unit (NICU) or statistical prognostic tools, nominally aimed at counseling parents of vulnerable infants. Now, neonatal follow-up has been transformed as a critical means to achieving the best possible outcomes for infants born at high risk and their families. As the wider import of long-term follow-up has become more broadly accepted, the complexities involved in providing exemplary follow-up have become clear as well. The providers dedicated to caring for these vulnerable families must necessarily integrate multiple disciplines and areas of expertise to meet their needs, including social work; case management; implementation science; occupational, physical, and speech therapies; psychology; and nutrition and feeding. Despite these needs, there remain no clear guidelines for provision of neonatal follow-up. Resources and staff for follow-up provision vary widely— approximately 50% of eligible infants receive developmental follow-up, and there remain disparities in access to follow-up care based on social determinants of health.

In this issue of *Clinics in Perinatology*, experts in their fields review the state-of-the-evidence for follow-up care of high-risk infants and their families. They demonstrate how follow-up must involve guidelines requiring that all children born high risk receive multidisciplinary, evidence-based care, increased involvement of families in decision making, and a commitment to justice in care with screening for adverse social determinants of health. In addition, investments in new models of care, interventions to alleviate the impacts of delays, disabilities, and adverse SDS should continue, with implementation science in service of translating the newest research into practice. Furthermore, to ensure the best outcomes, support is needed for continued research into novel delivery models, networks, community partnerships, and interventions for

Clin Perinatol 50 (2023) xxi–xxii
https://doi.org/10.1016/j.clp.2022.12.002
0095-5108/23/© 2022 Published by Elsevier Inc.     **perinatology.theclinics.com**

the most common *outpatient* issues high-risk children and families face. Finally, as noted in multiple articles, the idea of follow through embraced by all staff and providers from prebirth to school age helps providers of neonatal care meet their responsibility of providing continuous equitable and excellent care. This care must consider the many care transitions and medical, developmental, and psychosocial needs that families face from the NICU to home to a societal environment. This issue aims to give an overview of these concepts across different types of high-risk infants, varied models of care and settings, and new approaches to evidence translation.

Nathalie L. Maitre, MD, PhD
Emory University School of Medicine
Children's Healthcare of Atlanta
1123 Zonolite Road, Suite 22
Atlanta, GA 30306, USA

Andrea F. Duncan, MD, MSClinRes
Children's Hospital of Philadelphia
3401 Civic Center Boulevard
2nd Floor main, Division of Neonatology
Philadelphia, PA 19104, USA

*E-mail addresses:*
n.maitre@emory.edu (N.L. Maitre)
duncana2@chop.edu (A.F. Duncan)

# Outcomes of Preterm Infants
## Shifting Focus, Extending the View

Susan R. Hintz, MD, MS[a],*, Raye-Ann deRegnier, MD[b],
Betty R. Vohr, MD[c]

## KEYWORDS

- Prematurity • Follow-up care • Parents

## KEY POINTS

- Integration of parents in care and research, supporting their mental health, and providing evidence-based neonatal intensive care unit environments can assist in defining and improving developmental outcomes.
- Screening for social determinants of health in the hospital and addressing disparities in community developmental services will ensure that the benefits of early intervention are available to all children.
- Use of quality improvement networks can allow for more rapid deployment of best practices and advance research.
- Understanding adult health and quality of life is an important part of the research in preterm follow-up and must be expanded.

## INTRODUCTION

The past decades have seen extraordinary advances in perinatal and neonatal care, leading to significant improvements in both survival and survival without major inneonatal intensive care unit (NICU) morbidities among infants born very preterm.[1–3] With improved survival rates of smaller and sicker infants, the importance of understanding and improving later outcomes is increasingly critical. Most studies involving preterm infants follow children only to 2 to 3 years corrected age and focus primarily on a composite outcome of "neurodevelopmental impairment (NDI)" combining cognitive, neurologic, and neurosensory endpoints. However, these limited early childhood outcomes provide a narrow and often inaccurate view of an individual's lifelong abilities

[a] Division of Neonatal and Developmental Medicine, Department of Pediatrics, Stanford University School of Medicine, 453 Quarry Road, 4th Floor, Palo Alto, CA 94304, USA; [b] Ann & Robert H. Lurie Children's Hospital of Chicago, Northwestern University Feinberg School of Medicine, 225 East Chicago Avenue, Box 45, Chicago, IL 60611, USA; [c] Division of Neonatology, Department of Pediatrics, Women & Infants Hospital, Alpert Medical School of Brown University, 101 Dudley Street, Providence, RI 02905, USA
* Corresponding author.
*E-mail address:* srhintz@stanford.edu

Clin Perinatol 50 (2023) 1–16
https://doi.org/10.1016/j.clp.2022.10.001          **perinatology.theclinics.com**

and quality of life.[4,5,6] Furthermore, the emergence of later challenges in executive function, behavior, mental health, respiratory and cardiometabolic health, and quality of life may not be evident until later childhood or beyond.[7,8] The impact of very preterm birth on parental mental health, and in turn, the influence of parental stress, anxiety, and trauma on childhood outcomes is increasingly recognized.[9,10,11,12] Similarly, the relative importance of social and environmental (SES) factors on outcomes of children and adults born preterm, and the relative value placed on functional life outcomes also shift over the life course.[13,14] These interconnected themes support reenvisioning a true continuum-of-care for children born preterm and their families that integrates parent and family voices, recognizes social determinants of health (SDH), provides support, values outcomes as trajectories, and moves beyond traditional neurodevelopmental endpoints. There are substantial opportunities for new constructs of comprehensive life-course interventions that begin in the NICU, connect across high-risk infant follow-up and community resources, and continue beyond toddlerhood.[15,16,17,18]

## A NEW CONTEXT—PRIORITIES, GOALS, AND OUTCOMES
### Parent and Family Perspective

There have been hundreds of publications related to neonatal clinical trials and studies that include outcomes of infants born extremely preterm (EPT). However, these outcomes have almost always been defined solely by investigators or providers, and rarely reflect priorities of parents or individuals who themselves were born preterm. Janvier and colleagues reported that outcomes—particularly composite outcomes—may be difficult to interpret. They may not be seen as correlating with the longer-term functional and quality of life outcomes that are valuable to families.[19] Further research by this group[20] revealed that a majority parents of children who were born EPT (18 months to 7 years) expressed priorities for improvements in the realm of development; however, these were mainly described as behavioral, emotional health, and communication concerns rather than strictly cognitive. Respiratory health and overall medical fragility as well as growth and feeding issues were also prioritized. In other family studies of priorities for research, themes have included support for parental mental health; communication around uncertain outcomes; focusing on ongoing medical and functional challenges for the child; improving education and communication with primary care and other health-care providers; creating parental support systems beyond the NICU; developing alternative visit and intervention platforms, and addressing "real life" challenges such as connecting with services and financial assistance programs.[21,22] Eeles and colleagues[23] deployed a 3-round Delphi survey of parents and patients with lived experience of neonatal intensive care designed to identify research priorities. High-priority research questions included exploring how the NICU experience influences parent mental health and how emotional and mental well-being can be maintained through childhood; improving parental support in bonding in the NICU and for transition home; impact of neonatal conditions on patient health, functional outcomes, and medical conditions through childhood to adulthood—and ameliorating the influence of these conditions. These and other studies suggest that commonly pursued research outcomes as well as communication around outcomes to families must be reconsidered. Integrating parents, families, and individuals who were preterm into the research and quality improvement design process is crucial. As described by Dahan and colleagues,[24] including these key stakeholders can drive optimized research question and outcomes selection, identify unanticipated challenges and barriers for families, and guide appropriate communication.

## Use of Developmental Testing to Categorize and Define Outcomes

A large proportion of outcome studies on preterm and other high-risk children over the span of decades have focused on the results of standardized developmental testing. This is understandable because such testing seems to provide an objective way to categorize outcomes and compare them over time between cohorts. Clinically, test scores may be used to qualify children for early intervention (EI) programs and to provide information to families about supporting developmental activities. Unfortunately, the seemingly objective practice of stratifying the severity of NDIs as mild, moderate, or severe using categories of test results reflects values placed on specific standard deviations above or below the mean with limited additional information about how these scores are related to a child's everyday function or the impact on the family. Luu and Pearce[25] noted that more than a child's exact developmental test scores, parents may be more interested in a child's ability to "be happy, healthy, have friends, and be able to eventually live an independent life."

This coupled with the parent and family perspectives discussed previously suggest that results of developmental testing should be used alongside other information to categorize outcomes. Vision and hearing abilities are typically categorized by the supports required to improve function (glasses or hearing aids). This is also true for neurologic impairments such as cerebral palsy (CP). For example, the Gross Motor Functional Classification (GMFCS)[26] has been used to identify the impact of CP on a child's ability to move in the community with or without the need for mobility devices. Although the developers of the GMFCS do not recommend its use for children who do not have CP,[27] it may be useful as a model for developing a high-risk infant functional outcome measure for NICU graduates and has been done for children with other diagnoses.[28] Parental input about new functional outcome measures would complement the results of developmental testing and increase the relevance for future parents and providers alike.

Standardization of outcome definitions should be a priority, and these definitions should reflect perspectives of providers, parents, and adults born preterm. Describing impairments as mild, moderate, or severe based on developmental test scores is problematic because the definition of these categories often varies. For example, outcome data from 2187 toddlers in the Canadian Neonatal Network were categorized according to standards used in the Canadian and several other worldwide neonatal networks.[29] Using the same outcome information, the composite of severe NDI ranged from 3.5% to 14.9% depending on which categorization standards were used. This shows that what constitutes a "severe" impairment is variable and subjective. This variability may be confusing to physicians who need to counsel parents making life and death decisions. Although parents may use outcome information in only a limited way to make these decisions,[30,31,32] neonatologists should be able to use similar terms to describe the same outcomes. It would be optimal to enlist parents and individuals born preterm to help understand what constitutes a severe outcome. This may be based on child abilities that are more easily translated into everyday life rather than requiring neonatologists and parents to interpret how developmental test scores might be applied to a child's future.

When thinking about using developmental test results to monitor the quality of neonatal care, it is apparent that although NICU practices evolve quickly, developmental outcomes take time to acquire, analyze, and publish. As neonatal care may change rapidly, outcomes reported today on cohorts who are several years old may not accurately reflect future outcomes of current NICU graduates. Research on identification of robust, evidence-based early assessments, such as the General Movements Assessment[33] may help us to understand neurodevelopmental consequences of changes in neonatal care practices closer to real time.

## Mental Health

Although most trials and studies seeking to improve short-term and long-term outcomes for children born preterm focus on NICU-based interventions specific to the infant, the impact of the parent and family environment and relationships over the long trajectory of a child's life are profound and cumulative.[34] Parental mental health issues are increasingly recognized as highly prevalent, with approximately half of NICU parents suffering from high rates of depression and anxiety, and 20% to 40% with trauma reactions consistent with acute stress disorder or posttraumatic stress disorder.[9,35,36] Parental mental health difficulties may persist for years, may be associated with barriers to responsive parenting and parent–infant bonding, contribute to the evolution of vulnerable child syndrome, and may be associated with other adverse childhood developmental outcomes.[11,12,35,36] Given the pervasive and impactful nature of these issues, routine parent mental health screening as part of family-integrated care in the NICU and in the antenatal period is warranted for all cases in which NICU admission is likely to be required. However, clearly, screening and identification of mental health symptoms and psychosocial risk is only the first step. Systems and processes to access evidence-based preventative interventions and treatment of parental mental health challenges is a critical component to comprehensive and multidimensional care in the NICU, continuing through transition to home and beyond.[37,38,39] The National Perinatal Association (NPA) convened an interdisciplinary group of stakeholders to develop guidelines for psychosocial support services for NICU parents, which were published in a special issue of *Journal of Perinatology*.[40] This study was envisioned as a road map to provide guidance and resources for psychosocial support for parents, families, and for NICU providers and is available online through a unique collaboration between the NPA, Patient + Family Care, and the Preemie Parent Alliance (www.support4nicuparents.org). Shaw and colleagues developed a 6-session intervention for mothers of preterm infants in the NICU based on the principles of trauma-focused cognitive behavior therapy, which was effective at long-term reduction of trauma, anxiety, and depression symptoms,[37,41] and has expanded to integrate fathers, moved to group and virtual settings, and has been deployed in other NICUs. A comprehensive textbook[42] with companion website including downloadable tools and resources (https://www.appi.org/shaw) to guide intervention components has been published.

## SOCIAL DETERMINANTS OF HEALTH, ADDRESSING DISPARITIES IN CARE

There is increasing evidence that, in addition to biologic risk factors, a wide spectrum of socioeconomic factors contribute to the outcomes of pregnant women and infants born preterm.[43] Families often experience the impact of multiple socioeconomic risk factors in conjunction with the stressors associated with parenting a vulnerable infant in the NICU.[44] There is increasing evidence of the need for family-centered care that includes dignity and respect, information sharing, participation of families in decision-making, and ongoing collaboration of staff and families to effectively address these needs to achieve health care quality and equity. Successfully addressing these needs will entail developing strong relationships with families, identifying their strengths and challenges, and expanding multidisciplinary NICU teams to support families by addressing health-care disparities, supporting parents with psychosocial and mental health challenges, and minimizing language barriers.[45,46,47,48,49,50,51,52,53,54,55,56,57]

Residing in a high-risk neighborhood has been shown to be a marker of a spectrum of medical morbidities and structural inequities. For example, NICU graduates residing in high-risk neighborhoods in Rhode Island had higher rates of socioeconomic risk factors and were at increased risk of emergency department use after discharge as well as adverse neurodevelopmental outcomes at 2 years of age.[48,49] Knowledge of neighborhood risk in an NICU population can inform targeted implementation of programs for socially disadvantaged infants that include social workers and other mental health providers as participants in the NICU care team. Discharge transition planning requires confirmation that the family has appointments with their primary care provider, medical specialists, home health care, and home equipment services or durable medical equipment providers. Families need to be transitioned to an NICU follow-up program and receive a referral for EI programs offered under the Individuals with Disabilities Education Act Part C.[45]

Although EI programs have been shown to be effective,[50,51,52,53,54] in many communities, there are barriers to service provision that have been linked to family race, ethnicity, non-English speaking language, public insurance, and poverty.[50,55,56,57,58,59,60,61] The complexity of referral processes[62] may create barriers for non-English speaking families or those with low literacy. To remedy these barriers, families with private insurance can obtain bridge services until EI is initiated but infants with public insurance may have financial or transportation difficulties accessing private therapy services. The use of telehealth therapy services may address some but not all of these issues.[63,64,65,66] Going forward, several researchers have reported novel programs to improve the transition from NICU services to EI.[67,68] However, for now, each NICU must ascertain potential barriers in their community and identify local resources, such as outpatient therapy providers who accept a variety of insurance plans, to provide individualized bridge therapy services until EI programs are in effect.

### Making a Broader Commitment to Change

Transition to home as a process involves more than referral for EI services. A recent series of publications and perspectives led by Horbar and colleagues[15] and other members of the Vermont Oxford Network (VON) present a more encompassing stance to "follow-up" for high-risk children and their families, expanding and shifting the concept to "follow through." All care providers, from prenatal care and NICU through childhood and beyond, must actively participate in addressing social determinants of health and systemic inequities that substantively influence the long-term outcomes of patients and families. Potentially Better Practices (PBPs) are proposed under umbrella topics including promoting a culture of equity, identifying social risks and developing mitigating interventions, taking action to assist families in transition to home, maintaining support for families through infancy and childhood, developing quality improvement efforts to ensure high-quality NICU and follow through by eliminating disparities, and advocating for social justice at the local through national level. The many PBPs may seem overwhelming but they recognize the profound life-course challenges and barriers that our patients and their families face, all of which influence our traditional concept of "outcome" for a child born preterm. Recommended resources for these efforts include the VON for Health Equity website (https://public.vtoxford.org/health-equity/) and the Prenatal-to-3 Policy Impact Center (https://pn3policy.org/pn-3-state-policy-roadmap-2021/).

## A NEW CONTEXT—FRAMEWORKS FOR CHANGE
### The Neonatal Intensive Care Unit Environment and Models of Care

Other chapters in this edition of Clinics of Perinatology have comprehensive review and commentary on the importance of the NICU environment and models of care; however, given their import in recontextualizing family-centered care for high-risk infants, they will be briefly highlighted here.

### Physical neonatal intensive care unit environment

Physical characteristics of an NICU can facilitate the successful provision of transition care. The single-family room (SFR) NICU has been increasingly adopted in the United States to improve both infant outcomes and family satisfaction. A recent meta-analysis demonstrated that SFRs are significantly associated with lower rates of sepsis, and increased breastfeeding at discharge, however no difference in other neonatal morbidities associated with prematurity or 2-year neurodevelopment were seen.[69,70,71,72,73,74,75,76] When considering the NICU environment, organizational needs and resources (such as staffing) and the needs and desires of the population served must be considered. It is critical the environment is accessible and inclusive, making visitation and communication with staff easy for families visiting during day-time hours, nights, and weekends.

### Neonatal intensive care unit-to-home and beyond interventions

Optimally, NICU-to-home and community interventions are developed to include a "multilayered" bundle of patient and parent care and support interventions in the NICU,[39] continuing through the key transitional period of discharge, and in the home and community as part of follow-up and follow through. An example of this approach was reported by O'Brien and colleagues from a multinational, multi-NICU randomized controlled trial of Family Integrated Care (FICare).[77] This study team included parents in a model extending the principles of Family Centered Care with a central objective being that parents are true partners in the care of their child in the NICU while they are interacting with their infant and gaining knowledge, skills, and confidence in caring for their infant. Pillars of the intervention focused on parent education, NICU environment, psychosocial support, and staff education. At discharge, FICare improved infant weight gain, exclusive breastfeeding, and reduced parent stress and anxiety.

The Women and Infants Hospital of Rhode Island created an expanded medical home care team called the Transition Plus Program that provides enhanced transitional support beginning in the NICU and continuing for 90 days postdischarge. Predischarge, the team assesses parental needs including addressing food and housing insecurity, mental health concerns, and discharge readiness. Postdischarge supports include a phone call within 48 hours of discharge, 24/7 provider availability, and a home visit by a study Nurse Practitioner within 7 days of discharge. The intervention resulted in fewer emergency department visits[78] fewer rehospitalizations,[79] and lower total Medicaid spending[80] than a comparison group

Finally, an ongoing study of great interest is the Coached, Coordinated, Enhanced Neonatal Transition study,[81] a randomized controlled superiority trial enrolling parents of infants born at less than 27 weeks of gestation from NICUs in 3 Canadian provinces. The intervention includes parental psychosocial support delivered by a nurse navigator that includes Acceptance and Commitment Therapy-based coaching, care coordination and anticipatory education for parents beginning in the NICU and continuing through 12 months. The primary outcome is parenting stress as measured by the Parenting Stress Index fourth edition; many of the secondary outcomes are similarly focused on the parent, including quality of life, empowerment, and mental health outcomes.

### Approaches to "Follow-Up" Visits

Although benefits of neonatal follow-up programs have been described,[82,83] the composition and goals of these programs vary widely in the United States. A survey of NICU follow-up clinic directors in 2011 to 2012 revealed variable and diverse services provided in follow-up clinics, including primary care services, medical follow-up, developmental and hearing assessment, social services, and nutrition support.[84] Some clinics have multidisciplinary teams to manage infants with medical complexity.[85]

Although the American Academy of Pediatrics (AAP) recommends developmental surveillance within pediatricians' offices[86] for all infants, there are few society recommendations for NICU graduates. The AAP's *Guidelines for Perinatal Care, eighth edition*[87] recommends ongoing neurologic and developmental assessments with formal evaluation of those at highest risk at 1 and 2 years at a minimum. For infants with congenital heart disease, the American Heart Association has stratified risk for developmental problems by diagnostic categories and recommended ages and types of assessments for developmental follow-up.[88] Although more specific neonatology-based recommendations seem to be forthcoming for high-risk NICU graduates, currently there is no uniform approach to follow-up of high-risk NICU graduates. As these recommendations are developed, it will be important to incorporate parental views of needs for neurosensory problems, developmental delays and health problems that might require subspecialty expertise not found in their pediatricians' offices, particularly during the transition to home.

Studies of high-risk follow-up clinics have shown that nonattendance and attrition over time are common problems.[89,90,91,92,93] This is problematic because infants may not receive timely diagnoses or prompt support for growth, health, and neurodevelopmental problems if they are not evaluated. Furthermore, the evaluation of outcomes in quality improvement projects or research studies requires a representative sample of patients. There are many potential reasons for nonattendance, including lack of understanding of the role of the clinic in supporting their infant's development, lack of support for parents (eg, single parenting or need for sibling care during appointments), language barriers, transportation difficulties including extended distance from clinic, and lack of insurance or financial resources for clinic visits.

An unexpected consequence of the coronavirus disease 2019 pandemic was the dramatic increase of the use of telehealth for follow-up visits. It was noted early on that the use of this alternate visit type alleviates some of the barriers to follow-up (principally transportation and distance to appointments) and allows examiners to meet families and assess children in a more relaxed home environment.[64] There is accumulating evidence to support the validity of telehealth assessments, although more research is needed.[63,64,94] It should be noted that some of the barriers to in-person visits also apply to telehealth visits (insurance coverage, clinic hours), and there may be additional barriers related to the variable availability of interpreter services, parental Internet services, or computer access. The future of neonatal follow-up likely will incorporate a mix of in-person and telehealth visits to allow programs to individualize visits to accommodate specific family needs and preferences. A full review of telehealth in NICU follow-up is presented by Darrah N. Haffner and Sarah L. Bauer Huang's article, "Utilizing Telemedicine to Overcome Barriers to Neurodevelopmental Care from the NICU to School Entry," in this issue.

### Leveraging Multicenter Frameworks

Although investigations of multidimensional NICU-to-home and follow through interventions are often performed by single sites or through creation of groups of NICU and follow-up sites specific to a study, there are opportunities to leverage existing multicenter, continuum of care quality improvement frameworks to advance research and to deploy evidence-based changes.

In 2016, high-risk infant follow-up programs from the 6 state New England region came together to establish the first multistate collaborative dedicated solely to quality improvement for High Risk Infant Follow Up (HRIF; the New England Follow-up Network [NEFUN]). In the initial years of experience, NEFUN reported variability across states and sites, including eligibility criteria, follow-up visits cadence and content, and clinic personnel.[95] Furthermore, only 52.0% of infants born weighing 1000 g or lesser or at less than 28 weeks of gestation had follow-up visits between 18 and 24 months of corrected age. They found high rates of postdischarge health service utilization and rehospitalization, significant unmet postdischarge service needs, missed neurosensory screening, and other challenges. Moving forward, NEFUN collaborators aim to use this information to standardize follow-up processes and outcome measures across NEFUN sites to improve service delivery and create novel interventions to improve clinical outcomes.[95]

The California Perinatal Quality Care Collaborative (CPQCC) is a population-based dataset of perinatal variables and NICU-based outcomes including greater than 90% of VLBW infants cared for in California. The CPQCC partnered with California Children's Services (CCS) to create the CPQCC CCS HRIF Quality of Care Initiative. The statewide CPQCC CCS HRIF has site-specific online tools and reports as well as California-wide data. The program provides for a series of visits through 3 years of age for high-risk infants meeting CCS eligibility criteria (https://www.cpqcc.org/). This system therefore provides a linked, population-based, continuum of care infrastructure from birth and NICU course through HRIF referral and follow-up visits through 3 years.

Initial investigations by the group revealed an 80% HRIF referral at discharge among infants with birth weights 1500 g or lesser even though all were eligible. Significant SES, patient-level, and site-level disparities in referral were identified,[96] as well as disparities in attendance at a first visit by 12 months corrected age.[97] A statewide quality and process improvement initiative was undertaken, which increased referral rates to 94.9%, with substantial improvement across all socioeconomic, perinatal, and clinical variables. In addition, both referral to HRIF and follow-up rates increased significantly among children with moderate-severe hypoxic ischemic encephalopathy (HIE), and variation in follow-up rates by HRIF clinic decreased.[98]

Linking NICUs and follow-up systems in diverse, population-based, regional networks dedicated to quality improvement can begin to address issues of health equity in neonatal follow-up and service provision, provide opportunities for expanded family and community engagement, and promote statewide education and advocacy.

## EXTENDING OUR VIEW

Looking forward, as preterm survivors continue to age, it will be important to understand the impact of prematurity on both individuals and population health. In the Global Burden of Disease Study 2010,[99] neonatal disorders were associated with 8.1% of all disability-adjusted years due to high neonatal mortality and rates of lifelong disabilities. As the initial cohorts of infants with extreme prematurity become adults, there is increasing evidence that most, but not all, adults born preterm are free of disabling conditions and report a quality of life similar to full-term peers. It is also apparent that preterm birth has long-term consequences on many, if not most aspects of health and the ability to work, live independently, marry, and have children.[8]

In young adults, Eves[100] reported combined outcomes of 8 very preterm or very-low birth weight cohorts at a mean age of 24.6 years. In unadjusted analyses, lower gestational age, lower birth weight z-scores, neonatal bronchopulmonary dysplasia, any grade of intraventricular hemorrhage and lower maternal education were all significantly associated with lower intelligence quotients in adulthood. Recent studies have also identified that children born preterm have high rates of mental health disorders beginning at school age[101,102] and extending to adulthood.[103]

Although most follow-up studies focus on EPT (<28 weeks), some studies have expanded to moderate preterm (MPT: 29–33 weeks) or late preterm (LPT: 34–36 weeks) births. This is based on research showing that MPT survivors are at increased risk of adverse cognitive, executive function and behavioral outcomes[104,105,106,107,108] because they are born during a critical period of brain development.[109] Heinonen and colleagues addressed the subject of life-long brain vulnerability in LPT infants with assessments completed at a mean age of 68.1 years of age[110] and found that LPT seniors showed an almost 3-fold increased risk of Mild Cognitive Impairment suggesting early onset Alzheimer's. A positive finding was that the outcome was mediated by higher level of education attainment, informing the importance of equitable access to intervention and educational supports for former preterm adults. It also clearly demonstrates the important role of longitudinal population-based databases.

What is the future of neonatal follow-up for individuals born preterm? We must expand our vision both within the NICU and farther into the future with our patients. To achieve this, the following goals are proposed for comprehensive care: (1) Substantively integrate parents into their infants' care, starting in the NICU and continuing through follow-up; (2) Identify ways to support parents during the NICU stay, at discharge, and in the community as they navigate their future with their child; (3) Identify best practices for neonatal follow-up, incorporating parent perspectives and advocating for equitable care at all ages; (4) Define standardized, evidence-based outcomes that are meaningful to parents, families, and individuals born preterm at all ages; (5) Identify earlier outcomes that can allow us to monitor the quality of NICU care in more rapid fashion and at the same time, support further research on adults born preterm; and (6) Expand the vision and scope of "follow-up" for children born preterm and high-risk, with a goal to assure a more equitable and brighter future for individuals born preterm, their parents, and families.

## REFERENCES

1. Bell EF, Hintz SR, Hansen NI, et al. Eunice Kennedy Shriver national Institute of child health and Human development neonatal research network. Mortality, in-hospital morbidity, care practices, and 2-year outcomes for extremely preterm infants in the US, 2013-2018. JAMA 2022;327(3):248–63.

2. Norman M, Hallberg B, Abrahamsson T, et al. Association between Year of birth and 1-year survival among extremely preterm infants in Sweden during 2004-2007 and 2014-2016. JAMA 2019;321(12):1188–99.

3. Lee HC, Liu J, Profit J, et al. Survival without major morbidity among very low birth weight infants in California. Pediatrics 2020;146(1):e20193865.

4. Kilbride HW, Aylward GP, Doyle LW, et al. Prognostic neurodevelopmental testing of preterm infants: do we need to change the paradigm? J Perinatol 2017;37:475–9.

5. Serenius F, Ewald U, Farooqi A, et al. Neurodevelopmental outcomes among extremely preterm infants 6.5 Years after active perinatal care in Sweden. JAMA Pediatr 2016;170:954–63.

6. Roberts G, Anderson PJ, Doyle LW. Victorian Infant Collaborative Study Group. The stability of the diagnosis of developmental disability between ages 2 and 8 in a geographic cohort of very preterm children born in 1997. Arch Dis Child 2010;95:786–90.

7. Kajantie E, Johnson S, Heinonen K, et al. Common core assessments in follow-up studies of adults born preterm-Recommendation of the adults born preterm International collaboration. Paediatr Perinat Epidemiol 2021;35:371–87.

8. Marlow N, Johnson S, Hurst JR. The extremely preterm young adult - state of the art. Semin Fetal Neonatal Med 2022;27:101365.

9. Shaw RJ, Bernard RS, Storfer-Isser A, et al. Parental coping in the neonatal intensive care unit. J Clin Psychol Med Settings 2013 Jun;20:135–42.

10. Pace CC, Anderson PJ, Lee KJ, et al. Posttraumatic stress symptoms in mothers and fathers of very preterm infants over the first 2 years. J Dev Behav Pediatr 2020;41:612–8.

11. Treyvaud K, Lee KJ, Doyle LW, et al. Very preterm birth influences parental mental health and family outcomes seven years after birth. J Pediatr 2014; 164:515–21.

12. Brown RN, Pascoe L, Treyvaud K, et al. Early parenting behaviour is associated with complex attention outcomes in middle to late childhood in children born very preterm. Child Neuropsychol 2022;1–18. https://doi.org/10.1080/09297049.2022.2075334 [published online ahead of print, 2022 May 13].

13. Burnett AC, Cheong JLY, Doyle LW. Biological and social influences on the neurodevelopmental outcomes of preterm infants. Clin Perinatol 2018;45:485–500.

14. Saigal S. Preemie voices – young men and women born very Prematurely describe their lives, challenges and Achievements. Victoria, BC: Friesen Press; 2014.

15. Horbar JD, Edwards EM, Ogbolu Y. Our Responsibility to follow through for NICU infants and their families. Pediatrics 2020;146:e20200360.

16. Litt JS, Hintz SR. Quality improvement for NICU graduates: Feasible, relevant, impactful. Semin Fetal Neonatal Med 2021;26:101205.

17. van Wassenaer-Leemhuis AG, Jeukens-Visser M, van Hus JW, et al. Rethinking preventive post-discharge intervention programmes for very preterm infants and their parents. Dev Med Child Neurol 2016;58(Suppl 4):67–73.

18. McKenzie K, Lynch E, Msall ME. Scaffolding parenting and health development for preterm Flourishing across the life course. Pediatrics 2022;149(Suppl 5). e2021053509K.

19. Janvier A, Farlow B, Baardsnes J, et al. Measuring and communicating meaningful outcomes in neonatology: a family perspective. Semin Perinatol 2016; 40:571–7.

20. Jaworski M, Janvier A, Lefebvre F, et al. Parental perspectives regarding outcomes of very preterm infants: toward a balanced approach. J Pediatr 2018; 200:58–63.e1.

21. Petty J, Whiting L, Green J, et al. Parents' views on preparation to care for extremely premature infants at home. Nurs Child Young People 2018. https://doi.org/10.7748/ncyp.2018.e1084.

22. Lakshmanan A, Kubicek K, Williams R, et al. Viewpoints from families for improving transition from NICU-to-home for infants with medical complexity at a safety net hospital: a qualitative study. BMC Pediatr 2019;19:223.

23. Eeles AL, Burnett AC, Cheong JL, et al. Identifying research priorities in newborn medicine: a Delphi study of parents' views. BMJ Open 2021;11: e044836.

24. Dahan S, Bourque CJ, Reichherzer M, et al. Beyond a Seat at the table: the added value of family stakeholders to improve care, research, and education in neonatology. J Pediatr 2019;207:123–9.e2.

25. Luu TM, Pearce R. Parental voice-what outcomes of preterm birth matter most to families? Sem Perinatol 2022;46:151550.

26. Rosenbaum PL, Palisano RJ, Bartlett DJ, et al. Development of the gross motor function classification system for cerebral palsy. Dev Med Child Neurol 2008;50: 249–53.

27. Towns M, Rosenbaum P, Palisano R, et al. Should the Gross Motor Functional Classification System be used for children who do not have cerebral palsy? Dev Med Child Neurol 2018;60:147–54.

28. Kehrer C, Blumenstock G, Raabe C, et al. Development and reliability of a classification system for gross motor function in children with metachromatic leucodystrophy. Dev Med Child Neurol 2011;53:156–60.

29. Haslam MD, Lisonkova S, Creighton D, et al. Canadian Neonatal Network and the Canadian Neonatal Follow-up Network. Severe neurodevelopmental impairment in neonates born preterm: impact of varying definitions in a Canadian cohort. J Pediatr 2018;197:75–81.e4.

30. Boss R, Hutton N, Sulpar LJ, et al. Values parents apply to decision-making regarding delivery room resuscitation for high-risk newborns. Pediatrics 2008; 122:583–9.

31. French KB. Care of extremely small premature infants in the neonatal intensive care unit: a parent's perspective. Clin Perinatol 2017;44:275–82.

32. Janvier A, Lorenz JM, Lantos JD. Antenatal counselling for parents facing an extremely preterm birth: limitations of the medical evidence. Acta Paediatr 2012;101:800–4.

33. Peyton C, Einspieler C. General movements: a behavioral biomarker of later motor and cognitive dysfunction in NICU graduates. Pediatr Ann 2018;47: e159–3164.

34. Guralnick MJ. Preventive interventions for preterm children: effectiveness and developmental mechanisms. J Dev Behav Pediatr 2012;33:352–64.

35. Yildiz PD, Ayers S, Phillips L. The prevalence of posttraumatic stress disorder in pregnancy and after birth: a systematic review and meta-analysis. J Affect Disord 2017;208:634–45.

36. Erdei C, Liu CH, Machie M, et al. Parent mental health and neurodevelopmental outcomes of children hospitalized in the neonatal intensive care unit. Early Hum Dev 2021;154:105278.

37. Bernardo J, Rent S, Arias-Shah A, et al. Parental stress and mental health symptoms in the NICU: Recognition and interventions. Neoreviews 2021;22: e496–505.

38. Sabnis A, Fojo S, Nayak SS, et al. Reducing parental trauma and stress in neonatal intensive care: systematic review and meta-analysis of hospital interventions. J Perinatol 2019;39:375–86.

39. Treyvaud K, Spittle A, Anderson PJ, et al. A multilayered approach is needed in the NICU to support parents after the preterm birth of their infant. Early Hum Dev 2019;139:104838.

40. Hynan MT, Hall SL. Psychosocial program standards for NICU parents. J Perinatol 2015;35(Suppl 1):S1–4.

41. Shaw RJ, St John N, Lilo E, et al. Prevention of traumatic stress in mothers of preterms: 6-month outcomes. Pediatrics 2014;134:e481–8.

42. Shaw RJ, Horwitz SM, editors. Treatment of Psychological Distress in parents of premature infants: PTSD in the NICU. Washington DC: American Psychiatric Association Publishing, Inc.; 2020.

43. Howard K, Roberts G, Lim J, et al. Biological and environmental factors as predictors of language skills in very preterm children at 5 years of age. J Dev Behav Pediatr 2011;32:239–49.

44. Ortenstrand A, Westrup B, Brostrom EB, et al. The Stockholm neonatal family centered care study: effects on length of stay and infant morbidity. Pediatrics 2010;125:e278–85.

45. Vohr BR. NICU discharge preparation and transition planning: editorial. J Perinatol 2022;42:1–2.

46. McGowan EC, Abdulla LS, Hawes KK, et al. Maternal immigrant status and readiness to transition to home from the NICU. Pediatrics 2019;143:e 20182657.

47. McGowan EC, Du N, Hawes K, et al. Maternal mental health and neonatal intensive care unit discharge readiness in mothers of preterm infants. J Pediatr 2017; 184:68–74.

48. Manickam S, Vivier PM, Rogers ML, et al. Neighborhood inequality and emergency department use in neonatal intensive care unit graduates. J Pediatr 2020;226:294–8.

49. Nwanne OY, Rogers ML, McGowan EC, et al. High-risk neighborhoods and neurodevelopmental outcomes in infants born preterm. J Pediatr 2022;245:65–71.

50. Richardson ZS, Kehtani MA, Scully E, et al. Social and functional characteristics of receipt and service use intensity of core early intervention services. Acad Pediatr 2019;19:722–32.

51. Morgan C, Fetters L, Adde L, et al. Early intervention for children age 0 to 2 Years with or at hgh risk of cerebral palsy: International Clinical Practice Guideline based on systematic reviews. JAMA Pediatr 2021;175:846–58.

52. Spittle A, Orton J, Anderson PJ, et al. Early intervention programmes provided post hospital discharge to prevent motor and cognitive impairment in preterm infants. Cochrane Database Syst Rev 2015;2015(11):CD005495.

53. Dusing SC, Tripathi T, Marcinowski EC, et al. Supporting play exploration and early developmental intervention versus usual care to enhance development outcomes during the transition from the neonatal intensive care unit to home: a pilot randomized controlled trial. BMC Pediatr 2018;18:46.

54. Litt JS, Glymour MM, Hauser-Cram P, et al. Early intervention services improve school-age functional outcome among neonatal intensive care unit graduates. Acad Pediatr 2018;18:468–74.

55. Romo ML, McVeigh KH, Jordan P, et al. Birth characteristics of children who used early intervention and special education services in New York City. J Public Health (Oxf) 2020;42:e401–11.

56. Khetani MA, Richardson Z, McManus BM. Social disparities in early intervention service Use and provider-reported outcomes. J Dev Behav Pediatr 2017;38: 501–9.

57. Feinberg E, Silverstein M, Donahue S, et al. The impact of race on participation in part C early intervention services. J Dev Behav Pediatr 2011;32:284–91.
58. Barfield WD, Clements KM, Lee KG, et al. Using linked data to assess Patterns of early intervention (EI) referral among very low birth weight infants. Matern Child Health J 2008;12:24–33.
59. Wang CJ, Elliott MN, Rogowski J, et al. Factors influencing the enrollment of eligible extremely-low-birth-weight children in the Part C early intervention program. Acad Pediatr 2009;9:83–287.
60. McManus BM, Richardson Z, Schenkman M, et al. Timing and intensity of early intervention service use and outcomes among a aafety-net population of children. JAMA Netw Open 2019;2:e187529.
61. Atkins KL, Duvall SW, Dolata JK, et al. Part C early intervention enrollment in low birth weight infants at-risk for developmental delays. Matern Child Health J 2017;21:290–6.
62. Sanders BW, Zuckerman KE, Ash JS, et al. Early intervention referral information, transmission, and sources-A survey of state part C coordinators and analysis of referral forms. J Dev Behav Pediatr 2022;48:153–e161.
63. Valentine AZ, Hall SS, Young E, et al. Implementation of telehealth services to assess, monitor and treat neurodevelopmental disorders: systematic review. J Med Internet Res 2021;23:e22619.
64. DeMauro SB, Duncan AF, Hurt H. Telemedicine use in neonatal follow-up programs-What we can do and what we can't-Lessons learned from COVID-19. Semin Perinatol 2021;45:151430.
65. Quinton JK, Ong MK, Vangala S, et al. The association of broadband internet access and telemedicine utilization in rural western Tennessee: an observational study. BMC Health Serv Res 2021;21:765.
66. Sachs JW, Graven P, Gold JA, et al. Disparities in telephone and video telehealth engagement during the COVID-19 pandemic. JAMIA Open 2021;4:ooab056.
67. Baggett KM, Davis B, Landry SH, et al. Understanding the steps toward mobile early intervention for mothers and their infants exiting the neonatal intensive care unit: Descriptive examination. J Med Internet Res 2020;22:318519.
68. Pineda R, Heiny E, Roussin J, et al. Implementation of the Baby Bridge Program reduces timing between NICU discharge and therapy activation. J Early Interv 2020;42:275–96.
69. van Veenendaal NR, Heideman WH, Limpens J, et al. Hospitalising preterm infants in single family rooms versus open bay units: a systematic review and meta-analysis. Lancet Child Adolesc Health 2019;3(3):147–57.
70. Lester BM, Hawes K, Abar B, et al. Single-family room care and neurobehavioral and medical outcomes in preterm infants. Pediatrics 2014;134:754–60.
71. Lester BM, Salisbury AL, Hawes K, et al. 18-Month follow-up of infants cared for in a single-family room neonatal intensive care Unit. J Pediatr 2016;177:84–9.
72. Vohr B, McGowan E, McKinley L, et al. Differential effects of the single-family room neonatal intensive care Unit on 18- to 24-month Bayley scores of preterm infants. J Pediatr 2017;185:42–48 e41.
73. Feeley N, Robins S, Genest C, et al. A comparative study of mothers of infants hospitalized in an open ward neonatal intensive care unit and a combined pod and single-family room design. BMC Pediatr 2020;20(1):38.
74. Meredith JL, Jnah A, Newberry D. The NICU environment: Infusing single-family room benefits into the open-bay setting. Neonatal Netw 2017;36(2):69–76. https://doi.org/10.1891/0730-0832.36.2.69.

75. Adatsafavi H, Niknejad B, Shepley M, et al. Probabilistic Return-on-Investment analysis of single-family versus open-bay rooms in neonatal intensive care units-Synthesis and evaluation of early evidence on Nosocomial Infections, length of stay, and Direct Cost of care. J Intensive Care Med 2019;34(2):115–25.

76. Winner-Stoltz R, Lengerich A, Hench AJ, et al. Staff nurse Perceptions of open-pod and single family room NICU designs on work environment and patient care. Adv Neonatal Care 2018;18(3):189–98.

77. O'Brien K, Robson K, Bracht M, et al, FICare Study Group and FICare Parent Advisory Board. Effectiveness of Family Integrated Care in neonatal intensive care units on infant and parent outcomes: a multicentre, multinational, cluster-randomised controlled trial. Lancet Child Adolesc Health 2018;2:245–54. Erratum in: *Lancet Child Adolesc Health*. 2018;2:e20.

78. Vohr B, McGowan E, Keszler L, et al. Effects of a transition home program on preterm infant emergency room visits within 90 days of discharge. J Perinatol 2017;38:185–90.

79. Vohr B, McGowan E, Keszler L, et al. Impact of a transition home program on rehospitalization rates of preterm infants. J Pediatr 2016;181:86–92 e81.

80. Liu Y, McGowan E, Tucker R, et al. Transition Home Plus Program reduces medicaid spending and health care use for high-risk infants admitted to the neonatal intensive care unit for 5 or more days. J Pediatr 2018;200:91–97 e93.

81. Orkin J, Major N, Esser K, et al. Coached, Coordinated, Enhanced Neonatal Transition (CCENT): protocol for a multicentre pragmatic randomised controlled trial of transition-to-home support for parents of high-risk infants. BMJ Open 2021;11:e046706.

82. Seppanen A-V, Draper ES, Petrou S, et al, SHIPS Research Group. High health-care use at age 5 years in a European cohort of children born very preterm. J Pediatr 2022;243:69–77.

83. Novak I, Morgan C. High-risk follow-up:Early intervention and rehabilitation. Handb Clin Neurol 2019;162:483–510.

84. Bockli K, Andrews B, Pellerite M, et al. Trends and challenges in United States neonatal intensive care units follow-up clinics. J Perinatol 2014;34:71–4.

85. Connors J, Havranek T, Campbell D. Discharge of medically complex infants and developmental follow-up. Pediatr Rev 2021;42:316–28.

86. Lipkin PH, Macias MM. Council on Children with Disabilities, Section on Developmental and Behavioral Pediatrics. Promoting optimal development: identifying infants and young children with developmental disorders through developmental surveillance and screening. Pediatrics 2020;145:320193449.

87. American Academy of Pediatrics and American College of Obstetricians and Gynecologists. In: Kilpatrick SJ, Papile L, editors. Guidelines for perinatal care. Eighth edition. Washington DC): American Academy of Pediatrics (Elk Grove Village, IL) and American College of Obstetricians and Gynecologists; 2017. p. 472.

88. Marino BS, Lipkin PH, Newburger JW, et al. American heart association congenital heart Defects Committee, Council on Cardiovascular disease in the young, Council on Cardiovascular nursing and Stroke Council. Neurodevelopmental outcomes in children with congenital heart disease: evaluation and management: a scientific statement from the American heart association. Circulation 2012;126:1143–72.

89. Hintz SR, Gould JB, Bennett MV, et al. Factors associated with successful first high-risk infant clinic visit for very low birth weight infants in California. J Pediatr 2019;210:91–98e1.

Outcomes of Preterm Infants**15**

90. Lakshmanan A, Rogers EE, Lu T, et al. Disparities and early engagement associated with the 18- to 36- month high-risk infant follow-up visit among very low birth weight infants in California. J Pediatr 2022;248:30–8.e3.
91. Fraiman YS, Steward JE, Litt JS. Race, language, and neighborhood predict high-risk preterm infant follow-up program participation. J Perinatol 2022;42: 217–22.
92. Ballantyne M, Stevens B, Guttman A, et al. Maternal and infant predictors of attendance at neonatal follow-up programmes. Child Care Health Dev 2014; 40:250–8.
93. Ballantyne M, Benzies K, Rosenbaum P, et al. Mothers' and health care providers' perspectives of the barriers and facilitators to attendance at Canadian neonatal follow-up programs. Child Care Health Dev 2015;41:722–33.
94. Maitre NL, Benninger KL, Neel ML, et al. Standardized neurodevelopmental surveillance of high-risk infants using telehealth: implementation study during COVID-19. Pediatr Qual Saf 2021;28:3439.
95. Litt JS, Edwards EM, Lainwala S, et al. Optimizing high-risk infant follow-up in Nonresearch-based Paradigms: the new England follow-up network. Pediatr Qual Saf 2020;5(3):e287.
96. Hintz SR, Gould JB, Bennett MV, et al. Referral of very low birth weight infants to high-risk follow-up at neonatal intensive care unit discharge varies widely across California. J Pediatr 2015;166(2):289–95.
97. Pai VV, Kan P, Bennett M, et al. Improved referral of very low birthweight infants to high-risk infant follow-up in California. J Pediatr 2020;216:101–8.e1.
98. Pai VV, Kan P, Lu T, et al. Factors associated with follow-up of infants with hypoxic-ischemic encephalopathy in a high-risk infant clinic in California. J Perinatol 2021;41:1347–54.
99. Murray CJL, Vos T, Lozano R, et al. Disability-adjusted life years (DALYs) for 291 diseases and injuries in 21 regions, 1990-2010: a systematic analysis for the Global Burden of Disease Study 2010. Lancet 2012;380:2197–223.
100. Eves R, Mendonca M, Baumann N, et al. Association of very preterm birth or very low birth weight with intelligence in adulthood: an individual participant data meta-analysis. JAMA Pediatr 2021;175(8):e211058.
101. Lean RE, Lessov-Shlaggar CN, Gerstein ED, et al. Maternal and family factors differentiate profiles of psychiatric impairments in very preterm children at age 5-years. J Child Psychol Psychiatry 2020;61:157–66.
102. Treyvaud K, Ure A, Doyle LW, et al. Psychiatric outcomes at age seven for very preterm children: rates and predictors. J Child Psychol Psychiatry 2013;54(7): 772–9.
103. Johns CB, Lacadie C, Vohr B, et al. Amygdala functional connectivity is associated with social impairments in preterm born young adults. Neuroimage Clin 2019;21:101626.
104. Chyi LJ, Lee HC, Hintz SR, et al. School outcomes of late preterm infants: special needs and challenges for infants born at 32 to 36 weeks gestation. J Pediatr 2008;153:25–31.
105. Morse SB, Zheng H, Tang Y, et al. Early school-age outcomes of late preterm infants. Pediatrics 2009;123:e622–9.
106. Petrini JR, Dias T, McCormick MC, et al. Increased risk of adverse neurological development for late preterm infants. J Pediatr 2009;154(2):169–76.
107. Baron IS, Erickson K, Ahronovich MD, et al. Cognitive deficit in preschoolers born late-preterm. Early Hum Dev 2011;87:115–9.

108. Baron IS, Litman FR, Ahronovich MD, et al. Late preterm birth: a review of medical and neuropsychological childhood outcomes. Neuropsychol Rev 2012;22: 438–50.
109. Huppi PS, Warfield S, Kikinis R, et al. Quantitative magnetic resonance imaging of brain development in premature and mature newborns. Ann Neurol 1998;43: 224–35.
110. Heinonen K, Eriksson JG, Kajantie E, et al. Late-preterm birth and lifetime socioeconomic attainments: the Helsinki birth cohort study. Pediatrics 2013;132: 647–55.

# Neonatal Opioid Withdrawal Syndrome

## An Update on Developmental Outcomes

Kristen L. Benninger, MD, MSc[a],*, Jennifer M. McAllister, MD[b],
Stephanie L. Merhar, MD, MS[b]

## KEYWORDS

- Neonatal opioid withdrawal syndrome (NOWS)
- Neonatal abstinence syndrome (NAS) • Opioid • Neurodevelopment
- Developmental outcomes

## KEY POINTS

- Recent trends in care for opioid-exposed infants include an increased emphasis on non-pharmacologic management and decreased postnatal pharmacotherapy for clinical symptoms of withdrawal.
- The neurodevelopmental effects of prenatal opioid exposure are nearly impossible to disentangle from confounding socioeconomic, environmental, and genetic and epigenetic factors.
- Children with prenatal opioid exposure are at higher risk for developmental and behavioral concerns and poorer school performance.
- Care for the opioid-exposed child and family should be multi-disciplinary, comprehensive, and non-judgmental and focus on strengthening the caregiver–child relationship, providing social support, and positive developmental experiences.

## INTRODUCTION AND IMPORTANCE OF THE PROBLEM

Although there is evidence that rates of maternal opioid use during pregnancy have stabilized in the past several years, prenatal opioid exposure is still common, with one infant born exposed to opioids every 15 min in the United States.[1,2] Recent expert opinion has attempted to standardize the definition of neonatal opioid withdrawal,[3] but currently available literature uses a wide variety of definitions of prenatal opioid exposure/neonatal opioid withdrawal syndrome (NOWS)/neonatal abstinence syndrome

[a] Center for Perinatal Research, The Abigail Wexner Research Institute, Nationwide Children's Hospital, 575 Children's Crossroad, WB 5203, Columbus, OH 43215, USA; [b] Cincinnati Children's Hospital Perinatal Institute, University of Cincinnati College of Medicine, 3333 Burnet Ave, ML 7009, Cincinnati, OH 45229, USA
* Corresponding author.
*E-mail address:* Kristen.Benninger@nationwidechildrens.org

Clin Perinatol 50 (2023) 17–29
https://doi.org/10.1016/j.clp.2022.10.007
0095-5108/23/© 2022 Elsevier Inc. All rights reserved.

(NAS), complicating our understanding of outcomes. Recent trends in care for opioid-exposed infants include an increased emphasis on non-pharmacologic management and decreased postnatal pharmacotherapy for clinical symptoms of withdrawal.[4,5] However, prenatal opioid exposure itself may affect later development and behavior regardless of postnatal pharmacologic treatment.[6,7]

There is a paucity of well-controlled, prospective longitudinal studies comparing the neurodevelopment of children exposed to opioids prenatally and unexposed children. Some studies demonstrate differences between exposed and unexposed infants, but sample sizes are small and the influence of other factors that might affect neurodevelopment are rarely accounted for. The neurodevelopmental effects of prenatal opioid exposure are nearly impossible to disentangle from socioeconomic, environmental, and genetic and epigenetic factors (**Fig. 1**).[8,9] In addition, women on medication for opioid use disorder (MOUD) may use additional illicit substances or other prescribed medications that affect both short- and long-term outcomes.[10–13]

Even well-designed studies with strict inclusion criteria and high internal validity have limited generalizability to many real-world clinical scenarios, including maternal polysubstance use and adverse childhood experiences. Most published studies evaluate neurodevelopment at age 2 or younger. Unfortunately, assessment at toddler age, before the emergence of complex cognitive and behavioral processes, is likely inadequate to describe the full neurodevelopmental impact of prenatal opioid exposure and NOWS.[14] Finally, attrition bias due to difficulty following a large longitudinal cohort is especially problematic in a population disproportionately affected by socioeconomic hardship.

We provide a review of key findings by developmental domain. We include literature published in the past 10 years (with data collected in the past 20 years) including prenatal opioid exposure (+/− other substances), with or without pharmacologic treatment of NOWS. We attempt to provide a cohesive narrative, however, significant heterogeneity in definitions of NAS/NOWS, study type, presence of an unexposed comparison group, and type and timing of developmental assessments exist in the current literature.

## NEURAL BASIS OF POTENTIAL ALTERATIONS IN NEURODEVELOPMENT

Preclinical studies reveal potential mechanisms for alterations in neurodevelopment and behavior due to prenatal opioid exposure. In rodent and organoid models,

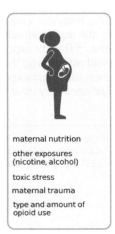
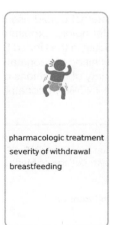
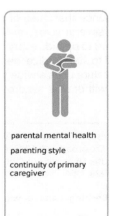
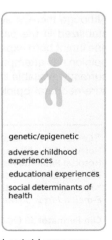

| | | | |
|---|---|---|---|
| maternal nutrition | pharmacologic treatment | parental mental health | genetic/epigenetic |
| other exposures (nicotine, alcohol) | severity of withdrawal | parenting style | adverse childhood experiences |
| toxic stress | breastfeeding | continuity of primary caregiver | educational experiences |
| maternal trauma | | | social determinants of health |
| type and amount of opioid use | | | |

**Fig. 1.** Factors affecting neurodevelopmental outcome after prenatal opioid exposure.

prenatal opioid exposure affects neurogenesis, neuronal development, glial cell development, and myelination as well as memory and behavior.[15] It is unknown whether these differences translate to humans, but neuroimaging studies demonstrate differences in brain volumes,[16,17] punctate white matter injury,[18] altered white matter microstructure,[19] altered network connectivity,[20–22] and increased cerebral perfusion[23] in infants and children exposed to opioids prenatally.

## COGNITIVE OUTCOMES
### Infants

In the ethanol, neurodevelopment, infant and child health (ENRICH) prospective cohort, Bayley Scales of Infant and Toddler Development, 3rd edition (Bayley-III) cognitive scores at 5 to 8 months were not different between MOUD (n = 42) and unexposed control (n = 36) groups or between infants who received pharmacologic treatment of NOWS and infants who did not.[24] Similarly, Labella and colleagues[25] report a study evaluating a parenting program for mothers on MOUD (n = 85) with scores in the normal range on Ages and Stages Questionnaire-3rd Edition (ASQ-3) at 3 and 6 months (Problem-Solving and Personal-Social domains). Conversely, in a prospective cohort study of 81 infants with prenatal opioid exposure, at 6 months of age, the opioid-exposed group scored lower than the unexposed matched comparison group in all Griffiths Scales of Child Development domains (Griffiths Scales) after correcting for maternal smoking and alcohol consumption (all $P < .001$).[26] Infants who received pharmacologic treatment of NOWS and infants with in-utero polysubstance exposure scored lower than those without pharmacologic treatment or polysubstance exposure.[26] In a small, retrospective cohort of infants with NOWS requiring pharmacologic treatment, Beckwith and Burke observed lower Bayley-III cognitive scores at 1 to 3 months compared with the test standard sample.[27] Infants receiving methadone had lower cognitive scores than those treated with morphine for NOWS.[28]

### Toddlers

In two retrospective studies (n = 285, n = 87) infants with pharmacologically treated NOWS had significantly lower Bayley-III cognitive scores at 15 to 24 months compared with population norms, but still within the normal range.[29,30] A small study of infants prenatally exposed to methadone demonstrated Bayley-III cognitive scores lower than controls at 18 to 24 months (mean ± SD, 83.30 ± 16.40 vs 97.60 ± 10.90, $P < .05$).[31] A recent, multi-site randomized study of morphine versus methadone for treatment of NOWS found no difference in Bayley-III cognitive scores between treatment groups at 18 months.[32] Infants discharged on phenobarbital had lower cognitive scores than those not receiving phenobarbital at discharge.[32] Infants from the maternal opioid treatment: human experimental research (MOTHER) randomized controlled trial (RCT) had Bayley-III cognitive scores within the normal range at 24 and 36 months (estimated marginal mean [95% CI], 96.3 [93.30, 99.33]; 98.5 [95.41, 101.57]).[33] There were no differences in cognitive scores between children with prenatal exposure to methadone compared with buprenorphine or in those who received pharmacologic treatment of NOWS compared with infants who did not.[33]

A longitudinal cohort of 100 opioid-exposed infants and 110 unexposed controls born in Christchurch, New Zealand (NZ) was followed from birth to 9.5 years.[34–40] At 2 years, opioid-exposed children had lower Bayley-II cognitive scores compared with controls (mean ± SD, 77.48 ± 18.04 vs 92.35 ± 16.30, $P < .0001$) with a higher proportion in the opioid-exposed group with cognitive delay (51.1% vs 13.9%, $P < .001$, OR 6.48).[34,38] The between-group differences in cognitive development remained after adjustment for covariates. However, postnatal parental and family factors explained 41% of the between-group differences in cognitive outcomes.[38]

### Preschool to School Age

In the Christchurch, NZ cohort, at 4.5 years, opioid-exposed children had higher rates of impairment across all outcome domains including verbal, auditory, and perceptual processing, and cognition/IQ (total IQ: mean ± SD, opioid-exposed 97.9 ± 15, control 112.2 ± 14.5, $P < .001$). Opioid-exposed children were three times more likely to have any learning or processing impairment (38% vs 12%, OR 4.7 [2.2–9.8]) and cognitive delay (39% vs 13%, OR 4.5 [2.2–9.2]).[35]

In a prospective, longitudinal study (BLINDED cohort) at 4 years, children in both opioid-exposed and unexposed control groups scored within the normal range on cognitive testing. However, children in the opioid-exposed group scored significantly lower on memory, attention, and executive functioning, and sensorimotor subtests of the NEPSY (A Developmental Neuropsychological Assessment) and on visual-spatial and vocabulary subtests of the Wechsler Preschool & Primary Scale of Intelligence.[41,42]

### Academic Achievement and Support

Two large studies using linked administrative and health data demonstrated increased need for special education services[43] and lower standardized test scores[44] in children with a history of NOWS. However, both are limited by unmeasured confounding factors and reliance on International Classification of Disease and Related Problems (ICD) codes for NOWS diagnosis. In a study by Fill and colleagues, compared with matched controls (n = 5,441), children with NOWS (n = 1,815) were more likely to be referred for a disability evaluation, meet criteria for a disability, and require classroom therapies or services in early childhood (all $P < .0001$).[43] Developmental delay (5.3% vs 3.5%; $P = .001$) and speech/language impairment (10.3% vs 8.3%; $P = .009$) were more likely among children with a history of NOWS. A multivariable analysis controlling for confounding variables showed similar findings.[43] A linked analysis of health and curriculum-based test data for children from Australia revealed lower test scores in grades 3,5, and 7 for all domains (reading, writing, numeracy, spelling, grammar/punctuation) in children with NOWS (n = 2234) compared with matched controls (n = 4330) and other local children (n = 598,265) with progressive worsening over time.[44] NOWS was independently associated with a risk of not meeting National Minimum Standards (aOR 2.5, 95% CI 2.2–2.7).[44]

In the Christchurch, NZ cohort, at 9.5 years, opioid-exposed children scored lower on all reading and mathematics subtests of the Woodcock Johnson-III Tests of Achievement and had higher rates of any educational delay (57% vs 15%, OR 7.47 [3.71–15.02]).[39]

## SPEECH AND LANGUAGE OUTCOMES
### Infants

In the ENRICH prospective cohort, Bayley-III language scores at 5 to 8 months were not different between MOUD-exposed and control groups or between infants who received pharmacologic treatment of NOWS and infants who did not.[24] Similarly, Labella and colleagues[25] reported communication scores in the normal range on ASQ-3 at 3 and 6 months. Conversely, in the Beckwith and Burke retrospective cohort, mean Bayley-III language scores were significantly lower in the NOWS group compared with the test standard sample.[27]

### Toddlers

In two retrospective studies (n = 285, n = 87), infants with pharmacologically treated NOWS had significantly lower Bayley-III language scores at 15 to 24 months compared with population norms, but mean scores were still within the normal range.[29,30] In a large retrospective study by Hall and colleagues (total n = 15,544), infants with prenatal opioid exposure (+/− NOWS) were more likely to be diagnosed with speech disorders (13.8% vs 6.5%, $P$ = .0005) than those without exposures.[6] Conversely, a small study of infants prenatally exposed to methadone demonstrated Bayley-III language scores similar to controls at 18 to 24 months (mean ± SD, 78.30 ± 16.10 vs 85.80 ± 13.60).[31]

The multi-site RCT of morphine or methadone for the treatment of NOWS found no difference in Bayley-III language scores between treatment groups at 18 months (mean ± SD, methadone: 96.0 ± 16.9, morphine: 94.2 ± 18.2).[32] However, 26% to 33% of infants scored <85 on the Bayley-III language composite, more than twice that in the normative sample, suggesting a higher risk of language delays.[32] Infants discharged on phenobarbital had lower language scores than those not receiving phenobarbital at discharge. In an adjusted analysis, infants with higher NOWS severity had lower Bayley-III language scores (high severity 84.8 ± 5.2 vs low severity 96.2 ± 3.9, $P$ = .013).[45]

Infants from the MOTHER trial had Bayley-III language scores within the normal range at 24 and 36 months (estimated marginal mean [95% CI], 92.7 [89.62, 95.73]; 98.4 [95.25, 101.47]). There were no differences in Bayley-III language scores between those with prenatal exposure to methadone compared with buprenorphine or in those who received pharmacologic treatment of NOWS compared with those who did not.[33]

In the Christchurch, NZ cohort, at 2 years, opioid-exposed children had lower scores for all components of language development compared with control children, with a higher proportion classified as having language problems (24.1% vs 10.9%, $P$ = .016, OR 2.6).[38] However, after adjustment for covariates, the differences in language development between groups were no longer present.[38]

### Preschool to School Age

In the Christchurch, NZ cohort, at 4.5 years, opioid-exposed children had scores on the Clinical Evaluation of Language Fundamentals Preschool (CELF-P) below the control group (mean ± SD, total 83.62 ± 14.85 vs 100.46 ± 15.97, $P$ < .001) and were three times more likely to have language delay/impairment (33% vs 11%, OR 4 [1.9–8.7]).[35,37] After adjustment for multiple confounding variables, opioid exposure remained a significant independent predictor of preschool language development.[37] Important positive mediators included the quality of parenting, home environment, and early childhood education participation.[37]

## MOTOR OUTCOMES

The literature from the past 10 years on motor outcomes in children with prenatal opioid exposure is mixed. In several studies, infants with prenatal opioid exposure had lower motor scores than population means, although still within the normal range. In the Beckwith and Burke[27] retrospective cohort, infants with NOWS had lower Bayley-III motor scores at 1 to 3 months compared with the test standard sample (96.25 vs 100, $P$ = .033). In a prospective study from Scotland, at 6 months, the opioid-exposed group (n = 81) scored lower than matched comparison (n = 26) on the Griffiths Scales after correcting for maternal smoking and alcohol consumption (102 vs 111, $P$ < .001).[26] Two studies suggest infants with higher-dose opioid exposure may have lower motor scores. Bier and colleagues[46] found infants exposed to high-dose methadone, compared with low-dose, had significantly lower Alberta Infant Motor Scale scores at 4 months of age. Labella and colleagues[25] report motor scores in the normal range on the ASQ-3 at 3 and 6 months. Finally, in a retrospective study published by Benninger and colleagues,[29] infants with NOWS had normal motor scores on the Test of Infant Motor Performance at 3 to 4 months and on the Bayley-III at 9 to 12 and 15 to 18 months of age.

Two studies in toddlers also showed lower motor scores in opioid-exposed children but with scores still falling in the normal range. In the Christchurch, NZ cohort, at 2 years, methadone-exposed children had lower Bayley-II motor scores compared with controls.[38] The between-group differences in motor development remained after adjustment for covariates but after additional parent and family factors were considered, these differences were no longer significant.[38] In a retrospective cohort study (n = 87) by Merhar and colleagues,[30] infants with pharmacologically treated NOWS had lower Bayley-III motor scores than the normative population (94 vs 100, $P < .03$) at 2 years but still scored within the normal range.

Only one study published in the past 10 years describes motor function in older children with prenatal opioid exposure. In a small study from Sweden, opioid-exposed children (n = 25) scored significantly lower on the motor scale of the McCarthy Scales of Children's Abilities compared with population norms ($P < .001$) at 5 to 6 years.[47]

Several studies evaluate the impact of different pre- and postnatal opioids on motor outcomes. Burke and Beckwith[28] found infants treated with morphine had higher Bayley-III motor scores at 2.5 months than those treated with methadone (96.3 vs 89.6, $P = .0149$). In an RCT of morphine versus methadone for treatment of NOWS, Czynski and colleagues[32] found no differences in Bayley-III motor scores at 18 months between the two groups. Infants with higher NOWS severity had lower Bayley-III motor scores ($P = .041$).[45] After adjustment for site, Child Protective Services involvement, sex, and head circumference, the differences in motor development between groups were no longer present. Finally, infants from the MOTHER trial had Bayley-III motor scores within the normal range at 24 and 36 months with no differences for those exposed prenatally to methadone versus buprenorphine.[33]

## BEHAVIORAL OUTCOMES

Several studies describe behavior problems in children with prenatal opioid exposure. Hall and colleagues found children exposed to opioids prenatally were more likely to have an ICD diagnosis of behavioral or emotional problem compared with unexposed children ($P = .0008$).[6] In the Christchurch, NZ cohort, Jaekel and colleagues[40] assessed children with prenatal opioid exposure at 2, 4.5, and 9 years using the Strengths and Difficulties Questionnaire (SDQ). Across all timepoints, opioid-exposed children had higher total difficulties scores compared with controls and the difficulties increased from ages 2 to 9 years.[40] Opioid-exposed children had more inattention/hyperactivity (mean difference [95% CI] 1.02 [0.33, 1.7]) and peer problems (0.53 [0.07, 0.99]) compared with controls at 2 years. By 4.5 years, opioid-exposed children had worse scores on all 4 SDQ domains and these trajectories worsened over time compared with unexposed children.[40] Children with higher risk scores in biological, maternal social, and postnatal rearing environment risk categories had higher total difficulty scores.[40]

## VISUAL OUTCOMES
### Visual Evoked Potentials

Visual Evoked Potentials (VEPs) test the health of the visual pathway from the retina to the occipital cortex by measuring changes in brain wave electrical activity.[48,49] VEP latency measures processing speed from the visual stimulus in the primary visual cortex; a slower latency suggests less visual maturation.[48,50] In a study by McGlone et al., at 6 months of age, 70% of methadone-exposed infants (n = 81) had at least one abnormal VEP response to different check sizes and slower median VEP peak times compared with controls.[50,51]

In an Australian cohort, methadone-exposed infants had significantly longer VEP latencies at 4 months than control infants.[52] At 36 months, no significant differences between groups remained.[48] The initial slow latencies at 4 months in the methadone-exposed group normalized by 36 months, indicating that visual maturation continues to develop into childhood.[48]

### Visual Acuity

Studies evaluating visual acuity in children with prenatal opioid exposure are limited. A study by Walhovd and colleagues demonstrated significantly lower left eye visual acuity at 4.5 years in children with prenatal opioid exposure compared with controls (P = .029) with a trend toward lower binocular visual acuity.[53]

### Strabismus/Eye Muscle/Binocular Movement

Most reports of disorders of the eye muscle and eye movement in children with prenatal opioid exposure describe nystagmus and strabismus in this population.[54–57] In the large retrospective study by Hall and colleagues,[6] opioid-exposed infants who required pharmacologic treatment of NOWS had the highest rates of strabismus (10.9%) compared with those with prenatal opioid exposure without pharmacologic treatment (3.4%) and unexposed infants (1%). In a longitudinal cohort study of infants with prenatal substance exposure, compared with infants with prenatal cocaine or cannabis exposure or unexposed infants, opioid-exposed infants had a higher risk of hospitalization for eye disorders and a 3.15x higher risk of ocular muscle disorders.[58] Co-exposure to maternal cigarette smoking, also associated with strabismus,[59] is a confounding factor in some studies.

### Visual Attention and Smooth Pursuit

The coordination of smooth pursuit with catch-up, fast saccadic eye movements allows accurate tracking of moving objects and is susceptible to effects of in-utero exposures.[60] Melinder and colleagues[60] found no differences in the number of saccades/s or with smooth pursuit for slow-moving object evaluations between opioid-exposed and unexposed 4-year-old children. After controlling for maternal employment, opioid-exposed children had slower smooth pursuit for fast-moving object evaluations.[60] However, this difference was not sustained when controlling for maternal education or birthweight.

Melinder and Konijnenberg investigated visual selective attention using a special negative priming (SNP) paradigm.[61] The opioid-exposed children had a reduced SNP effect and did not inhibit the prime distractor location compared with controls.[61] Pharmacologic treatment of NOWS and prenatal marijuana were risk factors for poorer performance.[61]

## MEDICAL COMORBIDITIES

Infants with prenatal opioid exposure have higher rates of health care utilization and hospital readmissions than the general population, even beyond the known risk of neonatal hospitalization for withdrawal.[62–65] Most studies evaluating later medical complications and rehospitalizations have relied on ICD codes. Several of these

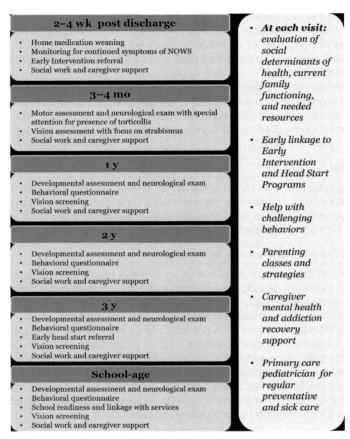

**2–4 wk post discharge**
- Home medication weaning
- Monitoring for continued symptoms of NOWS
- Early Intervention referral
- Social work and caregiver support

**3–4 mo**
- Motor assessment and neurological exam with special attention for presence of torticollis
- Vision assessment with focus on strabismus
- Social work and caregiver support

**1 y**
- Developmental assessment and neurological exam
- Behavioral questionnaire
- Vision screening
- Social work and caregiver support

**2 y**
- Developmental assessment and neurological exam
- Behavioral questionnaire
- Vision screening
- Social work and caregiver support

**3 y**
- Developmental assessment and neurological exam
- Behavioral questionnaire
- Early head start referral
- Vision screening
- Social work and caregiver support

**School-age**
- Developmental assessment and neurological exam
- Behavioral questionnaire
- School readiness and linkage with services
- Vision screening
- Social work and caregiver support

- *At each visit: evaluation of social determinants of health, current family functioning, and needed resources*
- *Early linkage to Early Intervention and Head Start Programs*
- *Help with challenging behaviors*
- *Parenting classes and strategies*
- *Caregiver mental health and addiction recovery support*
- *Primary care pediatrician for regular preventative and sick care*

**Fig. 2.** Recommended visit schedule and points of focus.

studies report higher rates of rehospitalization for infectious causes in opioid-exposed children compared with the general population.[62,63,66,67] However, a population-based study from Nordic countries demonstrated no difference in antibiotic prescription or infection diagnoses in opioid-exposed compared with unexposed children.[68]

Two studies report higher rates of torticollis (11.1% and 24.9%)[69,70] in infants with a history of pharmacologic treatment of NOWS compared with the general population (8%).[71] Most cases of torticollis in these reports are attributed to positional/postural causes related to hypertonicity and plagiocephaly.

## RECOMMENDATIONS

Neurodevelopmental follow-up of infants with NOWS is important to ensure adequate social support, developmental and behavioral surveillance, and early referral to appropriate developmental services. We provide a recommended visit schedule and points of focus in **Fig. 2**.

## SUMMARY AND FUTURE DIRECTIONS

Prenatal opioid exposure, with or without NOWS, is associated with developmental effects. However, it is unknown whether prenatal opioid exposure *causes* such effects or reflects a *correlation*, because of the significant confounding factors of polysubstance exposure, family trauma, and mental health disorders, and other environmental influences. Regardless, children exposed to opioids prenatally seem to be at higher risk for developmental and behavioral issues and should be followed closely after hospital discharge, ideally until at least school age. Care for the opioid-exposed child and family should be comprehensive and non-judgmental and should focus on strengthening the caregiver–child relationship, providing social support, and positive developmental experiences.

---

**Best practices**

*What is the current practice for neurodevelopmental follow-up of NOWS?*

Children with prenatal opioid exposure are at higher risk of developmental and behavioral concerns and poorer school performance than unexposed peers. Despite this, wide variability exists in practices for neurodevelopmental follow-up of infants and children with NOWS. Prenatal opioid exposure is not an automatic qualification for early intervention services in many states.

*What changes in current practice are likely to improve outcomes?*

Routine and regular neurodevelopmental follow-up of infants and children with NOWS until at least school age is important to ensure adequate social support, developmental and behavioral surveillance, and early referral to appropriate developmental services.

*Major Recommendations*

Prenatal opioid exposure is associated with developmental and behavioral problems, although it is not clear if the opioid exposure itself is causative. Pediatricians and neonatologists following children with prenatal opioid exposure should be aware of this higher risk, monitoring closely for developmental and behavioral problems and providing social support in the context of supportive, non-judgmental care.

---

## CLINICS CARE POINTS

---

- Prenatal opioid exposure is associated with developmental and behavioral problems, although it is not clear if the opioid exposure itself is causative.

- Pediatricians and neonatologists following children with prenatal opioid exposure should be aware of this higher risk, monitoring closely for developmental and behavioral problems and providing social supports in the context of supportive, non-judgmental care.

---

## DISCLOSURE

The authors have nothing to disclose.

## REFERENCES

1. Honein MA, Boyle C, Redfield RR. Public health surveillance of prenatal opioid exposure in mothers and infants. Pediatrics 2019;143(3).
2. Leech AA, Cooper WO, McNeer E, et al. Neonatal abstinence syndrome in the United States, 2004-16. Health Aff (Millwood) 2020;39(5):764–7.
3. Jilani SM, Jones HE, Grossman M, et al. Standardizing the clinical definition of opioid withdrawal in the neonate. J Pediatr 2022;243:33–39 e31.

4. Blount T, Painter A, Freeman E, et al. Reduction in length of stay and morphine use for NAS with the "eat, sleep, console" method. Hosp Pediatr 2019;9(8): 615–23.

5. Pahl A, Young L, Buus-Frank ME, et al. Non-pharmacological care for opioid withdrawal in newborns. Cochrane Database Syst Rev 2020;12(12):CD013217.

6. Hall ES, McAllister JM, Wexelblatt SL. Developmental disorders and medical complications among infants with subclinical intrauterine opioid exposures. Popul Health Manag 2019;22(1):19–24.

7. Leyenaar JK, Schaefer AP, Wasserman JR, et al. Infant mortality associated with prenatal opioid exposure. JAMA Pediatr 2021;175(7):706–14.

8. Jones HE, Kaltenbach K, Benjamin T, et al. Prenatal opioid exposure, neonatal abstinence syndrome/neonatal opioid withdrawal syndrome, and later child development research: shortcomings and solutions. J Addict Med 2019; 13(2):90–2.

9. Konijnenberg C. Methodological issues in assessing the impact of prenatal drug exposure. Subst Abuse 2015;9(Suppl 2):39–44.

10. Singal D, Chateau D, Struck S, et al. In Utero antidepressants and neurodevelopmental outcomes in kindergarteners. Pediatrics 2020;145(5):e20191157.

11. Jacobson JL, Akkaya-Hocagil T, Ryan LM, et al. Effects of prenatal alcohol exposure on cognitive and behavioral development: findings from a hierarchical meta-analysis of data from six prospective longitudinal U.S. cohorts. Alcohol Clin Exp Res 2021;45(10):2040–58.

12. Salzwedel AP, Grewen KM, Vachet C, et al. Prenatal drug exposure affects neonatal brain functional connectivity. J Neurosci 2015;35(14):5860–9.

13. Corsi DJ, Donelle J, Sucha E, et al. Maternal cannabis use in pregnancy and child neurodevelopmental outcomes. Nat Med 2020;26(10):1536–40.

14. Wong HS, Santhakumaran S, Cowan FM, et al. Medicines for neonates investigator G. Developmental assessments in preterm children: a meta-analysis. Pediatrics 2016;138(2).

15. Boggess T, Risher WC. Clinical and basic research investigations into the long-term effects of prenatal opioid exposure on brain development. J Neurosci Res 2020;100(1):396–409.

16. Merhar SL, Kline JE, Braimah A, et al. Prenatal opioid exposure is associated with smaller brain volumes in multiple regions. Pediatr Res 2020;90(2):397–402.

17. Hartwell ML, Croff JM, Morris AS, et al. Association of prenatal opioid exposure with precentral gyrus volume in children. JAMA Pediatr 2020;174(9):893–6.

18. Merhar SL, Parikh NA, Braimah A, et al. White matter injury and structural anomalies in infants with prenatal opioid exposure. AJNR Am J Neuroradiol 2019; 40(12):2161–5.

19. Monnelly VJ, Anblagan D, Quigley A, et al. Prenatal methadone exposure is associated with altered neonatal brain development. Neuroimage Clin 2018;18:9–14.

20. Jiang W, Merhar SL, Zeng Z, et al. Neural alterations in opioid-exposed infants revealed by edge-centric brain functional networks. Brain Commun 2022;4(3): fcac112.

21. Radhakrishnan R, Vishnubhotla RV, Guckien Z, et al. Thalamocortical functional connectivity in infants with prenatal opioid exposure correlates with severity of neonatal opioid withdrawal syndrome. Neuroradiology 2022;64(8):1649–59.

22. Radhakrishnan R, Vishnubhotla RV, Zhao Y, et al. Global brain functional network connectivity in infants with prenatal opioid exposure. Front Pediatr 2022;10: 847037.

23. Benninger KL, Peng J, Ho ML, et al. Cerebral perfusion and neurological examination characterise neonatal opioid withdrawal syndrome: a prospective cohort study. Arch Dis Child Fetal Neonatal Ed 2021;107(4):414–20.

24. Bakhireva LN, Holbrook BD, Shrestha S, et al. Association between prenatal opioid exposure, neonatal opioid withdrawal syndrome, and neurodevelopmental and behavioral outcomes at 5-8 months of age. Early Hum Dev 2019;128:69–76.

25. Labella MH, Eiden RD, Tabachnick AR, et al. Infant neurodevelopmental outcomes of prenatal opioid exposure and polysubstance use. Neurotoxicol Teratol 2021;86:107000.

26. McGlone L, Mactier H. Infants of opioid-dependent mothers: neurodevelopment at six months. Early Hum Dev 2015;91(1):19–21.

27. Beckwith AM, Burke SA. Identification of early developmental deficits in infants with prenatal heroin, methadone, and other opioid exposure. Clin Pediatr (Phila) 2015;54(4):328–35.

28. Burke S, Beckwith AM. Morphine versus methadone treatment for neonatal withdrawal and impact on early infant development. Glob Pediatr Health 2017;4. 2333794X17721128.

29. Benninger KL, Borghese T, Kovalcik JB, et al. Prenatal exposures are associated with worse neurodevelopmental outcomes in infants with neonatal opioid withdrawal syndrome. Front Pediatr 2020;8:462.

30. Merhar SL, McAllister JM, Wedig-Stevie KE, et al. Retrospective review of neurodevelopmental outcomes in infants treated for neonatal abstinence syndrome. J Perinatol 2018;38(5):587–92.

31. Serino Ma D, Peterson Md BS, Rosen Md TS. Psychological functioning of women taking illicit drugs during pregnancy and the growth and development of their offspring in early childhood. J Dual Diagn 2018;14(3):158–70.

32. Czynski AJ, Davis JM, Dansereau LM, et al. Neurodevelopmental outcomes of neonates randomized to morphine or methadone for treatment of neonatal abstinence syndrome. J Pediatr 2020;219:146–151 e141.

33. Kaltenbach K, O'Grady KE, Heil SH, et al. Prenatal exposure to methadone or buprenorphine: early childhood developmental outcomes. Drug Alcohol Depend 2018;185:40–9.

34. Levine TA, Woodward LJ. Early inhibitory control and working memory abilities of children prenatally exposed to methadone. Early Hum Dev 2018;116:68–75.

35. Lee SJ, Pritchard VE, Austin NC, et al. Health and neurodevelopment of children born to opioid-dependent mothers at school entry. J Dev Behav Pediatr 2020; 41(1):48–57.

36. Wouldes TA, Woodward LJ. Neurobehavior of newborn infants exposed prenatally to methadone and identification of a neurobehavioral profile linked to poorer neurodevelopmental outcomes at age 24 months. PLoS One 2020;15(10): e0240905.

37. Kim HM, Bone RM, McNeill B, et al. Preschool language development of children born to women with an opioid use disorder. Children 2021;8(4).

38. Levine TA, Davie-Gray A, Kim HM, et al. Prenatal methadone exposure and child developmental outcomes in 2-year-old children. Dev Med Child Neurol 2021; 63(9):1114–22.

39. Lee SJ, Woodward LJ, Henderson JMT. Educational achievement at age 9.5 years of children born to mothers maintained on methadone during pregnancy. PLoS One 2019;14(10):e0223685.

40. Jaekel J, Kim HM, Lee SJ, et al. Emotional and behavioral trajectories of 2 to 9 Years old children born to opioid-dependent mothers. Res Child Adolesc Psychopathol 2021;49(4):443–57.

41. Konijnenberg C, Sarfi M, Melinder A. Mother-child interaction and cognitive development in children prenatally exposed to methadone or buprenorphine. Early Hum Dev 2016;101:91–7.

42. Konijnenberg C, Melinder A. Executive function in preschool children prenatally exposed to methadone or buprenorphine. Child Neuropsychol 2015;21(5): 570–85.

43. Fill M-MA, Miller AM, Wilkinson RH, et al. Educational disabilities among children born with neonatal abstinence syndrome. Pediatrics 2018;142(3).

44. Oei JL, Melhuish E, Uebel H, et al. Neonatal abstinence syndrome and high school performance. Pediatrics 2017;139(2):e20162651.

45. Flannery T, Davis JM, Czynski AJ, et al. Neonatal abstinence syndrome severity index predicts 18-month neurodevelopmental outcome in neonates randomized to morphine or methadone. J Pediatr 2020;227:101–107 e101.

46. Bier JB, Finger AS, Bier BA, et al. Growth and developmental outcome of infants with in-utero exposure to methadone vs buprenorphine. J Perinatol 2015;35(8): 656–9.

47. Sundelin Wahlsten V, Sarman I. Neurobehavioural development of preschool-age children born to addicted mothers given opiate maintenance treatment with buprenorphine during pregnancy. Acta Paediatr 2013;102(5):544–9.

48. Whitham JN, Spurrier NJ, Baghurst PA, et al. Visual evoked potential latencies of three-year-old children prenatally exposed to buprenorphine or methadone compared with non-opioid exposed children: the results of a longitudinal study. Neurotoxicol Teratol 2015;52(Pt A):17–24.

49. Lambert JE, Peeler CE. Visual and oculomotor outcomes in children with prenatal opioid exposure. Curr Opin Ophthalmol 2019;30(6):449–53.

50. McGlone L, Hamilton R, McCulloch DL, et al. Neonatal visual evoked potentials in infants born to mothers prescribed methadone. Pediatrics 2013;131(3):e857–63.

51. McGlone L, Hamilton R, McCulloch DL, et al. Visual outcome in infants born to drug-misusing mothers prescribed methadone in pregnancy. Br J Ophthalmol 2014;98(2):238–45.

52. Whitham JN, Spurrier NJ, Sawyer MG, et al. The effects of prenatal exposure to buprenorphine or methadone on infant visual evoked potentials. Neurotoxicol Teratol 2010;32(2):280–8.

53. Walhovd KB, Bjørnebekk A, Haabrekke K, et al. Child neuroanatomical, neurocognitive, and visual acuity outcomes with maternal opioid and polysubstance detoxification. Pediatr Neurol 2015;52(3):326–32, e321-323.

54. Gill AC, Oei J, Lewis NL, et al. Strabismus in infants of opiate-dependent mothers. Acta Paediatr 2003;92(3):379–85.

55. Gupta M, Mulvihill AO, Lascaratos G, et al. Nystagmus and reduced visual acuity secondary to drug exposure in utero: long-term follow-up. J Pediatr Ophthalmol Strabismus 2012;49(1):58–63.

56. Hamilton R, McGlone L, MacKinnon JR, et al. Ophthalmic, clinical and visual electrophysiological findings in children born to mothers prescribed substitute methadone in pregnancy. Br J Ophthalmol 2010;94(6):696–700.

57. Mulvihill AO, Cackett PD, George ND, et al. Nystagmus secondary to drug exposure in utero. Br J Ophthalmol 2007;91(5):613–5.

58. Auger N, Rheaume MA, Low N, et al. Impact of prenatal exposure to opioids, cocaine, and cannabis on eye disorders in children. J Addict Med 2020;14(6): 459–66.
59. Yang Y, Wang C, Gan Y, et al. Maternal smoking during pregnancy and the risk of strabismus in offspring: a meta-analysis. Acta Ophthalmol 2019;97(4):353–63.
60. Melinder A, Konijnenberg C, Sarfi M. Deviant smooth pursuit in preschool children exposed prenatally to methadone or buprenorphine and tobacco affects integrative visuomotor capabilities. Addiction 2013;108(12):2175–82.
61. Konijnenberg C, Melinder A. Visual selective attention is impaired in children prenatally exposed to opioid agonist medication. Eur Addict Res 2015;21(2):63–70.
62. Uebel H, Wright IM, Burns L, et al. Reasons for rehospitalization in children who had neonatal abstinence syndrome. Pediatrics 2015;136(4):e811–20.
63. Milliren CE, Melvin P, Ozonoff A. Pediatric hospital readmissions for infants with neonatal opioid withdrawal syndrome, 2016-2019. Hosp Pediatr 2021;11(9): 979–88.
64. Shrestha S, Roberts MH, Maxwell JR, et al. Post-discharge healthcare utilization in infants with neonatal opioid withdrawal syndrome. Neurotoxicol Teratol 2021; 86:106975.
65. Percy Z, Brokamp C, McAllister JM, et al. Subclinical and overt newborn opioid exposure: prevalence and first-year healthcare utilization. J Pediatr 2020;222: 52–8.e51.
66. Skurtveit S, Nechanská B, Handal M, et al. Hospitalization of children after prenatal exposure to opioid maintenance therapy during pregnancy: a national registry study from the Czech Republic. Addiction 2019;114(7):1225–35.
67. Kelty E, Hulse G. A retrospective cohort study of the health of children prenatally exposed to methadone, buprenorphine or naltrexone compared with non-exposed control children. Am J Addict 2017;26(8):845–51.
68. Mahic M, Hernandez-Diaz S, Wood M, et al. In Utero opioid exposure and risk of infections in childhood: a multinational Nordic cohort study. Pharmacoepidemiol Drug Saf 2020;29(12):1596–604.
69. McAllister JM, Hall ES, Hertenstein GER, et al. Torticollis in infants with a history of neonatal abstinence syndrome. J Pediatr 2018;196:305–8.
70. Towers CV, Knapper A, Gaylord M, et al. Torticollis in infants with neonatal abstinence syndrome. J Perinatol 2021;41(3):615–8.
71. Boere-Boonekamp MM, van der Linden-Kuiper LL. Positional preference: prevalence in infants and follow-up after two years. Pediatrics 2001;107(2):339–43.

# Hypoxic-Ischemic Encephalopathy

## Changing Outcomes Across the Spectrum

Athina Pappas, MD[a], Gina Milano, MD[b],
Lina F. Chalak, MD, MSCS[b],*

### KEYWORDS

- HIE • CP • Bayley • Hypothermia • Neurodevelopmental outcomes

### KEY POINTS

- Therapeutic hypothermia significantly improves outcomes in hypoxic-ischemic encephalopathy (HIE), although infants with mild HIE are not well studied in trials.
- The loss of clinical equipoise regarding treatment of mild HIE is primarily due to overlapping definitions, a narrow therapeutic window for hypothermia and misclassifications during the early dynamic phase of encephalopathy.
- Standardizing the definition and cause of encephalopathy may help confirm HIE and exclude other causes.

### INTRODUCTION

The prevalence of HIE is estimated at 0.5 to 1 per 1000 live births in the United States and developed nations and may be significantly higher in low-source and midresource settings where precise figures remain unknown but are likely higher.[1–3] Hypoxic-ischemic encephalopathy (HIE) is a form of neonatal encephalopathy that occurs in term and late-preterm neonates who have evidence of severe acidosis or need for resuscitation at birth followed by (1) direct evidence of an abnormal neurobehavioral state characterized by seizures or abnormalities in consciousness, tone, posture, and reflexes, (2) evidence of an acute perinatal or sentinel event, (3) characteristic neuroimaging findings, and (4) exclusion of other causes of neonatal encephalopathy. Meeting all the above criteria is not always feasible, particularly in the immediate postnatal period. Neonates with most of these findings often are treated with hypothermia as "presumptive HIE"—early recognition being paramount to the initiation of

Financial disclosure. The authors have no financial relationships to disclose.
Conflict of interest: The other authors have no conflicts of interest.
[a] Wayne Medical school, Detroit, MI, USA; [b] University of Texas Southwestern Medical Center, 5323 Harry Hines, Dallas, Texas 75390, USA
* Corresponding author.
*E-mail address:* Lina.chalak@utsouthwestern.edu

perinatology.theclinics.com

neuroprotective therapies within a narrow therapeutic window. This review will focus on the spectrum of HIE, from mild to severe, and on the changing landscape of outcomes associated with therapeutic interventions. We will not address the other contributing causes of neonatal encephalopathy, which is beyond the scope of this article.

## Pathophysiology

The pathophysiology of HIE is extrapolated from human neuropathological studies and from preclinical models with measurable hypoxic-ischemic insults (consisting of systemic hypoxemia, cerebral hypoperfusion, or both) that are characterized at the cellular level by a biphasic process of primary and secondary energy failure.[3,4] The initial phase consists of the triggering hypoxic-ischemic insult that leads to primary energy failure (a reduction in high-energy phosphorylated metabolites and intracellular pH). This phase may be so severe that it results in permanent brain injury or if subacute may be responsive to resuscitation and neuroprotective strategies. Approximately 6 to 24 hours later, secondary energy failure ensues characterized by the activation of proteases and endonucleases, neuronal apoptosis, microglial activation, reduction of growth factors and protein synthesis, and further accumulation of excitatory neurotransmitters. Neuronal cell death may be immediate or delayed and result from neuronal apoptosis or necrosis. In human neonates, the pathway to brain injury is not always clearly understood. Many factors such as the triggering event, the degree of brain maturation, the extent and timing of hypoxia-ischemia, the metabolic energy substrates, cerebral blood flow patterns, and the preinjury health status of the fetus can impact brain and multiorgan injury.[5] In addition, repetitive insults may contribute to more severe pathologic outcomes and brain injury than isolated insults.

Risk Factors. Risk factors contributing to the neurotoxic cascade that leads to HIE include a multitude of perinatal conditions associated with the need for neonatal resuscitation.[6,7] Perinatal events may fail to predict risk in some cases. Maternal factors associated with a higher risk of HIE include hypertension, cardiopulmonary abnormalities, hypovolemic or cardiovascular collapse, and status epilepticus among others. Uteroplacental factors include uterine rupture, placental abruption, infarction, fibrosis, underperfusion, and placenta previa. Umbilical cord factors include umbilical cord prolapse, cord entanglement or compression, a tight nuchal cord or a true knot in the cord, and abnormalities of umbilical vessels. Intrapartum and fetal factors include abnormal presentation, abnormal fetal heart rate monitor patterns, thick meconium, prolonged labor, precipitous delivery, outborn birth, difficult delivery requiring instrumentation (forceps, vacuum), prolonged pregnancy, fetomaternal hemorrhage, severe isoimmune hemolytic disease, arrhythmias, twin-to-twin transfusion syndrome, and others.

## Identification of Neonates with Hypoxic-Ischemic Encephalopathy

Newborns with HIE present with characteristic signs and symptoms soon after birth that are characterized by physiologic and biochemical findings, neurologic examination abnormalities and electroencephalographic abnormalities. All neonates greater than 36 weeks' gestational age with a history of poor respiratory effort at birth and a need for resuscitation or evidence of neonatal encephalopathy should be carefully evaluated. The specific blood gas criteria that define HIE and are associated with neurologic compromise remain unknown.

Threshold blood gas criteria reported in trials to institute therapeutic hypothermia (TH) include the following: pH $\leq$ 7.0 or a base deficit of 16 mmol/L or more in umbilical cord blood or any blood sample within the first hour of life[8–12] and pH between 7.01

*and 7.15, base deficit 10 to 15.9 mmol/L* within the first hour with any of the following: an *acute perinatal event*, a *10-minute Apgar score of 5 or lesser, assisted ventilation initiated at birth and continued for at least 10 minutes.*[9,13] *Neurologic examination findings* include seizures and evidence of neonatal encephalopathy (**Table 1**) or other signs of central nervous system dysfunction (eg, jitteriness, clonus, apnea, abnormal posturing, and movements).[14,15] Other clinical findings include clinical signs or symptoms of multiorgan injury. *Electroencephalographic findings* include electrographic seizures or abnormalities in background pattern, reactivity, organization of states, and maturation. In addition, amplitude integrated electroencephalogram (EEG) (aEEG) may reveal electrographic seizures or abnormalities in background pattern (discontinuous background, burst suppression, continuous low voltage, or flat/iso-electric background). The sensitivity of aEEG for identifying isolated seizures is poor[16,17]; short seizures, focal discharges, and low-amplitude seizures may not be detected.

The encephalopathy varies from mild to severe and is more likely a spectrum with overlap in the definition (see **Table 1**. Modified Sarnat criteria for the designation of HIE stage of encephalopathy).[14,15] Defining "mild HIE" is challenging because of the need to categorize the severity within the therapeutic window of 6 hours, despite the evolving nature of neonatal encephalopathy in the first week after birth and heterogeneity in the timing of the insult. Further adding to the complexity is the dynamic evolution of the disease process and clinical overlap of presenting signs as well as a lack of an accepted definition for what constitutes mild in the first 6 hours of life whereby decisions regarding therapies are made. Notably, the modified Sarnat Examination—the gold standard for staging HIE—did not distinguish between mild and normal status on the examination form for decades.[18]

The Prospective Research in Mild HIE (PRIME), an international multicenter observational cohort (NCT01747863) at 6 academic centers,[19] provides the first empirically validated definition of mild HIE within 6 hours using 2 steps, as in prior cooling trials: first, screening for fetal acidosis and acute perinatal events per neonatal institute of child health development (NICHD) criteria and second, a certified examination performed using a modified Sarnat scoring system, which is expanded to include mild in addition to the moderate and severe abnormalities (see **Table 1**). PRIME shows that a substantial proportion of infants with this definition of mild HIE have abnormal outcomes when treated without hypothermia. Specifically, 41% have abnormal neurologic findings at discharge, whereas 16% have a disability using established NICHD criteria and 40% have delays in cognitive and language development (<85 Bayley Scales of Infant Development [Bayley]-3 at 18–22 months).[20]

For moderate–severe HIE, medical management in the neonatal intensive care unit (NICU) includes supportive intensive care and hypothermia (whole body or selective head cooling with systemic hypothermia). For mild HIE, therapeutic interventions remain more controversial. However, recent reports suggest that treatment with TH have increased substantially; in a UK population study, 35.8% of newborns with mild HIE underwent cooling.[21] Optimization of TH and adjuvant therapies is under investigation.[22] Following stabilization and treatment of life-threatening conditions in the newborn period, physical, occupational, and developmental care should be initiated as soon as possible. Neonates with HIE should be enrolled in early intervention, follow-up and developmental care programs before discharge. Despite hypothermia to 33°C to 35°C for 72 hours, more than 40% of infants with HIE develop poor outcomes. In a recent meta-analysis of hypothermia trial data (of 1216 newborns), 26% of neonates offered hypothermia died, 26% developed major disability and 19% developed cerebral palsy at 18 to 24 months of age.[23] This has widespread

**Table 1**
Modified Sarnat criteria for designation of hypoxic-ischemic encephalopathy stage of encephalopathy

| Categories | Normal | Mild | Moderate | Severe |
|---|---|---|---|---|
| Level of consciousness | Alert, responsive | Hyperalert, stare, exaggerated response to minimal stimuli, jitteriness, inconsolable | Lethargic | Stupor, coma |
| Spontaneous activity | Normal | Decreased, with or without periods of excessive activity | Decreased | No activity |
| Posture | Predominantly flexed when quiet | Mild flexion of distal joints (fingers, wrist) | Strong distal flexion, complete extension | Intermittent decerebration |
| Tone | Flexor tone in all extremities | Slightly increased peripheral tone | Hypotonia or hypertonia | Flaccid, rigid |
| Primitive Reflexes | | | | |
| • Suck | Strong, easy to elicit | Weak, poor | Weak or has bite | Absent |
| • Moro | Strong, easy to elicit | Low threshold to elicit | Incomplete | Absent |
| Autonomic nervous system | | | | |
| • Pupils | Normal size, reactive to light | Mydriasis | Miosis | Skew deviation/dilated, nonreactive/nonreactive |
| • Heart rate | Normal heart rate | Tachycardia (>160) | Bradycardia (<100) | Variable heart rate |
| • Respirations | Normal | Hyperventilation (>80) | Periodic breathing | Apnea on ventilator with or without spontaneous respiration |

**Table 2**
**Two-year outcomes among survivors of hypoxic-ischemic encephalopathy in randomized control trials of hypothermia**

| | Outcomes Among All Trial Participants | | | | | | | | |
| --- | --- | --- | --- | --- | --- | --- | --- | --- | --- |
| Death or Neurodevelopment Impairment (NDI) | | | Death | | | Major NDI (Among All) | | | |
| Study | N | Total | % | N | Total | % | N | Total | % |
| Gunn et al 1998[95] | 7 | 18 | 39 | 3 | 18 | 17 | 4 | 18 | 22 |
| Cool Cap Study 2005[11] | 59 | 108 | 55 | 36 | 108 | 33 | 23 | 108 | 21 |
| NICHD Study 2005[9] | 45 | 102 | 44 | 24 | 102 | 24 | 21 | 102 | 21 |
| TOBY Study 2009[8] | 74 | 163 | 45 | 42 | 163 | 26 | 32 | 163 | 20 |
| neo.nEURO Study 2010[10] | 27 | 53 | 51 | 20 | 53 | 38 | 7 | 53 | 13 |
| Zhou 2010[12] | 31 | 100 | 31 | 20 | 100 | 20 | 11 | 100 | 11 |
| ICE Study 2011[72] | 55 | 107 | 51 | 27 | 108 | 25 | 28 | 107 | 26 |
| All | 298 | 651 | **46** | 172 | 652 | **26** | 126 | 651 | **19** |

| | Outcomes Among Survivors | | | | | | | | |
| --- | --- | --- | --- | --- | --- | --- | --- | --- | --- |
| | Major NDI | | | MDI >2SD Below Mean | | | CP | | |
| Study | N | Total | % | N | Total | % | N | Total | % |
| Gunn et al 1998[95] | 4 | 15 | 27 | 3 | 13 | 23 | 3 | 15 | 20 |
| Cool Cap Study 2005[11] | 23 | 72 | 32 | 21 | 70 | 30 | 23 | 72 | 32 |
| NICHD Study 2005[9] | 21 | 78 | 27 | 19 | 75 | 25 | 15 | 77 | 19 |
| TOBY Study 2009[8] | 32 | 120 | 27 | 28 | 115 | 24 | 33 | 120 | 28 |
| neo.nEURO Study 2010[10] | 7 | 33 | 21 | | | | 4 | 32 | 13 |
| Zhou 2010[12] | 11 | 80 | 14 | | | | 10 | 80 | 13 |
| ICE Study 2011[72] | 28 | 80 | 35 | 17 | 73 | 23 | 21 | 79 | 27 |
| All | 126 | 478 | **26** | 88 | 346 | **25** | 109 | 475 | **23** |

implications for the children affected, their families, and the developmental care and assessment of these children at follow-up (**Table 2**).

## Follow-up Care

All neonates with moderate–severe neonatal encephalopathy should undergo long-term follow-up because they are at heightened risk for poor outcomes including cerebral palsy, cognitive impairment, feeding issues, growth failure, postneonatal epilepsy, neurosensory impairment, and neuropsychiatric and behavioral problems.[24]

## Cerebral Palsy Following Hypoxic-Ischemic Encephalopathy

Cerebral palsy is a term that describes a group of disorders characterized by abnormalities in muscle tone, movement, and/or posture associated with the loss of function presumed to be due to a nonprogressive lesion or abnormality in the developing fetal or infant brain.[25] Although a variety of perinatal risk factors (including HIE) are attributed to cerebral palsy (CP), in many cases, the true cause may be difficult if not impossible to ascertain.[7] Fewer than 10% of cases of cerebral palsy globally are attributable to HIE.[26] Nonetheless, cerebral palsy related to HIE has gained considerable attention because it may be amenable to postnatal therapies. In a meta-analysis of randomized

**Table 3**
**Cerebral palsy among survivors of hypoxic-ischemic encephalopathy in randomized control trials of hypothermia**

| Trial | Hypothermia (%) | Normothermia (%) | Or (95% CI) |
|---|---|---|---|
| Cool Cap Study 2005[11] | 32 | 43 | 0.75 (0.48–1.16) |
| NICHD Study 2005[9] | 19 | 30 | 0.68 (0.38–1.22) |
| TOBY Study 2009[59] | 28 | 41 | 0.67 (0.47–0.96) |
| Neo.nEURO Study 2010[10] | 12 | 48 | 0.15 (0.04–0.60) |
| Zhou Study 2010[12] | 14 | 28 | 0.40 (0.17–0.92) |
| ICE Study 2011[72] | 27 | 29 | 0.92 (0.54–1.59) |

controlled trials of hypothermia for HIE, 19% of neonates offered hypothermia developed disabling cerebral palsy at 18 to 24 months of age as compared with 31% of those treated with intensive care alone (**Table 3**).[23] Similar rates are reported at school age (17% and 29%, respectively).[27] Risk factors may include clinical variables (eg, initial severity and persistence of encephalopathy[28]) and other intrinsic factors (eg, genetic susceptibility, genetic polymorphisms[29]).

Two major CP subtypes are commonly associated with the mechanisms of HIE[7] (although other CP-subtypes are reported in the literature[30]). These include spastic quadriparesis (often observed following a watershed pattern of brain injury) and dyskinetic CP (often observed following injury to the basal ganglia, deep gray structures, and perirolandic cortex). Early detection may be feasible in high-risk infants using neonatal MRI,[31] neurologic examination, and the General Movements Assessment.[32–34] Definitive diagnosis typically is possible by 5 years (the age selected by CP registries to ensure diagnostic accuracy[35]). Presenting signs and symptoms may include abnormal muscle tone and deep tendon reflexes, gross motor developmental delay, abnormalities in postural or protective reflexes, and coordination of movement. Early detection allows for timely access to support services and early intervention.

Spastic cerebral palsy is characterized by increased or *spastic* passive tone of a clasp-knife character, increased deep tendon reflexes, pyramidal signs (eg, persistence of Babinski response) and sustained clonus.[25] Dyskinetic or athetoid cerebral palsy is characterized by spontaneous changes in muscle tone (dystonia), involuntary movements, and persistence of postural reflexes.[36] Other brain and nervous system symptoms may coexist. These include cognitive impairment, speech and language impairment, delays in developmental milestones, hearing or vision impairment and seizure disorders.[37] Orthopedic issues, contractures and dislocations of the hips and other joints may develop in severe cases, mainly between 3 and 6 years.[38]

Cerebral palsy may vary in severity from mild to severe; the risk of comorbidities increases with the extent of functional motor impairment.[39] Several developmental instruments may assist in grading the level of impairment such as the Gross Motor Function Classification System[25] and the Pediatric Evaluation of Disability Inventory.[40–42] Functional assessment tools for manual function and communication skills also exist (eg, Bimanual Fine Motor Function Scale, Manual Ability Classification System, Communication Function Classification System).[43,44]

Diagnosis is made by neurologic examination. Algorithms for the categorization of cerebral palsy may facilitate diagnosis (eg, the Surveillance for Cerebral Palsy in Europe Hierarchical Classification).[45,46] The following additional tests may be performed: neuroimaging (preferably MRI of the brain), electroencephalogram, vision, and hearing testing. Management requires a team approach including a primary care physician; pediatric neurologist; neurodevelopmental specialist; physical medicine and rehabilitation physician; occupational, physical, and speech therapists; nurse; social workers; and other specialists (eg, gastroenterologist and/or orthopedic specialist). Prognosis varies depending on the severity of cerebral palsy and the response to therapeutic interventions aimed at minimizing functional impairment.[39] Cerebral palsy is a lifelong disorder that may require long-term care. Among children with CP following HIE, there is a high concordance between 18-month and 24-month level of functioning and school age outcomes.[27,47] Although there is no cure for cerebral palsy, treatment improves overall function, daily living and quality of life. Numerous effective interventions are available including casting, bimanual training, constraint-induced movement therapy, goal-directed training, hippotherapy, environmental enrichment, literacy interventions, oral stimulation, sensorimotor electrical stimulation, botulinum toxin, intrathecal baclofen, anticonvulsants, scoliosis correction, selective dorsal rhizotomy, and so forth.[48]

### Cognitive Impairment Following Hypoxic-Ischemic Encephalopathy

Despite hypothermia and critical care management, cognitive impairment remains an acute and chronic problem for the survivors of neonatal encephalopathy. Greater than 50% of neonates with HIE have subnormal IQ scores (IQ < 85), and 27% have scores in the extremely low range (IQ < 70) even after hypothermia.[27] Cognitive deficits may exist with or without cerebral palsy or other neuromotor impairments.[49-51] Risk factors include severity of encephalopathy, poor head growth, neurologic comorbidities, parental IQ, environmental, and socioeconomic factors. Presenting signs and symptoms may include developmental delay, school difficulties, impaired memory and attention/executive function, lower school achievement, and special educational needs.[51,52] Cognitive impairment occurs over a spectrum ranging from mild learning disabilities to profound impairment.[27,53-55] Diagnosis is best achieved with formal testing using developmental instruments such as the Bayley, Griffith's Mental Development, NEPSY, or Wechsler intelligence scales. The spectrum of cognitive outcomes attributed to neonatal encephalopathy among infants treated with and without hypothermia is summarized in **Table 4**.

Management of cognitive impairment requires referral to early intervention (0–3 years) followed by school-based programs guided by an individualized educational plan.[56] Early therapy that includes the parents[57] and addresses the psychosocial needs of the child and family is paramount. Assistive devices may aid with communication and learning: glasses, hearing aids/cochlear implants, assistive communication devices, other adaptive equipment, and student or caregiver assistants.[58] These are vital to the optimal functioning of the child. Ongoing neurodevelopmental assessment, follow-up and intervention to address the special needs of children born with HIE, and any related comorbidities may positively affect outcomes. Prognosis depends on the severity of impairment and the presence of other comorbidities.[27,56] Severe cognitive impairment typically remains static throughout the life span.[27,47,59] Mild–moderate impairment without cerebral palsy or other neuropsychological comorbidities may be more amenable to therapeutic intervention; in these cases, cognitive scores observed in early infancy or childhood may improve with time (18–2 years vs school age).[60]

### Cognitive Outcomes of Infants with Mild Hypoxic-Ischemic Encephalopathy

Definitions ascribed to mild HIE are not specific to the first 6 hours of age and use variable psychometric follow-up measures (**Table 5**). Studies reporting outcomes of

**Table 4**
**Long-term cognitive and behavioral outcomes following moderate-to-severe hypoxic-ischemic encephalopathy**

| Author, Year | Study Type | Primary Outcome | Mean Age (Range) | Cohort Details | N | Sex (Boys/N) | Characteristic Controls | Measures | Results |
|---|---|---|---|---|---|---|---|---|---|
| Marlow et al,[51] 2005 | Observational, case-control | Cognition and Behavior | 7 y, 2 mo (6.5–9 y) | GA ≥ 35 wk, identified from the Trent Neonatal Survey database of babies born 1992–1994 | 65 participants, 50 without CP (N = 18 with severe NE) | 31/50 | N = 49 Children attending mainstream school were compared with a child from same school, matched for sex, age, ethnic group and first language | Cognitive BAS-II; NEPSY Behavior: SDQ (parental and teacher) | Cognitive outcomes: Moderate NE: No significant difference in general IQ or subscale scores on BAS; significantly lower scores on language, sensorimotor, narrative memory and sentence repetition domains on NEPSY Severe NE: Significantly lower scores compared with control group in general cognitive ability on BAS and multiple domains of NEPSY (attention, executive function, language, visuospatial, memory and learning, memory for names, narrative memory, orientation, and everyday memory) Behavioral outcomes: Moderate NE: no significant difference compared with control group. Severe NE: Significantly higher overall behavioral scores and hyperactivity compared with other comparison groups |

| Lindstrom et al,[96] 2006 | Observational, cohort study | Cognition and Behavior | 16 y, 1 mo (15–19 y 1, mo) | Term born Swedish cohort, born 1985 | 43 participants, 28 without CP | 18/28 | N = 15 siblings for comparison of behavior outcome | Cognitive (11/28): WISC-III Behavior (28/28): Parental questionnaires via telephone interview consisting of Connors 10-item scale, ADHD Rating Scale IV, Asperger Syndrome Screening Questionnaire | Cognitive outcomes: 4/11 with IQ ≤ 70; 3/11 with IQ 71–85 Behavioral outcomes: Significant differences compared with siblings on the Connors scale (P < .003), the inattention subscale of the ADHD Rating Scale IV (P < .006) and the Asperger Syndrome Screening Questionnaires |
| Steinman et al,[55] 2009 | Observational, cohort study | Cognition | 4 y | | 81 participants completed follow-up; 64 without neuromotor impairment | 35/64 (55%) | NA | Cognitive: Wechsler Preschool and Primary Scale of Intelligence – Revised | Cognitive outcomes: Findings included an independent association between the degree of watershed injury on neonatal MRI and future verbal abilities measured by the WPPSI-R (11% with a verbal IQ score <70). There was no association between the degree of basal ganglia injury and verbal abilities |

(continued on next page)

**Table 4**
*(continued)*

| Author, Year | Study Type | Primary Outcome | Mean Age (Range) | Cohort Details | N | Sex (Boys/ N) | Characteristic Controls | Measures | Results |
|---|---|---|---|---|---|---|---|---|---|
| Van Kooij et al,[97] 2010 | Observational, case-control | Cognition | 9–10 y | Full-term infants born 1993–1997 and admitted to local NICU | 80 survivors with mild or moderate NE. 69 children without CP | Unknown | 52, matched for sex and age | Cognitive: WISC-III IQ estimated with subtests (Similarities, Vocabulary, Block Patterns, and Object Assembly) | Cognitive outcomes: control children had significantly higher mean estimate IQ scores as compared with the children with mild or moderate NE without CP. 17.4% of children without CP scored 1–2 SD less than the mean and 7.2% of children without CP scored less than 2 SD |
| Pappas 2015[98] | Observational, cohort study | Cognition and Behavior | 6–7 y | School-aged survivors of the NICHD Neonatal Research Network RCT of whole body Hypothermia; participants were recruited between 2000 and 2003 | 110 participants, 86 without CP | 61/110 | NA | Cognitive: Wechsler intelligence scales, NEPSY Behavior: Parental report | Cognitive outcomes: Subnormal IQ scores were identified in more than a quarter of the children: 96% of survivors with CP had an IQ < 70, 9% of children without CP had an IQ < 70, and 31% had an IQ of 70–84. 20% of children with normal IQ and 28% of those with IQ scores 70–84 received special educational support services or were held back ≥1 grade. Behavior outcomes: Behavior problems occurred in 21% of children at 18 mo (as |

| Study | Study type | Focus | Age | Birth/Data | Participants | | | Assessment | Outcomes |
|---|---|---|---|---|---|---|---|---|---|
| | | | | | | | | | indicated by the BSID-II Behavior Rating Scale) and 7% of children at 6–7 y of age (by parental report) among those treated with hypothermia |
| Van Schie et al,[99] 2015 | Observational, cohort study | Behavior | 7 y, 6 mo (6 y, 4 mo–8 y, 2 mo) | Born 1999–2002 | 25 participants, 17 without CP | 19/25 | NA | Behavior: Child Checklist (parents) | Behavior outcomes: 4/17 children had a total score in subclinical (n = 3) or clinical (n = 1) range; proportion not much higher than in reference sample |
| Hayes et al,[100] 2018 | Observational, cohort study | Cognition and Behavior | 5 y, 8 mo (3 y, 8 mo–8 y, 10 mo) | Born 2001–2005 retrospective data collection; 2005–2008 prospective assessments | 68 participants without CP (N = 47 with mild HIE; N = 21 with moderate HIE) | NA | NA | Cognitive: NEPSY-2 (58/68), Behavior Rating Inventory of Executive function (40/68) Behavior: Child Behavior Checklist (66/68) | Cognitive outcomes: Difficulties observed (>1 SD less than the mean) in 16/24 NEPSY-2 subtests and on timed assessments using Movement ABC-2. Abnormalities were observed in the "control" aspects of cognition (attention and memory) Behavior outcomes: Behavioral problems, particularly internalizing behaviors were higher than expected among survivors of HIE |

**Table 5**
Characteristics of studies including mild hypoxic-ischemic encephalopathy not cooled

| Author, Year | Center/Country/Dates | Number Mild HIE | Normal/Abnormal Outcome | Inclusion Criteria | Outcome Definition | Follow-up mo/y | Standardized Follow-up Tools |
|---|---|---|---|---|---|---|---|
| Nadgyman et al, 2003 | Berlin/Germany/1998-1999 | 14 | 10/4 | 37-42 wk GA Asphyxia | Mild = a DQ being 1-2 SD (91.8-97.8) | 20 mo | Griffiths |
| Van Schie et al, 2015 | Amsterdam/Netherlands/1999-2002 | 6 | 4/2 | 38-42 wk GA Diagnosis of HIE I, II, or III | BSID-II Normal ≥85 Mild delay 70-84 | 7 y | M-ABC/CBCL Bayley@ 2 y |
| Liauw et al, 2009 | Netherlands/2001-2003 | 3 | 2/1 | >37 wk GA MRI to assess brain injury due to perinatal asphyxia | Category 3 + 4 = adverse | 2 y and 5 y Van Weichen | Gessell and Towen |
| El-Ayouty et al, 2007 | Mansoura/Egypt/2002-2004 | 3 | 3/0 | 38-42 wk GA Diagnosis of HIE I, II, or III | Abnormal = abnormal neurologic examination or Denver screening | 18 mo | Denver Developmental Screen |
| Alderliesten et al, 2011 | Utrecht/Netherlands/2002-2008 | 2 | 2/0 | >36 wk GA Perinatal asphyxia, MRI, outcome | A composite death during the neonatal period, cerebral palsy, or Griffiths <85 | 18-46 mo | Griffiths |
| Murray et al, 2016 | Cork/Ireland/2003-2005 | 22 | 16/6 | ≥37 wk GA Diagnosis of HIE I, II, or III EEG | Abnormal outcome at 5 y of age | 5 y | WPPSI-III |
| Polat et al, 2013 | Manisa/Turkey/2006-2008 | 11 | 10/1 | 37-41 wk GA Diagnosis of HIE I, II, or III | | 44-48 mo | Denver Developmental Screen |
| Gardiner et al, 2014 | Perth/Australia/2008-2010 | 9 | 7/2 | ≥35 wk GA (mean 40 wk)<6 h old Asphyxia and or HIE II, III | Mild delay = 1 SD less than OR severe <2 SD | 24 mo | Bayley-III |

| | | | | | Abnormal outcome ≤85 18–36 mo | Bayley-III Ages and Stages (ASQ3) |
|---|---|---|---|---|---|---|
| Looney et al, 2015 | Cork/Ireland/2009–2011 | 15 | 9/6 | >36 wk GA Perinatal asphyxia and HIE with matched controls | | |
| Belet et al, 2004 | Ankara/Turkey/Not reported | 2 | 2/0 | ≥37 wk GA Diagnosis of HIE I, II, III | Bayley score and Denver score 3.5–4 y | Bayley Denver Developmental Screen |
| Lally et al, 2014 | Kerala/India/Not reported | 24 | 22/2 | >36 wk GA encephalopathy who underwent MRI | Cerebral Palsy, or composite score <85 3.5 y | Bayley-III |

infants treated for mild HIE are plagued by bias inherent to retrospective reports and a lack of systematic assessments after discharge.[61–68] Six studies conducted in Europe, 3 in Asia, 1 in Africa, and 1 in Australia have focused on mild HIE. All but one study provides infants intensive care alone without cooling. In the cooled non-RCT study 65 participants in total were enrolled, 9 had mild HIE and 2 (22%) had abnormal outcomes, the same percentage (22%) as in the noncooled outcome group. A meta-analysis including 558 participants, 111 of which had mild HIE, reports that 24 (22%) participants have abnormal outcomes at 18 months of age or older.[69]

*Prehypothermia*. Robertson and colleagues showed that no studied infants among those with mild HIE developed any major disability. The mean Stanford-Binet Intelligence Scale score was 101.5 (±14.0), and the mean developmental quotient using the Peabody Picture Vocabulary Test was 104.1 (±13.7)[70]; at 8 years of age, their school performance was similar to that of matched controls.[53] Subsequently, Van Handel and colleagues examined behavioral functioning at 9 to 10 years of age. Children with mild HIE had similar IQ compared with control children but social and attention problem scores were higher among the children with mild HIE.[71] Murray and colleagues evaluated cognitive outcomes at 5 years of age among 22 infants with mild HIE and reported that they had lower scores than control infants on full-scale IQ tests [99 (94–112) versus 117 (110–124), $P = .001$], verbal IQ [105 (99–111) versus 116 (112–125), $P = .001$], and performance IQ [103 (98–112) versus 115 (107–124), $P = .004$].[62] A systematic review summarized prehypothermia outcomes in a total of 250 mild HIE infants, with atypical results at greater than 18 months of age in 56 (22%).[63]

### Outcome of Mild Hypoxic-Ischemic Encephalopathy in the Hypothermia Epochs

Four RCTs included infants with mild HIE due to their intent-to-treat analysis design.[63] Jacobs *and colleagues* enrolled 42 participants with mild HIE, and although not powered to examine the significance of the comparison, noted a rate of death or major sensorineural disability of 38% among those who received hypothermia versus 25% in those allocated to normothermia.[72] Zhou and colleagues[73] included 34 participants with mild HIE (19 hypothermia vs 15 control); abnormal outcomes were reported in 6/19 cooled and 7/15 controls. Battin *and colleagues*[74] enrolled 9 infants with mild HIE, abnormal outcomes occurred in 1/4 cooled and 2/2 controls. Wyatt and colleagues RCT[75] enrolled 8 infants with mild HIE and showed abnormal outcomes in 2/5 cooled and 0/3 in control. The pooled participants in these RCT studies were summarized in a recent systematic review, reporting an abnormal outcome in 29% of those receiving hypothermia versus 37% of controls, with an odds ratio of 0.67 (95% CI: 0.28–1.61, $P = .59$).[63] The trend was not significant and none of the studies were individually powered to detect a clinical effect of hypothermia for mild HIE.

### Feeding Issues and Growth Failure

Feeding issues, dysphagia, and growth failure are common following HIE and may persist to school age.[76] Important risk factors include cranial nerve dysfunction leading to impaired swallowing, pharyngeal reflexes, and abnormalities in gastrointestinal motility.[77] Presenting signs and symptoms may include difficulty in sucking or swallowing, frequent choking, vomiting, aspiration, excessive drooling, and slower than normal growth.[78] In addition, irregular breathing, constipation, and urinary incontinence may be observed among severely affected children. Feeding issues may vary from absent to severe impairment requiring gastrostomy tube placement. Additionally, Nissen fundoplication may be required for children with severe gastroesophageal reflux.[79] Medical management should target both feeding issues and optimizing growth. Referral to occupational therapy, a registered dietitian or a specialized multidisciplinary feeding clinic for a comprehensive evaluation and treatment plan is recommended.[80] The prognosis is child-dependent and is directly related to the severity of underlying hypoxic-ischemic brain injury.

### Sleep and Altered Circadian Rhythm

In addition to neurodevelopmental impairment and growth failure, newborns with HIE are at risk for sleep-related circadian dysfunction that may further influence neurodevelopmental outcomes and family functioning; amplitude integrated aEEG may predict these abnormalities.[81]

### Neonatal Seizures and Postnatal Epilepsy Following Hypoxic-Ischemic Encephalopathy

HIE is a common cause of seizures in the newborn period and beyond.[82] Whether seizures directly or indirectly contribute to brain injury among the survivors of HIE is controversial, due to the difficulty in separating the severity of the underlying brain injury from the impact of the seizures themselves. Treatment of seizures is also controversial. In a recent study by Hunt and colleagues, the treatment of electrographic and clinical seizures with commonly used antiepileptic drugs did not significantly improve outcomes beyond the neonatal period.[83] However, a study by Kharoshankaya and colleagues found an association between total neonatal seizure burden greater than 40 minutes with a more than 9-fold risk of abnormal neurodevelopmental outcomes (OR 9.56, 95% CI 2.43–37.67); this finding is independent of HIE severity at 6 hours, or of treatment with TH.[84] The presence of seizures alone is not associated with worse outcomes. TH decreases total seizure burden and has an antiepileptic effect.[85]

The incidence of repeated seizures beyond the newborn period is reported to be 10% to 16% at both 18 to 24 months[8,11] and 6 to 7 years of age.[27] Clinical presentation may vary from child to child in terms of severity and frequency of postnatal seizures. Seizures may lead to impaired control of muscle tone, movement, posture, thinking, speech, vision, gaze and/or bowel, and bladder function.[86] Postnatal seizures may range from none to intractable epilepsy (eg, infantile spasms)[87,88] and may be predicted by neuroimaging and neurophysiological measures (such as EEG and evoked potentials).[88] Early identification is critical to optimal management. Antiepileptic medications and close follow-up by a pediatric neurologist are recommended. The risk and benefit profiles of antiepileptic drugs used in this population are currently under investigation.[89,90]

### Neuropsychiatric Comorbidities and Behavioral Problems

Children with a history of HIE are reported to have more special educational needs, memory and behavioral problems (see **Table 4**). Data are primarily from single center cohort studies of children treated with intensive care without hypothermia. One study reports severe behavioral problems in 8% of children with moderate HIE and 23% of children with severe HIE.[51] Another study reports more behavioral problems even among neonates with mild encephalopathy as compared with controls; children with mild or moderate encephalopathy manifest more social problems, anxiety, depression, attention deficit, autism symptomatology, and thought problems.[71] A few studies also suggest higher rates of hyperactivity among children with a history of moderate HIE.[51,71,91]

### Neurosensory Impairment

Deafness occurs in 4% to 6% of children with moderate–severe HIE; blindness defined as (<20/200 vision) occurs in 6% to 14% of affected children.[8–12,23,72] Regular assessment and prompt intervention for hearing and vision problems is important to the follow-up care of these children.

### Parent and Family Well-Being

In children with neonatal encephalopathy due to HIE, parent mental health and social context are important contributing factors to cognitive and language functioning and neurodevelopmental outcomes.[92] Addressing the psychosocial needs of the family is an important part of follow-up care.

Involving families is essential and integral to the treatment care plan and to the long-term outcome of neonates affected by HIE.[93,94]

## SUMMARY

Neonatal HIE is a leading cause of death and neurodevelopmental impairment in neonates. Standardizing the definition and cause of encephalopathy may help confirm HIE and exclude other causes. Understanding the stage and severity of encephalopathy and the long-term outcomes may affect treatment decisions and influence the choice to initiate TH. Traditionally, infants with mild HIE were treated with intensive care alone due to the perceived low risk for impairment. Recently, multiple studies suggest that infants treated for mild HIE without hypothermia may be at significant risk of abnormal neurodevelopmental outcomes. This review summarizes the spectrum of HIE presentations and their long-term implications.

---

**Best practices**

*What is the current practice for defining HIE?*

Newborns with HIE present with signs and symptoms soon after birth that are characterized by physiologic and biochemical findings, neurologic examination abnormalities and electroencephalographic abnormalities. Collectively, these criteria are used to define the stages of encephalopathy. Standardization of the definition of encephalopathy may help to confirm HIE and exclude other causes. This has implications on therapeutic interventions.

*Best Practice/Guideline/Care Path Objective(s):*

Presently, TH is the accepted best treatment modality for moderate–severe neonatal encephalopathy. Research is underway to determine whether TH may also benefit neonates with mild HIE. Challenges remain in defining mild HIE due to the need to categorize severity within the therapeutic window of 6 hours, the evolving nature of neonatal encephalopathy in the first week after birth and the heterogeneity in the timing of the insult. Further adding to the complexity is the dynamic disease process and clinical overlap of presenting signs, as well as a lack of an accepted definition for what constitutes mild in the first 6 hours of life whereby decisions regarding therapies are made.

*What changes in current practice are likely to improve outcomes?*

Clarification of the definition of HIE across the spectrum and further study of long-term outcomes is likely to improve the care of neonates with HIE.

Major Recommendations: Comprehensive follow-up care of neonates affected by HIE should include assessments of neuromotor outcomes, cognition, seizures neurosensory outcomes, behavior, sleep, growth, nutrition, functional impairment, and the influence on the family. Due to the high risk of potential adverse outcomes, follow-up should continue to school age and beyond.

Bibliographic Source(s): This is important: list current sources/references to support info above.

## REFERENCES

1. Lawn JE, Cousens S, Zupan J. 4 million neonatal deaths: when? Where? Why? Lancet 2005;365(9462):891–900.
2. Lawn J, Shibuya K, Stein C. No cry at birth: global estimates of intrapartum still-births and intrapartum-related neonatal deaths. Bull World Health Organ 2005; 83(6):409–17.
3. Higgins RD, Shankaran S. Hypothermia for hypoxic ischemic encephalopathy in infants > or =36 weeks. Early Hum Dev 2009;85(10 Suppl):S49–52.
4. Laptook AR. Use of therapeutic hypothermia for term infants with hypoxic-ischemic encephalopathy. Pediatr Clin North America 2009;56(3):601–16. Table of Contents.
5. Gunn AJ, Bennet L. Fetal hypoxia insults and patterns of brain injury: insights from animal models. Clin perinatology 2009;36(3):579–93.
6. Locatelli A, Lambicchi L, Incerti M, et al. Is perinatal asphyxia predictable? BMC pregnancy and childbirth 2020;20(1):186.
7. Executive summary: neonatal encephalopathy and neurologic outcome, second edition. Report of the American College of Obstetricians and Gynecologists' Task Force on neonatal encephalopathy. Obstet Gynecol 2014;123(4):896–901.
8. Azzopardi DV, Strohm B, Edwards AD, et al. Moderate hypothermia to treat peri-natal asphyxial encephalopathy. New Engl J Med 2009;361(14):1349–58.
9. Shankaran S, Laptook AR, Ehrenkranz RA, et al. Whole-body hypothermia for neonates with hypoxic-ischemic encephalopathy. New Engl J Med 2005; 353(15):1574–84.
10. Simbruner G, Mittal RA, Rohlmann F, et al. Systemic hypothermia after neonatal encephalopathy: outcomes of neo.nEURO.network RCT. Pediatrics 2010;126(4): e771–8.
11. Gluckman PD, Wyatt JS, Azzopardi D, et al. Selective head cooling with mild systemic hypothermia after neonatal encephalopathy: multicentre randomised trial. Lancet 2005;365(9460):663–70.
12. Zhou WH, Cheng GQ, Shao XM, et al. Selective head cooling with mild systemic hypothermia after neonatal hypoxic-ischemic encephalopathy: a multicenter randomized controlled trial in China. J Pediatr 2010;157(3):367–72, 372 e361-363.
13. Yeh P, Emary K, Impey L. The relationship between umbilical cord arterial pH and serious adverse neonatal outcome: analysis of 51,519 consecutive vali-dated samples. BJOG : Int J Obstet Gynaecol 2012;119(7):824–31.
14. Sarnat HB, Sarnat MS. Neonatal encephalopathy following fetal distress. A clin-ical and electroencephalographic study. Arch Neurol 1976;33(10):696–705.
15. Voorhies T, Vanucci R. In: Sarnat H, editor. Topics in neonatal Neurology. Or-lando, FL: Grune & Stratton; 1984. p. 61–82.
16. Shah DK, Mackay MT, Lavery S, et al. Accuracy of bedside electroencephalo-graphic monitoring in comparison with simultaneous continuous conventional electroencephalography for seizure detection in term infants. Pediatrics 2008; 121(6):1146–54.
17. Shellhaas RA, Soaita AI, Clancy RR. Sensitivity of amplitude-integrated electro-encephalography for neonatal seizure detection. Pediatrics 2007;120(4):770–7.
18. Chalak L. New Horizons in mild hypoxic-ischemic encephalopathy: a Standard-ized algorithm to Move past conundrum of care. Clin Perinatol 2022;49(1): 279–94.

19. Prempunpong C, Chalak LF, Garfinkle J, et al. Prospective research on infants with mild encephalopathy: the PRIME study. J Perinatol 2018;38(1):80–5.
20. Chalak LF, Nguyen KA, Prempunpong C, et al. Prospective research in infants with mild encephalopathy identified in the first six hours of life: neurodevelopmental outcomes at 18-22 months. Pediatr Res 2018;84(6):861–8.
21. Shipley L, Gale C, Sharkey D. Trends in the incidence and management of hypoxic-ischaemic encephalopathy in the therapeutic hypothermia era: a national population study. Arch Dis Child Fetal neonatal edition 2021;106(5): 529–34.
22. Robertson NJ, Tan S, Groenendaal F, et al. Which neuroprotective Agents are Ready for Bench to bedside Translation in the newborn infant? J Pediatr 2012; 160(4):544–52, e544.
23. Tagin MA, Woolcott CG, Vincer MJ, et al. Hypothermia for neonatal hypoxic ischemic encephalopathy: an updated systematic review and meta-analysis. Arch Pediatr Adolesc Med 2012;166(6):558–66.
24. Lemyre B, Chau V. Hypothermia for newborns with hypoxic-ischemic encephalopathy. Paediatr Child Health 2018;23(4):285–91.
25. Rosenbaum P, Paneth N, Leviton A, et al. A report: the definition and classification of cerebral palsy April 2006. Developmental Med child Neurol Suppl 2007; 109:8–14.
26. Nelson KB, Grether JK. Causes of cerebral palsy. Curr Opin Pediatr 1999;11(6): 487–91.
27. Shankaran S, Pappas A, McDonald SA, et al. Childhood outcomes after hypothermia for neonatal encephalopathy. New Engl J Med 2012;366(22):2085–92.
28. Shankaran S, Laptook AR, Tyson JE, et al. Evolution of encephalopathy during whole body hypothermia for neonatal hypoxic-ischemic encephalopathy. J Pediatr 2012;160(4):567–72, e563.
29. Gibson CS, Maclennan AH, Dekker GA, et al. Candidate genes and cerebral palsy: a population-based study. Pediatrics 2008;122(5):1079–85.
30. Shankaran S, Barnes PD, Hintz SR, et al. Brain injury following trial of hypothermia for neonatal hypoxic-ischaemic encephalopathy. Arch Dis Child 2012;97(6): F398–404.
31. Ouwehand S, Smidt LCA, Dudink J, et al. Predictors of outcomes in hypoxic-ischemic encephalopathy following hypothermia: a meta-analysis. Neonatology 2020;117(4):411–27.
32. King AR, Machipisa C, Finlayson F, et al. Early detection of cerebral palsy in high-risk infants: Translation of evidence into practice in an Australian hospital. J paediatrics child Health 2021;57(2):246–50.
33. Glass HC, Li Y, Gardner M, et al. Early identification of cerebral palsy using neonatal MRI and General movements assessment in a cohort of high-risk term neonates. Pediatr Neurol 2021;118:20–5.
34. Robinson H, Hart D, Vollmer B. Predictive validity of a qualitative and quantitative Prechtl's General Movements Assessment at term age: comparison between preterm infants and term infants with HIE. Early Hum Dev 2021;161: 105449.
35. Novak I, Morgan C, Adde L, et al. Early, Accurate diagnosis and early intervention in cerebral palsy: Advances in diagnosis and treatment. JAMA Pediatr 2017;171(9):897–907.
36. Monbaliu E, De La Pena MG, Ortibus E, et al. Functional outcomes in children and young people with dyskinetic cerebral palsy. Developmental Med child Neurol 2017;59(6):634–40.

37. Compagnone E, Maniglio J, Camposeo S, et al. Functional classifications for cerebral palsy: correlations between the gross motor function classification system (GMFCS), the manual ability classification system (MACS) and the communication function classification system (CFCS). Res Dev disabilities 2014;35(11): 2651–7.
38. Helenius IJ, Viehweger E, Castelein RM. Cerebral palsy with dislocated hip and scoliosis: what to deal with first? J Child Orthop 2020;14(1):24–9.
39. Natarajan G, Shankaran S, Pappas A, et al. Functional status at 18 months of age as a predictor of childhood disability after neonatal hypoxic-ischemic encephalopathy. Developmental Med child Neurol 2014;56(11):1052–8.
40. Vos-Vromans DC, Ketelaar M, Gorter JW. Responsiveness of evaluative measures for children with cerebral palsy: the gross motor function measure and the pediatric evaluation of disability Inventory. Disabil Rehabil 2005;27(20): 1245–52.
41. Berg M, Jahnsen R, Froslie KF, et al. Reliability of the pediatric evaluation of disability Inventory (PEDI). Phys Occup Ther Pediatr 2004;24(3):61–77.
42. Haley S, Coster W, Ludlow L, et al. Pediatric evaluation of disability Inventory (PEDI). Boston, MA: Trustees of Boston University; 1998.
43. Randall M, Harvey A, Imms C, et al. Reliable classification of functional profiles and movement disorders of children with cerebral palsy. Phys Occup Ther Pediatr 2013;33(3):342–52.
44. Hidecker MJ, Ho NT, Dodge N, et al. Inter-relationships of functional status in cerebral palsy: analyzing gross motor function, manual ability, and communication function classification systems in children. Developmental Med child Neurol 2012;54(8):737–42.
45. Surveillance of cerebral palsy in Europe: a collaboration of cerebral palsy surveys and registers. Surveillance of Cerebral Palsy in Europe (SCPE). Developmental Med child Neurol 2000;42(12):816–24.
46. Kuban KC, Allred EN, O'Shea M, et al. An algorithm for identifying and classifying cerebral palsy in young children. J Pediatr 2008;153(4):466–72.
47. Guillet R, Edwards AD, Thoresen M, et al. Seven- to eight-year follow-up of the CoolCap trial of head cooling for neonatal encephalopathy. Pediatr Res 2012; 71(2):205–9.
48. Novak I, Morgan C, Fahey M, et al. State of the evidence Traffic Lights 2019: systematic review of interventions for Preventing and treating children with cerebral palsy. Curr Neurol Neurosci Rep 2020;20(2):3.
49. Lee-Kelland R, Jary S, Tonks J, et al. School-age outcomes of children without cerebral palsy cooled for neonatal hypoxic-ischaemic encephalopathy in 2008-2010. Arch Dis Child Fetal neonatal edition 2020;105(1):8–13.
50. Perez A, Ritter S, Brotschi B, et al. Long-term neurodevelopmental outcome with hypoxic-ischemic encephalopathy. J Pediatr 2013;163(2):454–9.
51. Marlow N, Rose AS, Rands CE, et al. Neuropsychological and educational problems at school age associated with neonatal encephalopathy. Arch Dis Child Fetal neonatal edition 2005;90(5):F380–7.
52. van Handel M, de Sonneville L, de Vries LS, et al. Specific memory impairment following neonatal encephalopathy in term-born children. Dev Neuropsychol 2012;37(1):30–50.
53. Robertson CM, Finer NN, Grace MG. School performance of survivors of neonatal encephalopathy associated with birth asphyxia at term. J Pediatr 1989;114(5):753–60.

54. van Handel M, Swaab H, de Vries LS, et al. Long-term cognitive and behavioral consequences of neonatal encephalopathy following perinatal asphyxia: a review. Eur J Pediatr 2007;166(7):645–54.
55. Steinman KJ, Gorno-Tempini ML, Glidden DV, et al. Neonatal watershed brain injury on magnetic resonance imaging correlates with verbal IQ at 4 years. Pediatrics 2009;123(3):1025–30.
56. Robertson CM, Perlman M. Follow-up of the term infant after hypoxic-ischemic encephalopathy. Paediatr Child Health 2006;11(5):278–82.
57. Hutchon B, Gibbs D, Harniess P, et al. Early intervention programmes for infants at high risk of atypical neurodevelopmental outcome. Developmental Med child Neurol 2019;61(12):1362–7.
58. Lin SC, Gold RS. Assistive technology needs, functional difficulties, and services utilization and coordination of children with developmental disabilities in the United States. Assist Technol 2018;30(2):100–6.
59. Azzopardi D, Strohm B, Marlow N, et al. Effects of hypothermia for perinatal asphyxia on childhood outcomes. New Engl J Med 2014;371(2):140–9.
60. Marlow N, Wolke D, Bracewell MA, et al. Neurologic and developmental disability at six years of age after extremely preterm birth. New Engl J Med 2005;352(1):9–19.
61. Massaro AN, Murthy K, Zaniletti I, et al. Short-term outcomes after perinatal hypoxic ischemic encephalopathy: a report from the Children's Hospitals Neonatal Consortium HIE focus group. J Perinatol 2015;35(4):290–6.
62. Murray DM, O'Connor CM, Ryan CA, et al. Early EEG grade and outcome at 5 Years after mild neonatal hypoxic ischemic encephalopathy. Pediatrics 2016;138(4):e20160659.
63. Conway JM, Walsh BH, Boylan GB, et al. Mild hypoxic ischaemic encephalopathy and long term neurodevelopmental outcome - a systematic review. Early Hum Dev 2018;120:80–7.
64. Mir IN, Johnson-Welch SF, Nelson DB, et al. Placental pathology is associated with severity of neonatal encephalopathy and adverse developmental outcomes following hypothermia. Am J Obstet Gynecol 2015;213(6):849.e1-7.
65. Mir IN, Johnson-Welch SF, Nelson DB, et al. Placental pathology is associated with severity of neonatal encephalopathy and adverse developmental outcomes following hypothermia. Am J Obstet Gynecol 2015;213(6):849 e841–847.
66. Chalak L, Latremouille S, Mir I, et al. A review of the conundrum of mild hypoxic-ischemic encephalopathy: current challenges and moving forward. Early Hum Dev 2018;120:88–94.
67. Chalak LF. Best practice guidelines on management of mild neonatal encephalopathy: is it really mild? Early Hum Dev 2018;120:74.
68. Chalak L, Ferriero DM, Gressens P, et al. A 20 years conundrum of neonatal encephalopathy and hypoxic ischemic encephalopathy: are we closer to a consensus guideline? Pediatr Res 2019;86(5):548–9.
69. Conway JM, Walsh BH, Boylan GB, et al. Mild hypoxic ischaemic encephalopathy and long term neurodevelopmental outcome - a systematic review. Early Hum Dev 2018;120:80–7.
70. Robertson C, Finer N. Term infants with hypoxic-ischemic encephalopathy: outcome at 3.5 years. Dev Med Child Neurol 1985;27(4):473–84.
71. van Handel M, Swaab H, de Vries LS, et al. Behavioral outcome in children with a history of neonatal encephalopathy following perinatal asphyxia. J Pediatr Psychol 2010;35(3):286–95.

72. Jacobs SE, Morley CJ, Inder TE, et al. Whole-body hypothermia for term and near-term newborns with hypoxic-ischemic encephalopathy: a randomized controlled trial. Arch Pediatr Adolesc Med 2011;165(8):692–700.
73. Zhou WH, Cheng GQ, Shao XM, et al. Selective head cooling with mild systemic hypothermia after neonatal hypoxic-ischemic encephalopathy: a multicenter randomized controlled trial in China. J Pediatr 2010;157(3):367–72.
74. Battin MR, Dezoete JA, Gunn TR, et al. Neurodevelopmental outcome of infants treated with head cooling and mild hypothermia after perinatal asphyxia. Pediatrics 2001;107(3):480–4.
75. Wyatt JS, Gluckman PD, Liu PY, et al. Determinants of outcomes after head cooling for neonatal encephalopathy. Pediatrics 2007;119(5):912–21.
76. Vohr BR, Stephens BE, McDonald SA, et al. Cerebral palsy and growth failure at 6 to 7 years. Pediatrics 2013;132(4):e905–14.
77. Jensen PS, Gulati IK, Shubert TR, et al. Pharyngeal stimulus-induced reflexes are impaired in infants with perinatal asphyxia: Does maturation modify? Neurogastroenterol Motil 2017;29(7).
78. Arora I, Bhandekar H, Lakra A, et al. Filling the Gaps for feeding difficulties in neonates with hypoxic-ischemic encephalopathy. Cureus 2022;14(8):e28564.
79. Rothenberg SS. Laparoscopic Nissen procedure in children. Semin Laparosc Surg 2002;9(3):146–52.
80. Vyas SS, Ford MK, Tam EWY, et al. Intervention experiences among children with congenital and neonatal conditions impacting brain development: patterns of service utilization, barriers and future directions. Clin Neuropsychol 2021; 35(5):1009–29.
81. Tian Q, Pan Y, Zhang Z, et al. Predictive value of early amplitude integrated electroencephalogram (aEEG) in sleep related problems in children with perinatal hypoxic-ischemia (HIE). BMC Pediatr 2021;21(1):410.
82. Boylan GB, Kharoshankaya L, Wusthoff CJ. Seizures and hypothermia: importance of electroencephalographic monitoring and considerations for treatment. Semin Fetal neonatal Med 2015;20(2):103–8.
83. Hunt RW, Liley HG, Wagh D, et al. Effect of treatment of clinical seizures vs electrographic seizures in full-term and near-term neonates: a randomized clinical trial. JAMA Netw Open 2021;4(12):e2139604.
84. Kharoshankaya L, Stevenson NJ, Livingstone V, et al. Seizure burden and neurodevelopmental outcome in neonates with hypoxic-ischemic encephalopathy. Developmental Med child Neurol 2016;58(12):1242–8.
85. Guidotti I, Lugli L, Guerra MP, et al. Hypothermia reduces seizure burden and improves neurological outcome in severe hypoxic-ischemic encephalopathy: an observational study. Developmental Med child Neurol 2016;58(12):1235–41.
86. Berg AT, Berkovic SF, Brodie MJ, et al. Revised terminology and concepts for organization of seizures and epilepsies: report of the ILAE Commission on Classification and Terminology, 2005-2009. Epilepsia 2010;51(4):676–85.
87. Abu Dhais F, McNamara B, O'Mahony O, et al. Impact of therapeutic hypothermia on infantile spasms: an observational cohort study. Developmental Med child Neurol 2020;62(1):62–8.
88. Nevalainen P, Metsaranta M, Toiviainen-Salo S, et al. Neonatal neuroimaging and neurophysiology predict infantile onset epilepsy after perinatal hypoxic ischemic encephalopathy. Seizure : J Br Epilepsy Assoc 2020;80:249–56.
89. Shetty J. Neonatal seizures in hypoxic-ischaemic encephalopathy–risks and benefits of anticonvulsant therapy. Developmental Med child Neurol 2015; 57(Suppl 3):40–3.

90. Yozawitz E, Stacey A, Pressler RM. Pharmacotherapy for seizures in neonates with hypoxic ischemic encephalopathy. Paediatr Drugs 2017;19(6):553–67.
91. Robertson CM, Finer NN. Educational readiness of survivors of neonatal encephalopathy associated with birth asphyxia at term. J Dev Behav Pediatr 1988;9(5):298–306.
92. Danguecan A, El Shahed AI, Somerset E, et al. Towards a biopsychosocial understanding of neurodevelopmental outcomes in children with hypoxic-ischemic encephalopathy: a mixed-methods study. Clin Neuropsychol 2021;35(5):925–47.
93. Chalak L, Pilon B, Byrne R, et al. Stakeholder engagement in neonatal clinical trials: an opportunity for mild neonatal encephalopathy research. Pediatr Res 2022. https://doi.org/10.1038/s41390-022-02067-y.
94. Pilon B. Family reflections: hope for HIE. Pediatr Res 2019;86(5):672–3.
95. Gunn AJ, Gluckman PD, Gunn TR. Selective head cooling in newborn infants after perinatal asphyxia: a safety study. Pediatrics 1998;102(4 Pt 1):885–92.
96. Lindstrom K, Lagerroos P, Gillberg C, et al. Teenage outcome after being born at term with moderate neonatal encephalopathy. Pediatr Neurol 2006;35(4):268–74.
97. van Kooij BJ, van Handel M, Nievelstein RA, et al. Serial MRI and neurodevelopmental outcome in 9- to 10-year-old children with neonatal encephalopathy. J Pediatr 2010;157(2):221–227 e222.
98. Pappas A, Shankaran S, McDonald SA, et al. Cognitive outcomes after neonatal encephalopathy. Pediatrics 2015;135(3):e624–34.
99. van Schie PE, Schijns J, Becher JG, et al. Long-term motor and behavioral outcome after perinatal hypoxic-ischemic encephalopathy. Eur J paediatric Neurol 2015;19(3):354–9.
100. Hayes BC, Doherty E, Grehan A, et al. Neurodevelopmental outcome in survivors of hypoxic ischemic encephalopathy without cerebral palsy. Eur J Pediatr 2018;177(1):19–32.

# Neurodevelopmental Outcomes in Children with Congenital Heart Disease

## Ten Years After the American Heart Association Statement

Trisha Patel, MD[a,b], Dawn Ilardi, PhD[a,b],
Lazaros Kochilas, MD, MSCR[a,b,*]

### KEYWORDS

- Congenital heart disease • Neurodevelopment

### KEY POINTS

- Children with congenital heart disease (CHD) have risk factors for neurodevelopmental concerns, spanning from the genetic background, impaired in-utero and postnatal physiology, medical exposures, and residual chronic disease.
- Cyanotic heart disease and single ventricle physiology are the conditions with the highest risk of affecting most neurodevelopmental domains.
- Neurodevelopmental concerns range from infancy to adulthood and can lead to academic and psychological difficulties, delayed transition to adulthood, need for disability assistance, and underemployment.
- Early neurodevelopmental evaluation and intervention are essential for individuals with CHD; however, patient/family-related factors as well as health care access challenges remain barriers.

## INTRODUCTION

Congenital heart disease (CHD) is the most common birth defect, affecting approximately 1% of all live births in the United States.[1] Following improvements in medical and surgical care, childhood mortality from CHD has decreased in the last 30 years, with the largest decreases seen in patients with transposition of the great arteries (TGA), complete atrioventricular canal, and single ventricle CHD.[2,3] These

[a] Emory University School of Medicine, 1405 Clifton Road, Atlanta, GA 30322, USA; [b] Children's Healthcare of Atlanta, 1400 Tullie Road, Atlanta, GA 30329, USA
* Corresponding author. Children's Healthcare of Atlanta Cardiology, Emory University, 1760 Haygood Drive, Health Sciences Research Bldg (HSRB), W-468, Atlanta, Ga 30322.
*E-mail address:* lazaros.kochilas@emory.edu

Clin Perinatol 50 (2023) 53–66
https://doi.org/10.1016/j.clp.2022.10.002          **perinatology.theclinics.com**

improvements have led to an increased number of patients with CHD reaching adulthood; thus the long-term morbidities of CHD, including associated neurodevelopmental (ND) concerns, are increasingly important.[4] In 2012, writing groups from the American Heart Association (AHA) and the American Academy of Pediatrics (AAP) created a scientific statement to provide the first guidelines for the evaluation and management of ND outcomes associated with CHD.[5]

A decade later, using the 2012 AHA statement as an initial framework, this article aims to summarize the literature and current clinical practices related to ND follow-up of children with CHD. The specific areas of focus for this article are the (1) etiology and risk factors that predispose individuals with CHD to ND problems, (2) key ND areas of concern across development, (3) updates on the ND evaluation process and related interventions, and (4) challenges in facilitating and completing the ND evaluation.

## DISCUSSION
### Etiology and Risk Factors

There are a number of factors linked to CHD-related ND concerns, spanning from prenatal life to adulthood. An outline of the most important risk factors that predispose individuals with CHD to ND problems is summarized in **Table 1**. Genetic abnormalities such as Trisomy 21, Turner Syndrome, Williams syndrome, and 22q11.2 deletion are frequently associated with alterations of heart and brain health and have long been recognized among the highest risk factors for ND problems in the context of CHD.[6]

Impaired *in utero* hemodynamics further contribute to ND risks, as evidenced by delayed cortical development, decreased cerebral volumes, delayed sulcation, and reduction in global cerebral blood flow detected by fetal magnetic resonance imaging in fetuses with complex CHD.[7–9] Abnormal placental structure and function in mothers of infants with CHD were also shown to be associated with lower fetal cerebral oxygen and brain volume.[10]

After birth, cerebral blood flow and oxygen content continue to be abnormal before (and sometimes even after) medical or surgical intervention in infants with complex CHD and serve as additional risk factors for ND problems. Such risk factors include low cardiac output, diastolic steal in association with a patent ductus arteriosus or other form of aortopulmonary shunt, decreased pulmonary perfusion or mixing between the systemic and pulmonary venous return.[11] Hypoplastic left heart syndrome (HLHS) with intact atrial septum, obstructed total anomalous pulmonary venous return, and TGA with intact atrial and ventricular septum represent conditions at the highest risk for brain injury as they are associated with profound acidosis and hypoxemia.

Many infants with CHD will require some form of curative or palliative cardiac intervention, including cardiac surgery. Cardiac surgery frequently requires cardiopulmonary bypass (CPB), and at times deep hypothermic circulatory arrest (DHCA), which expose the brain to a period of global cerebral hypoperfusion followed by reperfusion injury. Both of these modalities lead to a host of physiologic abnormalities affecting brain tissue oxygenation on top of exposure to sedatives and anesthetics with potential effects on the developing brain.[12] Thanks in large part to the Boston Circulatory Arrest studies conducted in the 1980s and 1990s for patients with TGA and arterial switch operation, there is now a better understanding of the deleterious long-term effects of extended periods of DHCA and CPB on ND outcomes.[13] Since then, modifications to CPB techniques have been made, but contemporary studies continue to show that longer CPB times are a risk factor for deficits in cognitive, language, and motor domains for both two-ventricle and single-ventricle patients.[14,15]

| Table 1 |
| --- |
| Risk factors for neurodevelopmental concerns in the congenital heart disease population |

| Timeframe | Risk Factors for Neurodevelopmental Concerns |
| --- | --- |
| Prenatal | Genetic predisposition to CHD<br>Genetic abnormalities and syndromes<br>Impaired *in-utero* hemodynamics<br>Placental abnormalities |
| Neonatal transition | Prematurity (<37 weeks)<br>Neonatal transition<br>Acidosis and hypoxemia |
| Cardiac intervention | Exposure to CPB and DHCA<br>Use of ECMO and VAD<br>Use of volatile anesthetics |
| Postoperative recovery | Unstable hemodynamics and AP shunt steal<br>History of cardiopulmonary resuscitation<br>Prolonged hospitalization (>2 weeks)<br>Perioperative seizures<br>Psychological stress (separation from family; medical trauma) |
| Across the lifespan | Long-term cyanosis (with or without cardiac surgery)<br>Neuroimaging abnormalities<br>Microcephaly (<2 standard deviations)<br>Repeated hospitalizations, operations, and catheterizations<br>End-organ injury (ie, liver, kidneys)<br>Need for heart transplant<br>Pacemaker or ICD placement |

*Abbreviations:* AP, aortopulmonary shunt; CHD, congenital heart disease; CPB, cardiopulmonary bypass; DHCA, deep hypothermic circulatory arrest; ECMO, extracorporeal membrane oxygenation; ICD, implantable Cardioverter Defibrillator; VAD, ventricular assist device.

After cardiac surgery, children with CHD are vulnerable to further brain injury due to risk for low cardiac output, hypoxemia, and postoperative cardiac arrest. Common complications of postoperative cardiac arrest include prolonged hospitalization and use of volatile anesthetics, which are also linked to worse ND outcomes.[14] Children with complex CHD frequently suffer from chronically impaired circulation that is associated with complications to other organ systems and requires ongoing medical management, which further increases the risk for ND problems. Recurrent kidney failure following cardiac surgery is one such complication that has been associated with worse ND outcomes.[16]

More recently, the impact of psychosocial and environmental stressors has been recognized, with their effects being frequently more significant in predicting ND outcomes than medical and clinical factors. Such stressors can begin early; for example, with long hospital admissions, infants and family are frequently exposed to noxious stimuli during their stay in the intensive care unit (ICU). These infants may also be separated from their family, leading to poor caregiver-infant bonding, which is a crucial component of appropriate neurodevelopment.[17] Caregiver stress, anxiety, depression, and medical trauma in families of children with CHD have been well-documented during the ICU stay, with their effects lingering much longer and associated with lower cognitive outcomes and higher behavioral concerns.[18–20] Finally, newer research highlights the risks associated with social determinants of health, with variables such as race, ethnicity, and socioeconomic status predicting ND outcomes in the child with CHD.[21–23]

### Neurodevelopmental Outcomes

All ND domains have been implicated in the context of outcomes for children with CHD (**Fig. 1**). These include attention, executive functioning, intellectual functioning, learning and memory, language, visual-spatial and nonverbal, motor, social, emotional, and behavioral functioning. The reader is referred elsewhere for a comprehensive review, as each domain will be briefly reviewed below.[24]

In young children with CHD, ND concerns are most apparent in the domains of motor, speech, and language skills. Motor delays occur in about one-third of all children with CHD, and these delays involve fine and gross motor skills.[25] Severe motor impairments are most prevalent in the younger CHD population, but are present throughout childhood and adolescence.[25] In school-age children, problems related to visual motor integration skills are concerning, as these can impact functional skills such as handwriting. Prolonged CPB times and inability to establish oral feeding were associated with worse language skills when compared with a control population.[14] Similar to other neurocognitive domains, patients with cyanotic CHD and single ventricle lesions tend to have more pronounced language delays when compared with the non-CHD population.[26,27] These findings support the need for early ND evaluation, with ongoing monitoring for those areas affected.

As children with CHD get older, attention and executive functioning impairments are among the most reported areas of concern. Executive functioning is a complex construct that includes cognitive and behavioral skills associated with goal-directed behavior and higher-order thinking and reasoning. Depending on the measure, specific areas of executive functioning include inhibition, initiation, working memory, planning, problem-solving, organization, flexibility, problem-solving, and others. Weaknesses in

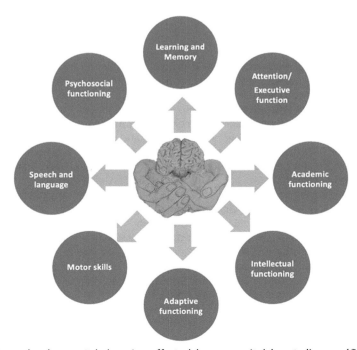

**Fig. 1.** Neurodevelopmental domains affected by congenital heart disease. (*Courtesy of* Jayur Patel, RDCS, Atlanta, Georgia.)

various skill areas of executive functioning have been reported across types of cyanotic CHD, with worse outcomes for those with single ventricle physiology.[27–29] Attention problems include difficulties with divided attention and conflict monitoring, as well as decreased ability to maintain alertness and vigilance in school-age children.[24] In pre-school children, attention skills were decreased in 40% to 65% of children with CHD compared with their peers.[30] Higher rates of inattention are evident in patients with cyanosis and single ventricle physiology.[31] Adolescents with single ventricle disease and tetralogy of Fallot (with and without a genetic disorder) present with higher rates of Attention Deficit Hyperactivity Disorder than the general population.[32] Given that attention and executive skills change across development, these domains need close monitoring based on CHD outcome literature.

Larger domains of ND skills also need to be monitored. For example, intellectual functioning is generally average to low average, but scattered weaknesses are apparent when separate subdomains are explored.[23] Children with cyanotic lesions and single ventricle physiology have been found to have lower overall intellectual functioning when compared with controls and children with acyanotic CHD.[27] Children with CHD and comorbid genetic syndromes are more likely to be diagnosed with an intellectual disability.[27]

In terms of academic functioning, studies show high rates of remedial school services, tutoring, grade retention, and special education services in the CHD population when compared with non-CHD peers.[24] Preschool children with CHD were found to have more delays than expected in pre-academic skills (like pre-reading and pre-spelling), although no difference was found between single ventricle or two ventricle patients.[21] A retrospective cohort study of school-age children in North Carolina found that children with CHD underachieved and did not reach standards in math and reading.[33] Patients with both severe and nonsevere CHD groups showed poor performance in reading and math and had frequent need for special education assistance.[33] A systematic review and meta-analysis also showed poor academic achievement in those with CHD when compared with non-CHD peers.[34]

Adaptive functioning, or the skill to learn age-appropriate proficiencies necessary for everyday life and independent living, is a specific area in which children with CHD have notable impairments. In a recent study, adolescents with CHD were found to have substantial functional impairments (<2nd percentile) with community use, functional academics (application of reading and math to everyday life), self-care, self-direction (responsibility and self-control), and social skills.[35] Adaptive functioning concerns can impact adult transition. Teenagers with CHD are also likely to miss more school days than peers without CHD (particularly in the 12 to 17 years range) and are 14 times more likely to have a disability that limits physical activity.[36] Memory and organizational difficulties also make the transition of medical care to the adult congenital world challenging. Approximately two-thirds of patients with CHD have been lost to follow up when they reach 18 years old; about 50% of them are lost in the late teenage transitional years.[37]

ND outcomes further show that social, emotional, and behavioral concerns need evaluation and monitoring. Studies show an increased risk for anxiety disorder, depression, and symptoms associated with internalizing (eg, anxiety, depression) and externalizing symptoms (eg, hyperactivity, aggression).[38,39] Individuals with CHD have also been found to have weaker social communication skills, as well as higher rates of autism spectrum disorder.[31,40]

The ND concerns experienced by the child with CHD can change across development, with some resolving and others becoming more apparent with age. To capture and screen for overarching ND concerns, health-related quality of life (HRQOL) survey tools have been used. HRQOL is a multifactorial concept that assesses physical, emotional, social, and cognitive or school functioning. Large-scale studies with parent and self-report measures of QOL in the United States and the United Kingdom showed lower HRQOL scores throughout all age categories in samples with CHD.[37] However, other studies, including a large multicenter study, showed that self-reported HRQOL was similar in both the CHD and control population in young children.[41] As children enter their teenage years, HRQOL scores continue to be low. Findings show lower psychologic scores and self-reports of cognitive problems and negative perception of physical appearance related to surgical scars, cyanosis, and short height.[42]

### Neurodevelopmental Evaluation

Given the variable ND concerns across development, it is important that providers treating children with CHD ensure early and ongoing ND evaluation as appropriate. Since 2012, the AHA/AAP high-risk referral criteria have served as guidelines for providers. There are a variety of ways that an ND evaluation can be completed. One such avenue is through a formal cardiac ND program. Referral to these programs often is the primary cardiologist's responsibility but other providers in the care team and even the child's parent can refer the child to these programs. In the absence of a cardiac ND program, evaluation usually takes place in schools or by a community psychologist, which can be associated with delays in care and increased financial burden.[43]

Following the AHA statement in 2012, a group of cardiac ND clinicians and researchers from the United States, Canada, and Europe formed in 2016 the Cardiac Neurodevelopmental Outcome Collaborative (CNOC; https://www.cardiacneuro.org/) with the mission to determine and implement best practices of ND and psychosocial services for individuals affected by CHD.[44] The CNOC helped facilitate institutional collaboration to support the needs of children with CHD and their families through clinical, research and quality of care initiatives. In an early survey with CNOC member institutions, 23 centers reported variable practices in timing and test administration.[45] Given rapid changes and growth, as well as variable practices since the initial AHA 2012 statement, CNOC developed detailed ND evaluation recommendations to guide care providers of children with CHD, including specific test batteries and clinical considerations.[46] For infants and preschool children, it is recommended that the ND evaluation includes a neurology consult, as well as assessment of early cognitive, language, nonverbal, social-emotional and behavioral, school-readiness, and adaptive skills as appropriate.[46] For the school-age children, assessment of intellectual, language, nonverbal, learning/memory, attention/executive function, fine motor, social-emotional and behavioral, academic, and adaptive skills are recommended as appropriate.[43]

### Psychosocial Intervention

In comparison with other populations of chronically ill children, there are few intervention programs directly tailored to children with CHD and their families. CNOC recently published a summary of the current state of psychosocial intervention literature, along with research agenda to inform future directions.[44,47] Much of the interventions currently in place are adapted from other patient population groups, including preterm infants.[47] Aspects of the preterm-centered Newborn Individualized Developmental Care and Assessment Program, specifically skin-to-skin contact, cue-based care, and family support, have been associated with improved ND outcomes in the CHD population.[47] Other intervention programs like peer support and therapeutic camp programs for oncology patients and interventions for addressing neurocognitive

**Table 2**
**Provider, patient, and family barriers to neurodevelopmental evaluation**

| Patient Factors | Family Factors | Provider Factors |
|---|---|---|
| Conflicts with other medical needs | Unawareness of the importance and need of ND | Limited access to qualified individuals for evaluation |
| Prolonged hospitalization | Insurance limitations or self-pay | Low priority compared with somatic disease |
| | Hesitation due to perceived stigma | Lengthy ND evaluation |

*Abbreviation:* ND, neurodevelopmental.

deficits have been shown to be effective in non-CHD chronically ill children, but there is limited information about how such adapted programs and interventions can benefit the CHD population.[47]

Currently, medical interventions, like skin-to-skin contact and multi-disciplinary feeding programs for infants with CHD, improve oral feeding, reduce length of stay and promote autonomic stability and early cognitive development.[48] The Congenital Heart Disease Intervention Program (CHIP), an intervention study with infant and school-aged children with CHD, has shown improvements in infant feeding practices, maternal anxiety, and increased school attendance.[49,50] These studies were comprised of six psychoeducational and coaching sessions delivered by a clinical psychologist and a cardiology nurse specialist, with session scopes including management of grief, exposure to medical equipment, and coaching on ways to optimize feeding success and soothing.

Although benefit has been noted in the infant and school-aged groups, the CHIP family-based workshop for parents, children with CHD, and siblings did not find a significant benefit for the child with CHD, when compared with the control group.[51] Notably in the CHIP studies, there was no improvement in school performance for the child, with similar ratings given by the parent and teacher pre and post-intervention.[52] In adolescents, an additional study evaluating improvement in working memory through the use of Cogmed (a computerized program designed to improve executive function, attention, and organization skills) found no significant change in working memory after three months but did find improvement in inhibitory control and attention.[53] Increasing HRQOL through increasing aerobic exercise in adolescents has also proven to be beneficial, with improvement noted in self-reported cognitive functioning and parent-reported social functioning.[54]

Intervention evaluation is especially lacking in the adolescent and adult populations with CHD.[55] Upon review of the current literature as of 2021, CNOC has identified adolescent and adult-targeted interventions, prospective randomized control trials with long-term follow-up of ND outcomes (and not just immediate pre-post evaluation outcomes), and large-scale, multi-centered studies evaluating ND interventions aimed to the executive function and visual-spatial processing domains, as additional areas of interest.[47]

## *Challenges*

Despite the need for ND evaluation for the CHD population, barriers and challenges exist (**Table 2**). Some of these challenges are system related, some are related to the patient or the family, but some may surprisingly exist within the provider's team itself. For example, in a survey distributed to primary care providers asking about

---

**Box 1**
**Categories of pediatric CHD patients at high risk for developmental disorders or disabilities**

1. Neonates or infants requiring open heart surgery (cyanotic and acyanotic types), for example, HlHS, IAA, PA/IVS, TA, TAPVC, TGA, TOF, tricuspid atresia.

2. Children with other cyanotic heart lesions not requiring open heart surgery during the neonatal or infact period, for example, TOF with PA and MAPCA(s), TOF with shunt without use of CPB, Ebstein anomaly.

3. Any combination of CHD and the following comorbidities:
   3.1. Prematurity (<37 wk)
   3.2. Developmental delay recognized in infancy
   3.3. Suspected genetic abnormality or syndrome associated with DD
   3.4. History of mechanical support (ECMO or VAD use)
   3.5. Heart transplantation
   3.6. Cardiopulmonary resuscitation at any point
   3.7. Prolonged hospitalization (postoperative LOS >2 wk in the hospital)
   3.8. Perioperative seizures related to CHD surgery
   3.9. Significant abnormalities on neuroimaging or microcephaly[a]

4. Other conditions determined at the discretion of the medical home providers

[a]Normative data by sex, including percentiles and z scores, are available from the World Health Organization (www.who.int/childgrowth; accessed February 2010).*Abbreviations:* CHD, indicates congenital heart disease; CPM, Cardio-pulmonary bypass; DD, developmental disorder or disability; ECMO, extracorporeal membrane oxygenation; HLHS, hypoplastic left heart syndrome; IAA, interrupted aortic arch; LOS, length of stay; MAPCA, major aortopulmonary collateral arterise; PA, pulmonary atresia; PA/IVS, pulmonary atresia with intact ventricular septum; TA, truncus arteriosus; TAPVC, total anomalous pulmonary venous connection; TGA, transposition of the great arteries; TOF, tertralogy of Fallot; and VAD, ventricular assist device.

*Adapted from* Marino BS, Lipkin PH, Newburger JW, et al. Neurodevelopmental outcomes in children with congenital heart disease: evaluation and management: a scientific statement from the American Heart Association. Circulation. 2012;126(9):1143-1172.

---

awareness of the 2012 AHA statement, 79% of providers were unaware of the statement, whereas 93% of them stated that an ND evaluation had not been included in the recommendations from the pediatric cardiologist.[56] Reduced awareness about the need for ND evaluation has also been reported among families. For example, 82% of parents of children with single ventricle CHD were unaware of the need for ND evaluation. Both medical providers and families may not always be able to identify children with ND concerns, and parents tend to overestimate their child's abilities.[57,58] These findings highlight the lack of consistency in cardiologists' referrals and counseling about the importance of ND evaluation.[59]

Family hesitation about the ND referral and difficulty connecting with an ND specialist were reported by one study.[56] Distance from the family's home to access clinical therapy is an important obstacle that limits access to ND specialists.[60] Poor insurance coverage for some locations providing ND evaluations can create financial hardship for families and discourage them from pursuing such evaluations.[60,61] The addition of a lengthy ND evaluation on the already busy medical schedule of families of children with CHD, who face multiple comorbidities, requires care coordination and can be another challenge for them to overcome.[61] Studies have shown that increased CHD complexity affects the compliance for outpatient ND appointments, with 25% of single ventricle patients returning for ND evaluation versus 63% of patients with two-ventricle lesions.[62] This may be due to the higher hospitalization rates for patients with single ventricle CHD, as a third of the patients who did not attend their ND appointment had recently been admitted or discharged from the hospital.[60]

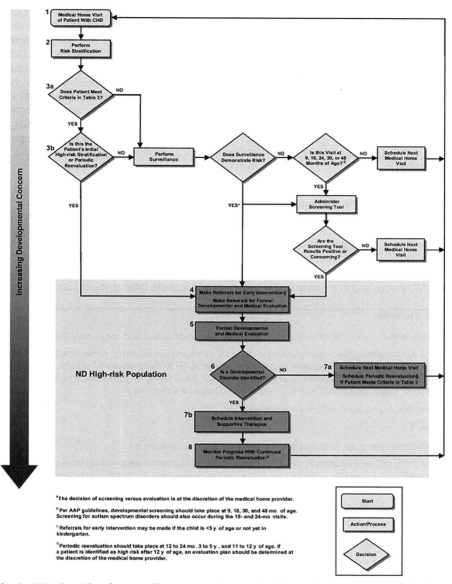

**Fig. 2.** CHD algorithm for surveillance, screening, evaluation, and management of developmental disorders and disabilities. ND indicates neurodevelopmental; AAP, American Academy of Pediatrics. B, Description of congenital heart disease algorithm for surveillance, screening, evaluation, and management of developmental disorders and disabilities. AAP indicates American Academy of Pediatrics, CHD, congenital heart disease; DD, developmental disorder or disability. (Reprinted with permission Circulation. 2012;126:1143-1172. © 2012 American Heart Association, Inc.)

Finally, there are limited resources to cover the ND evaluation needs of every child with CHD, and therefore, alternative approaches should be considered for the early screening of this population. Researchers in Europe developed the "Brief Developmental Assessment" (BDA) to cover important developmental domains and practical for use within inpatient and outpatient settings by pediatric cardiac care providers who are non-developmental specialists. Preliminary results were promising that BDA can detect children with a diagnosis associated with developmental delays and with acceptable sensitivity/specificity and reproducibility.[63,64] Feasibility and acceptance of remote videoconferencing for delivering the BDA will further enhance the ability of screening more children with CHD and lead to earlier identification of ND concerns.[65]

## SUMMARY

Children with CHD show abnormalities in brain development before birth, but the neurological insults continue throughout development. All domains of ND and psychosocial functioning can show areas of weakness in CHD, but outcomes are variable. These ND concerns can span into adulthood leading to challenges with the adult transition. Thus, referral for ND evaluation is of paramount importance using the 2012 AHA guidelines for high-risk CHD. Resources should be available, and programs need to be aware of and work to reduce the provider- and patient-specific barriers to completing the ND evaluation in a timely fashion, so that appropriate interventions can be initiated.

---

**Best practices**

*What is the current practice for neurodevelopment evaluation and congenital heart disease?*

The AHA outlined recommendations in 2012 for categories of pediatric patients with CHD who are at highest risk for neurodevelopmental concerns, with the purpose of optimizing early neurodevelopmental screening and evaluation for these children. Providers have been tasked to refer these individuals to early neurodevelopmental screening.

*Best Practice/Guideline/Care Path Objective(s)*

**Box 1**

*What changes in current practice are likely to improve outcomes?*

Early referral and education about the importance of neurodevelopmental screening to families and providers, including pediatric cardiologists, general pediatricians, and family medicine providers.

*Is there a Clinical Algorithm? If so, please include*

**Fig. 2**

*Pearls/Pitfalls at the point-of-care:*

1. Include a neurodevelopmental evaluation in the do list in the discharge summary after interventions for CHD or discharge after neonatal stabilization for children with at risk CHD

2. Encourage proactive communication between the family of a patient with CHD and any other caretakers, including teachers, to promote early recognition and early screening for neurodevelopmental concerns.

*Major Recommendations:*

- Children who meet AHA 2012 criteria for high-risk CHD population at risk for neurodevelopmental concerns require referral for evaluation and often time regular therapies and support.

- Providers who treat these individuals should refer patients for evaluation and should counsel families early on in their partnership on the importance of neurodevelopmental evaluation.

*Bibliographic Source(s):*

1. Marino BS, Lipkin PH, Newburger JW, Peacock G, Gerdes M, Gaynor JW, Mussatto KA, Uzark K, Goldberg CS, Johnson WH, Jr., Li J, Smith SE, Bellinger DC, Mahle WT. Neurodevelopmental outcomes in children with congenital heart disease: evaluation and management: a scientific statement from the American Heart Association. *Circulation.* 2012;126:1143-72.

## DISCLOSURE

The authors do not have any relationships relevant to the content of this article to disclose. All authors have approved the final version of the article.

## REFERENCES

1. Pace ND, Oster ME, Forestieri NE, et al. Sociodemographic factors and survival of infants with congenital heart defects. Pediatrics 2018;142(3):e20180302.
2. Gilboa SM, Salemi JL, Nembhard WN, et al. Mortality resulting from congenital heart disease among children and adults in the United States, 1999 to 2006. Circulation 2010;122(22):2254–63.
3. Spector LG, Menk JS, Knight JH, et al. Trends in long-term mortality after congenital heart surgery. J Am Coll Cardiol 2018;71(21):2434–46.
4. Gilboa SM, Devine OJ, Kucik JE, et al. Congenital heart defects in the United States: estimating the magnitude of the affected population in 2010. Circulation 2016;134(2):101–9.
5. Marino BS, Lipkin PH, Newburger JW, et al. Neurodevelopmental outcomes in children with congenital heart disease: evaluation and management: a scientific statement from the American Heart Association. Circulation 2012;126(9):1143–72.
6. Rollins CK, Newburger JW, Roberts AE. Genetic contribution to neurodevelopmental outcomes in congenital heart disease: are some patients predetermined to have developmental delay? Curr Opin Pediatr 2017;29(5):529–33.
7. Morton PD, Ishibashi N, Jonas RA. Neurodevelopmental abnormalities and congenital heart disease: insights into altered brain maturation. Circ Res 2017; 120(6):960–77.
8. Masoller N, Sanz-Cortes M, Crispi F, et al. Severity of fetal brain abnormalities in congenital heart disease in relation to the main expected pattern of in utero brain blood supply. Fetal Diagn Ther 2016;39(4):269–78.
9. Khalil A, Suff N, Thilaganathan B, et al. Brain abnormalities and neurodevelopmental delay in congenital heart disease: systematic review and meta-analysis. Ultrasound Obstet Gynecol 2014;43(1):14–24.
10. Andescavage NN, Limperopoulos C. Placental abnormalities in congenital heart disease. Transl Pediatr 2021;10(8):2148–56.
11. Wernovsky G, Licht DJ. Neurodevelopmental outcomes in children with congenital heart disease-what can we impact? Pediatr Crit Care Med 2016;17(8 Suppl 1): S232–42.
12. Veraar CM, Rinosl H, Kuhn K, et al. Non-pulsatile blood flow is associated with enhanced cerebrovascular carbon dioxide reactivity and an attenuated relationship between cerebral blood flow and regional brain oxygenation. Crit Care 2019; 23(1):426.
13. Bellinger DC, Wypij D, Rivkin MJ, et al. Adolescents with d-transposition of the great arteries corrected with the arterial switch procedure: neuropsychological assessment and structural brain imaging. Circulation 2011;124(12):1361–9.

14. Mussatto KA, Hoffmann RG, Hoffman GM, et al. Risk and prevalence of developmental delay in young children with congenital heart disease. Pediatrics 2014; 133(3):e570–7.

15. International Cardiac Collaborative on Neurodevelopment I. Impact of operative and postoperative factors on neurodevelopmental outcomes after cardiac operations. Ann Thorac Surg 2016;102(3):843–9.

16. Pande CK, Noll L, Afonso N, et al. Neurodevelopmental outcomes in infants with cardiac surgery associated acute kidney injury. Ann Thorac Surg 2022. In press.

17. Ryan KR, Jones MB, Allen KY, et al. Neurodevelopmental outcomes among children with congenital heart disease: at-risk populations and modifiable risk factors. World J Pediatr Congenit Heart Surg 2019;10(6):750–8.

18. Kasparian NA, Kan JM, Sood E, et al. Mental health care for parents of babies with congenital heart disease during intensive care unit admission: systematic review and statement of best practice. Early Hum Dev 2019;139:104837.

19. Williams TS, Deotto A, Roberts SD, et al. COVID-19 mental health impact among children with early brain injury and associated conditions. Child Neuropsychol 2022;28(5):627–48.

20. McWhorter LG, Christofferson J, Neely T, et al. Parental post-traumatic stress, overprotective parenting, and emotional and behavioural problems for children with critical congenital heart disease. Cardiol Young 2022;32(5):738–45.

21. Brosig CL, Bear L, Allen S, et al. Preschool neurodevelopmental outcomes in children with congenital heart disease. J Pediatr 2017;183:80–86 e81.

22. Bucholz EM, Sleeper LA, Sananes R, et al. Trajectories in neurodevelopmental, health-related quality of life, and functional status outcomes by socioeconomic status and maternal education in children with single ventricle heart disease. J Pediatr 2021;229:289–293 e283.

23. Cassidy AR, Newburger JW, Bellinger DC. Learning and memory in adolescents with critical biventricular congenital heart disease. J Int Neuropsychol Soc 2017; 23(8):627–39.

24. Cassidy AR, Ilardi D, Bowen SR, et al. [Formula: see text]Congenital heart disease: a primer for the pediatric neuropsychologist. Child Neuropsychol 2018; 24(7):859–902.

25. Liamlahi R, von Rhein M, Buhrer S, et al. Motor dysfunction and behavioural problems frequently coexist with congenital heart disease in school-age children. Acta Paediatr 2014;103(7):752–8.

26. Burns J, Varughese R, Ganigara M, et al. Neurodevelopmental outcomes in congenital heart disease through the lens of single ventricle patients. Curr Opin Pediatr 2021;33(5):535–42.

27. Nattel SN, Adrianzen L, Kessler EC, et al. Congenital heart disease and neurodevelopment: clinical manifestations, genetics, mechanisms, and implications. Can J Cardiol 2017;33(12):1543–55.

28. Cassidy AR, White MT, DeMaso DR, et al. Executive function in children and adolescents with critical cyanotic congenital heart disease. J Int Neuropsychol Soc 2015;21(1):34–49.

29. Schaefer C, von Rhein M, Knirsch W, et al. Neurodevelopmental outcome, psychological adjustment, and quality of life in adolescents with congenital heart disease. Dev Med Child Neurol 2013;55(12):1143–9.

30. Gaudet I, Paquette N, Bernard C, et al. Neurodevelopmental outcome of children with congenital heart disease: a cohort study from infancy to preschool age. J Pediatr 2021;239:126–135 e125.

31. Hansen E, Poole TA, Nguyen V, et al. Prevalence of ADHD symptoms in patients with congenital heart disease. Pediatr Int 2012;54(6):838–43.

32. DeMaso DR, Calderon J, Taylor GA, et al. Psychiatric disorders in adolescents with single ventricle congenital heart disease. Pediatrics 2017;139(3):e20162241.

33. Oster ME, Watkins S, Hill KD, et al. Academic outcomes in children with congenital heart defects: a population-based cohort study. Circ Cardiovasc Qual Outcomes 2017;10(2):e003074.

34. Glinianaia SV, McLean A, Moffat M, et al. Academic achievement and needs of school-aged children born with selected congenital anomalies: a systematic review and meta-analysis. Birth Defects Res 2021;113(20):1431–62.

35. Tan A, Semmel ES, Rodrigues N, et al. Adaptive functioning in adolescents with congenital heart disease referred for neurodevelopmental follow-up. J Pediatr Neuropsychol 2022;8:68–78.

36. Razzaghi H, Oster M, Reefhuis J. Long-term outcomes in children with congenital heart disease: national Health Interview Survey. J Pediatr 2015;166(1):119–24.

37. Marelli A, Miller SP, Marino BS, et al. Brain in congenital heart disease across the lifespan: the cumulative burden of injury. Circulation 2016;133(20):1951–62.

38. Bean Jaworski JL, Flynn T, Burnham N, et al. Rates of autism and potential risk factors in children with congenital heart defects. Congenit Heart Dis 2017; 12(4):421–9.

39. Abda A, Bolduc ME, Tsimicalis A, et al. Psychosocial outcomes of children and adolescents with severe congenital heart defect: a systematic review and meta-analysis. J Pediatr Psychol 2019;44(4):463–77.

40. Tan A, Semmel ES, Wolf I, et al. Implementing standard screening for autism spectrum disorder in CHD. Cardiol Young 2020;30(8):1118–25.

41. Abassi H, Huguet H, Picot MC, et al. Health-related quality of life in children with congenital heart disease aged 5 to 7 years: a multicentre controlled cross-sectional study. Health Qual Life Outcomes 2020;18(1):366.

42. Shearer K, Rempel GR, Norris CM, et al. "It's no big deal": adolescents with congenital heart disease. J Pediatr Nurs 2013;28(1):28–36.

43. Ilardi D, Sanz JH, Cassidy AR, et al. Neurodevelopmental evaluation for school-age children with congenital heart disease: recommendations from the cardiac neurodevelopmental outcome collaborative. Cardiol Young 2020;30(11):1623–36.

44. Sood E, Jacobs JP, Marino BS. The Cardiac Neurodevelopmental Outcome Collaborative: a new community improving outcomes for individuals with congenital heart disease. Cardiol Young 2020;30(11):1595–6.

45. Miller TA, Sadhwani A, Sanz J, et al. Variations in practice in cardiac neurodevelopmental follow-up programs. Cardiol Young 2020;30(11):1603–8.

46. Ware J, Butcher JL, Latal B, et al. Neurodevelopmental evaluation strategies for children with congenital heart disease aged birth through 5 years: recommendations from the cardiac neurodevelopmental outcome collaborative. Cardiol Young 2020;30(11):1609–22.

47. Cassidy AR, Butler SC, Briend J, et al. Neurodevelopmental and psychosocial interventions for individuals with CHD: a research agenda and recommendations from the Cardiac Neurodevelopmental Outcome Collaborative. Cardiol Young 2021;31(6):888–99.

48. Harrison TM, Brown R. Autonomic nervous system function after a skin-to-skin contact intervention in infants with congenital heart disease. J Cardiovasc Nurs 2017;32(5):E1–13.

49. McCusker CG, Doherty NN, Molloy B, et al. A controlled trial of early interventions to promote maternal adjustment and development in infants born with severe congenital heart disease. Child Care Health Dev 2010;36(1):110–7.

50. McCusker CG, Doherty NN, Molloy B, et al. A randomized controlled trial of interventions to promote adjustment in children with congenital heart disease entering school and their families. J Pediatr Psychol 2012;37(10):1089–103.

51. van der Mheen M, Meentken MG, van Beynum IM, et al. CHIP-Family intervention to improve the psychosocial well-being of young children with congenital heart disease and their families: results of a randomised controlled trial. Cardiol Young 2019;29(9):1172–82.

52. Calderon J, Bellinger DC. Executive function deficits in congenital heart disease: why is intervention important? Cardiol Young 2015;25(7):1238–46.

53. Calderon J, Wypij D, Rofeberg V, et al. Randomized controlled trial of working memory intervention in congenital heart disease. J Pediatr 2020;227:191–198 e193.

54. Dulfer K, Duppen N, Kuipers IM, et al. Aerobic exercise influences quality of life of children and youngsters with congenital heart disease: a randomized controlled trial. J Adolesc Health 2014;55(1):65–72.

55. Tesson S, Butow PN, Sholler GF, et al. Psychological interventions for people affected by childhood-onset heart disease: a systematic review. Health Psychol 2019;38(2):151–61.

56. Knutson S, Kelleman MS, Kochilas L. Implementation of developmental screening guidelines for children with congenital heart disease. J Pediatr 2016;176:135–141 e132.

57. Costello JM, Mussatto K, Cassedy A, et al. Prediction by clinicians of quality of life for children and adolescents with cardiac disease. J Pediatr 2015;166(3): 679–683 e672.

58. Mahle WT, Clancy RR, Moss EM, et al. Neurodevelopmental outcome and lifestyle assessment in school-aged and adolescent children with hypoplastic left heart syndrome. Pediatrics 2000;105(5):1082–9.

59. Alam S, Ilardi D, Cadiz E, et al. Impact of cardiac neurodevelopmental evaluation for children with congenital heart disease. Dev Neuropsychol 2021;47(1):32–41.

60. Loccoh EC, Yu S, Donohue J, et al. Prevalence and risk factors associated with non-attendance in neurodevelopmental follow-up clinic among infants with CHD. Cardiol Young 2018;28(4):554–60.

61. Glotzbach KL, Ward JJ, Marietta J, et al. The benefits and bias in neurodevelopmental evaluation for children with congenital heart disease. Pediatr Cardiol 2020;41(2):327–33.

62. Michael M, Scharf R, Letzkus L, et al. Improving neurodevelopmental surveillance and follow-up in infants with congenital heart disease. Congenit Heart Dis 2016; 11(2):183–8.

63. Brown KL, Ridout DA, Pagel C, et al. Validation of the Brief Developmental Assessment in pre-school children with heart disease. Cardiol Young 2018; 28(4):571–81.

64. Wray J, Brown KL, Ridout D, et al. Development and preliminary testing of the Brief Developmental Assessment: an early recognition tool for children with heart disease. Cardiol Young 2018;28(4):582–91.

65. Read JS, Brown K, Wray J. The feasibility and acceptability of remote videoconference use of the brief developmental assessment tool for young children with congenital heart disease. Telemed J E Health 2022. https://doi.org/10.1089/tmj. 2021.0609.

# Health Care Disparities in High-Risk Neonates

Yvette R. Johnson, MD, MPH[a],*, Charleta Guillory, MD, MPH[b], Sonia Imaizumi, MD[c]

## KEYWORDS

- Health disparities • Racial disparity • Structural racism
- Maternal and infant mortality • High-risk NICU follow-up/care of NICU graduate
- Quality of NICU care delivery

## KEY POINTS

- Long-standing health disparities in maternal reproductive health outcomes and infant morbidity and mortality are rooted in a foundation of structural racism.
- Black women die in pregnancy at rates 3 times higher than non-Hispanic white women. Black infant mortality is twice as high as non-Hispanic white infants within the 1st year of life.
- Black and Hispanic infants are more likely to receive neonatal intensive care unit (NICU) care in poorer quality NICUs and receive lower quality of care within NICUs, and are less likely to be referred for high-risk infants' follow-up after discharge, leading to higher rates of adverse neurodevelopmental outcomes.
- Implicit bias training, quality improvement initiatives, and antiracism interventions help to eliminate health disparities in neonatal care and long-term outcomes.
- Patient-provider relationships, family-centered care, individualized infant and family NICU care, and a diverse health care workforce will help to eliminate disparities.

## INTRODUCTION

Despite great advances in Neonatal-Perinatal Medicine in the past 4 decades, the United States has fallen from number 6 to number 26 in the world with regard to infant mortality. This state is even more shocking when considering the disparity between African American and White infant mortality, with the ratio increasing from 1.6 to 2.2 during the same period.[1,2] The National Institutes of Health defines health disparities as "differences in the incidence, prevalence, mortality, and burden of diseases and other adverse health conditions that exist among specific population

[a] Texas Christian University, Burnett School of Medicine, Cook Children's Medical Center, N.E.S.T. Developmental Follow-up Clinic, 1500 Cooper Street, Fort Worth, TX 76104, USA; [b] Baylor College of Medicine, Texas Children's Hospital, Section of Neonatology, 6621 Fannin, Houston, TX 77030, USA; [c] Newtown Square, MultiPlan.com, 18 Campus Boulevard, Suite 200, Newtown Square, PA 19073, USA
* Corresponding author.
*E-mail address:* yvette.johnson@cookchildrens.org

Clin Perinatol 50 (2023) 67–80
https://doi.org/10.1016/j.clp.2022.11.008
0095-5108/23/© 2022 Elsevier Inc. All rights reserved.

groups in the United States." Eliminating health disparities among different segments of the population is a major Healthy People 2030 goal.[3–6] Health disparities often arise from intentional or unintentional discrimination or marginalization, reinforcing social disadvantage and vulnerability.[1] Key drivers of these health disparities involve a complex interaction between health systems, societal factors, environmental factors, and economic factors (**Fig. 1**). These social determinants of health, often shaped by public policies, affect health outcomes (**Fig. 2**). Where high-risk infants are concerned, disparities are found in aspects of neonatal intensive care unit (NICU) care and early morbidity as well as in long-term outcomes and access. Disparities in NICU access and care are well documented throughout numerous networks and studies.[7–27] The NICU setting is uniquely positioned to implement interventions that achieve more equitable NICU care and quality outcomes for all infants, especially for Black and Hispanic infants, as well as others with adverse social determinants of health who comprise a disproportionate number of infants requiring NICU care. Equitable, high-quality NICU care during this critical phase of infant and familial development has great potential to affect long-term outcomes.[28] Although improvement in disparities in the NICU are critical, the purpose of this article is to describe the disparities found across the follow-up care continuum of high-risk infants and suggest possible solutions (see **Fig. 2**).

### Maternal Stress in the Neonatal Intensive Care Unit: an Additional Burden Affecting Disparities in Infant Outcomes

All mothers experience stress while having a child in the NICU setting; this seems to be a universal experience. Parents are uncertain whether their child will survive or not and start to wonder about long-term neurodevelopmental outcomes. This high level of stress manifests as higher rates of postpartum depression, anxiety, posttraumatic stress disorder, sleep disturbances, feelings of grief and isolation, helplessness, and

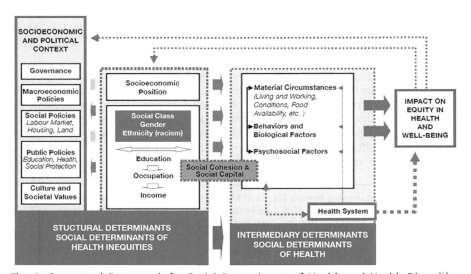

**Fig. 1.** Conceptual Framework for Social Determinants of Health and Health Disparities. (*From* Solar O and Irwin A. A, conceptual framework for action on the social determinants of health. Social Determinants of Health Discussion Paper 2 (Policy and Practice), WHO, 2010.).

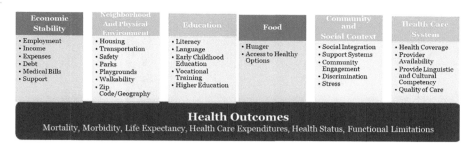

**Fig. 2.** Social determinants of health. (Artiga S, et al. Disparities in Health and Health Care: Five Key Questions and Answers. Kaiser Family Foundation Executive Summary 2020.)

an unhealthy parent-infant relationship.[29] A deeper understanding of the major sources of stress and appropriate interventions may suggest where interventions affecting parent-child interactions could lead to better long-term outcomes.

Black and Hispanic women are particularly vulnerable to chronic stress and disparities in care over the life course. A qualitative study using in-depth in-person interviews evaluated lived experiences of stress among Black women with very low-birth-weight infants hospitalized in the NICU. Identified sources of stress included (1) individual characteristics of the mother, (2) the hospital experience, and (3) the local community.[30] The Black women in this study disproportionately experienced personal stress, feeling overwhelmed and powerless. Stressors were superimposed on previous life events (eg, previous pregnancy loss, complex perinatal course). They also experienced hospital-specific stressors such as poorer quality of care (eg, nursing care), poor communication with provider, transportation, and parking concerns. Community-based sources of stress during their NICU stay included lack of social supports and financial resources, homelessness, and work-related challenges (eg, inadequate maternity leave). Other studies have demonstrated that Black, low-income mothers experience lower power and efficacy of voice when speaking with medical providers in the NICU.[31,32] Black and Hispanic women experienced stress differently than White women, suggesting a need for future screening with better measures of stress, to develop improved targeted interventions. Examples include the use of socioecological model, a theoretic framework to promote more equitable care for all mothers during the NICU stay.[33–53]

## Disparities in Outcomes

Despite well-documented racial disparities in health outcomes of high-risk infants, underlying causes have not been well studied. Research investigations often use race as a proxy measure—or even a confounder—to explain differences in outcomes by race. However, they do not explore the basis for these differences, instead attributing this to vague and multifactorial issues. The lack of direct mechanistic link between race and outcomes perpetuates the idea of race as a biological factor rather than a social construct. In reality, disparities in health outcomes by race/ethnicity (**Fig. 3**) often have racism or its downstream logistical consequences as a root cause of poor outcomes.[33,54–57]

There are 5 leading causes of infant mortality (**Figs. 4** and **5**) in the United States: preterm birth and low birth weight, sudden infant death syndrome, congenital anomalies, accidental injuries, and maternal pregnancy complications.[39,58] Understanding and implementing programs to address the disparities are critical to improving the lives of Black babies.

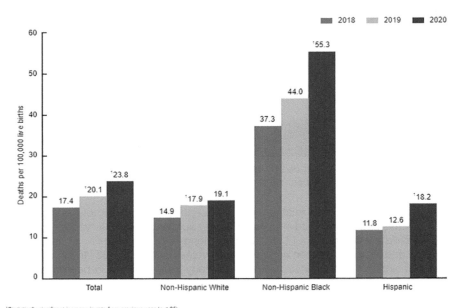

**Fig. 3.** Maternal mortality rates by race and ethnicity. (*From* Hoyert DL. Maternal mortality rates in the United States, 2020. NCHS Health E-Stats; 2022.).

New evidence suggests an improved survival rate of Black infants with "racial concordance" between the providing physician and the newborn patient. For example, the data suggest that the Black infant mortality rate could be decreased by half if Black infants are cared for by Black physicians. Furthermore, these findings seem more beneficial if the hospital delivers more Black infants and experience more

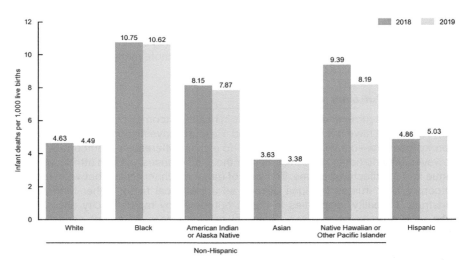

**Fig. 4.** Mortality trends by race/ethnicity. (Ely DM, Driscoll AK. Infant mortality in the United States, 2019: Data from the period linked birth/infant death file. National Vital Statistics Reports; vol 70 no 14. Hyattsville (MD): National Center for Health Statistics. 2021. DOI: https://dx.doi.org/10.15620/cdc:111053.).

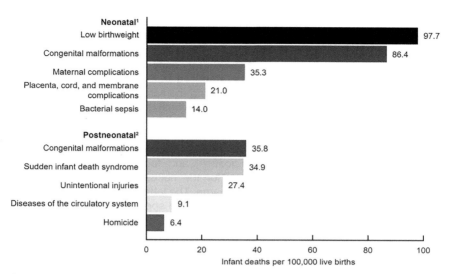

**Fig. 5.** Leading causes of Neonatal and postneonatal mortality in the United States. (*From Ely DM, Driscoll AK, Matthews TJ. Infant Mortality by Age at Death in the United States, 2016. NCHS Data Brief. 2018;(326):1–8.*)

birthing challenges. Although no examination of preterm birth or adverse birth event rates was provided, this presents an intriguing possibility when addressing disparities in Black infant perinatal outcomes.[41]

### Beyond the Neonatal Intensive Care Unit: Follow Through of High-Risk Infant Follow-up

The neonatal community does not exist in a social vacuum: the idea that health outcomes of this fragile population are inevitably linked to social determinants of health including race, ethnicity, income, immigration status, and neighborhood of residence alter access to the NICU, and NICU care also holds true for HRIF programs. An ethical responsibility of NICU providers to address these concerns was introduced by Horbar and colleagues, with the concept of "follow through... a more comprehensive approach that begins before birth and continues into childhood."[59] This approach requires collaboration among health professionals, families, and communities, who work together as partners in care to eliminate health disparities. Several "potentially better practices" for follow-through care can be implemented to reduce health disparities, provide equitable NICU and outpatient care, and improve long-term outcomes for all infants.

Disparities in NICU and newborn quality of care are extensively described and are not the focus of this article, but in contrast, their consequences on post-NICU discharge period and beyond are rarely described. Sigurdson[11] and colleagues studied family and clinician accounts that suggested that vulnerable populations may receive suboptimal NICU family-centered care, which involves family presence and development of trusting relationships between parents and the NICU staff. This type of care, along with comprehensive Community Care Programs is effective in reducing life-threatening illness in high-risk infants.[60–62] McPherson and colleagues found that children who required 3 or more appointments after discharge were more likely to miss some, and the primary care appointment was the one most likely to be completed.[63–71]

Disparities in outcomes may be minimized by early detection in the NICU: infants who will require follow-up need to be identified before discharge, with a medical home and care coordination established using the same principles used in cases of special health care needs. To this effect, the National Perinatal Association organized a multidisciplinary group to develop guidelines and recommendations for NICU transition to home. These guidelines include discharge readiness; clinical and other needs assessment; discharge education; a comprehensive discharge summary; anticipatory guidance; and a family, home, medication, and technology needs assessment, providing a comprehensive framework for the necessary interdisciplinary, family, and patient-centered transition and discharge. The latter emphasizes the importance of appointment confirmations for primary care and specialists, including neurodevelopmental follow-up.[72]

The postdischarge needs and care for NICU graduates are influenced (**Fig. 6**) by the same health care disparities and social determinants of health that affect an infant's and family's trajectory until the day of NICU discharge. Just as disparities have clearly been demonstrated in NICU care, disparities have been demonstrated in access to follow-up care and care delivery.

In a study of 237 infants, Swearingen[73] showed that 62% were lost to follow-up over a period of 2 years and associated factors were older gestational age, African American race, and maternal smoking. Less attrition was associated with older maternal age, diagnosis of bronchopulmonary dysplasia, and longer hospital stay. The investigators conclude that social disparities affect neonatal follow-up clinic attendance and suggest that efforts be made to identify and target high-risk infants during the initial hospitalization. Fraiman[74] found similar results in a study of 477 infants from a single Academic Level III NICU, in which 41.9% participated in a follow-up program, and participation was lower for Blacks than for Whites, especially when English was not the primary language and families were from neighborhoods with very low "child opportunity index." They also found that younger and smaller newborns with morbidities, and discharged home as opposed to transferred, participated in higher numbers.

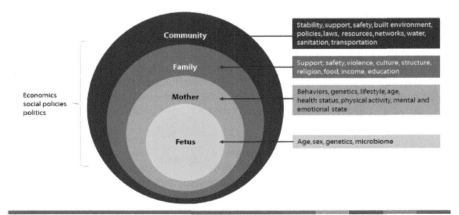

**Fig. 6.** The circle of influence in perinatal health. (*From* Barfield WD. Social disadvantage and its effect on maternal and newborn health. Semin Perinatol. 2021;45(4):151407.)

### Improvement Recommendations

Litt and Hintz[75,76] describe examples of quality improvement projects for high-risk infant follow-up programs that could ostensibly decrease disparities in outcomes. They outline 5 areas for care improvement: (1) establishment of evidence-based care delivery systems, (2) standardization of key outcomes and their measures, (3) utilization of a family centered care approach, and (4) prioritizing parent goals and (5) developing professional standards of care for high-risk infant follow-up. Horbar and colleagues[59] (Lorenz Curve for segregation by race-ethnicity in US-Horbar 2019 and Lorenz curve for inequality-Horbar 2019)[12,59] inspire us further with their aforementioned "follow-through" proposal to establish a comprehensive approach that begins before birth and continues into childhood involving health professionals, families, and communities. They provide a comprehensive list of 71 "Potentially Better Practices" that can be instituted to aid with increasing quality of care, addressing adverse social determinants of health, and decreasing inequities and resultant

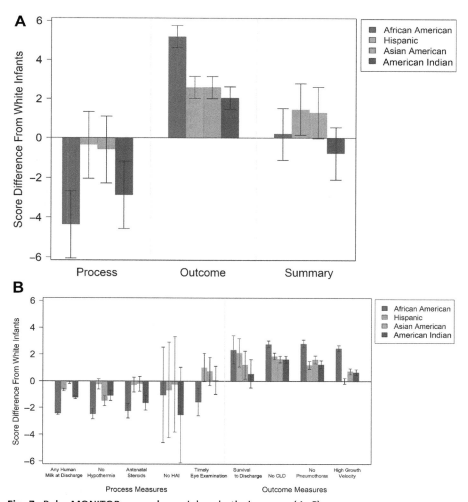

**Fig. 7.** Baby-MONITOR scores by racial and ethnic group (*A, B*).

disparities across the follow-through care spectrum, including during infancy and early school age. These suggested practices include key interventions including promoting a culture of equity via implicit bias training for trainees, faculty, and staff; bolstering NICU discharge planning with routine access to evidence-based early educational and developmental intervention programs for all high-risk infants after NICU discharge; universal screening for adverse social determinants of health in the follow-up clinics with inclusion of neighborhood level factors and continued surveillance of these factors throughout early childhood; inclusion of programs such as Reach Out and Read; partnering with pre-K programs; advocating for social justice at the local, state, and national levels; and developing robust quality improvement efforts with clear improvement metrics that include participation by parents— including those from diverse backgrounds—in improvement efforts.[59] Quality improvement initiatives undertaken should always include assessment of equity with aims that include eliminating disparities. In addition to quality improvement programs occurring at the time of hospitalization and discharge, increased medical education beyond the traditional technical medical education must occur, beginning at the earliest points in training to address implicit bias and increase understanding of the impact the social determinants of health. Quality improvement science has significant potential to help achieve equitable NICU care and quality. These initiatives should always include equity aims, open data sharing, and use of disparity dashboards to demonstrate consistent care across all racial and ethnic groups (**Fig. 7**) and meaningful improvement in the care of high-risk neonates.[77,78] The potentially better practices proposed by Horbar and colleagues are intended to serve as a starting point and will require engagement of hospital administration, as well as robust community partnerships to implement successfully (see **Table 1**).[59] The most important thing to do is to just get started. "Neonatal care providers play critical roles at life changing moments for infants and families and are poised to help change the lives of families through follow through."

Clinical research initiatives, prioritizing research studies aimed to evaluate effective interventions, and developing best practices to eliminate health disparities are vital. In addition, having a diverse medical workforce at all levels of NICU care and academic medicine aids in decreasing disparities in care, ensuring greater

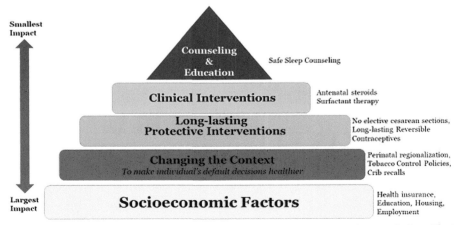

**Fig. 8.** The health impact pyramid for infant mortality prevention. *(From* Frieden TR. A Framework for Public Health Action: The Health Impact Pyramid. Am J Public Health 2010;100(4): 590-5.)

**Table 1**
**Potentially better practices proposed by Horbar and Edwards and colleagues to help eliminate disparities in follow-up care and outcomes[30,74]**

| | |
|---|---|
| Promote a Culture of Equity | Establish cultural sensitivity; acknowledge and manage implicit and explicit personal biases; facilitate nurse-led rounds |
| Identify social risks of families and provide interventions to prevent and mitigate those risks | Screen for social determinants of health; provide support when necessary, such as assistance with housing, meals, and transportation and counseling for mental health, drug or alcohol problems, or smoking cessation; include social workers and legal specialists on teams |
| Take action to assist families after discharge | Provide carefully tailored discharge teaching; use home visiting and social media; establish meaningful clinical-community partnerships |
| Maintain support for families through infancy | Use parent coaches and innovative medical visit structures; provide contraception, family planning, and evidence-based early intervention programs |
| Develop robust QI efforts to ensure equitable, high-quality follow-through care to all newborns by eliminating modifiable disparities | Establish measurable aims; engage all disciplines, parents, and primary care providers; obtain support from organizational leaders through a formal charter |
| Advocate for social justice at the local, state, and national levels | Ensure that social justice is part of every organization's mission; advocate that health care organizations accept and act on their responsibility for the populations and neighborhoods that they serve; speak out! |

*From* Beck AF, Edwards EM, Horbar JD, Howell EA, McCormick MC, Pursley DM. The color of health: how racism, segregation, and inequality affect the health and well-being of preterm infants and their families. Pediatr Res. 2020;87(2):227-234.

# STRATEGIES TO TACKLE RACISM AT EVERY LEVEL

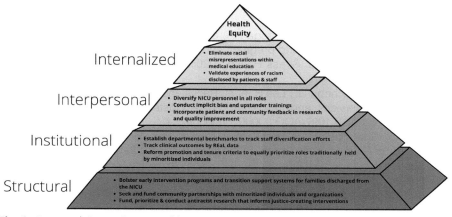

**Fig. 9.** Proposed Strategies to Tackle Racism at Every Level in Neonatology. (*Reproduced with permission from* Neoreviews, 23(1), e1-e12, Copyright © 2022 by the AAP.)

opportunities for patient-provider concordance and enhanced patient-provider relationships to help eliminate bias. Community engagement, interventions to diminish the effects of social disadvantage, and addressing social determinants of health are essential. An example of this is demonstrated by the public health impact pyramid.[79–82] This pyramid illustrates population level interventions and individual interventions that affect disparities; population interventions have a greater impact (**Fig. 8**).

Despite recommendations such as those put forth by the experts earlier, the dearth of standardized, evidence-based approaches to the postdischarge care of the high-risk infants compounds the existent disparities via solidifying the access and care inequities that influence the short- and long-term outcomes of our most fragile citizens.[30,74]

### Interventions in the Neonatal Intensive Care Unit to Decrease Health Disparities and Improve Outcomes

(**Table 1**).

| Best practices |
| --- |
| What are the current practices for health equity in Neonatology: |
| Although there are many outstanding approaches to dealing with health disparities in Neonatology, we currently have no formalized standards of practice. We are highlighting in this review the need for an organized standardized approach **Fig. 9**[72] (Proposed Strategies to Tackle Racism at Every Level in Neonatology). |

### DISCLOSURE

The authors have nothing to disclose.

### REFERENCES

1. Braveman PA, Kumanyika S, Fielding J, et al. Health disparities and health equity: the issue is justice. Am J Public Health 2011;101(S1):S149–55.
2. Artiga S, Orgera K, Pham O. Disparities in health and health care: five key questions and answers. Kaiser Family Foundation Executive Summary; 2020.
3. Jones CP. Levels of racism: a theoretic framework and a gardener's tale. Am J Public Health 2000;90:1212–5.
4. Chambers BD, Arabia SE, Arega HA, et al. Exposures to structural racism and racial discrimination among pregnant and early post-partum Black women living in Oakland, California. Stress Health 2020;36(2):213–9. https://doi.org/10.1002/smi.2922.
5. Sutton MY, Anachebe NF, Lee R, et al. Racial and ethnic disparities in reproductive health services and outcomes, 2020. Obstet Gynecol 2021;137:225–33. https://doi.org/10.1097/AOG.0000000000004224.
6. Lu MC, Kotelchuck M, Hogan V, et al. Closing the black-white gap in birth outcomes: a life-course approach. Ethn Dis 2010;20(1 0 2):S62–76.
7. Barfield WD, Cox S, Henderson ST. Disparities in neonatal intensive care: context matters. Pediatrics 2019;144(2). e20191688.
8. Barfield WD. Public health implications of very preterm birth. Clin Perinatol 2018; 45(3):565–77. https://doi.org/10.1016/j.clp.2018.05.007.
9. Blair IV, Steiner JF, Havranek EP. Unconscious (implicit) bias and health disparities: where do we go from here? Perm J 2011;15(2):71–8.

10. Boghossian NS, Geraci M, Edwards EM, et al. Changes in hospital quality at hospitals serving black and hispanic newborns below 30 weeks' gestation. J Perinatol 2022;42(2):187–94.

11. Sigurdson K, Mitchell B, Liu J, et al. Racial/ethnic disparities in neonatal intensive care: a systematic review. Pediatrics 2019;144(2):e20183114.

12. Horbar JD, Edwards EM, Greenberg LT. Racial segregation on inequality in neonatal intensive care unit care for very low birth weight and very preterm infants. JAMA Pediatr 2019;173(5):455–61.

13. Boghossian NS, Geraci M, Lorch SA, et al. Racial and ethnic differences over time and outcomes of infants born less than 30 weeks' gestation. Pediatrics 2019;144:e20191106.

14. Profit J, Gould JB, Bennett M, et al. Racial/ethnic disparity in NICU quality of care delivery. Pediatrics 2017;140(3):e20170918.

15. Howell EA, Hebert P, et al. Black/white differences in very low birth weight neonatal mortality rates among New York city hospitals. Pediatrics 2008;121:e407–15.

16. Profit J, Goldstein BA, Tamaresis Kan P, et al. Regional variation in antenatal corticosteroid use: a network-level quality improvement study. Pediatrics 2015;135:e397–404.

17. Dereddy NR, Talati AJ, Smith A, et al. A multipronged approach is associated with improved breast milk feeding rates in very low birth weight infants of an inner-city hospital. J Hum Lact 2015;31(1):43–6.

18. Patel AL, Johnson TJ, Meier PP. Racial and socioeconomic disparities in breast milk feedings in US neonatal intensive care units. Pediatr Res 2021;89:344–52.

19. Parker MG, Greenberg LT, Edwards EM, et al. National trends in the provision of human milk at hospital discharge among very low-birth-weight infants. JAMA Pediatr 2019;173(10):961–8. https://doi.org/10.1001/jamapediatrics.2019.2645.

20. Sigurdson K, Morton C, Mitchell B, et al. Disparities in NICU Quality Care: a qualitative study of family and clinician accounts. J Perinatol 2018;38:600–7.

21. Broyles RS, Tyson JE, Heyne ET, et al. Comprehensive follow-up care and life-threatening illnesses among high-risk infants: a randomized controlled trial. JAMA 2000;284(16):2070–6. https://doi.org/10.1001/jama.284.16.2070.

22. O'Shea TM, Nageswaran S, Hiatt DC, et al. Follow-up care for infants with chronic lung disease: a randomized comparison of community and center-based models. Pediatrics 2007;119(4):e947–57. https://doi.org/10.1542/peds.2006-1717.

23. McPherson ML, Lairson DR, O'Brien SE, et al. Non-compliance with medical follow-up after pediatric intensive care. Pediatrics 2002;109(6):e94. https://doi.org/10.1542/peds.109.6.e94.

24. Campbell D, Imaizumi SO, Bernbaun JC. Health and developmental outcomes of infants requiring NICU. In AAP-textbook of pediatric care; McInerny TK – Editor in chief-AAP-2009.

25. Smith VC, Cove K, Goyer E. NICU discharge preparation and transition planning: guidelines and recommendations. J Perinatol 2022;42(suppl 1):7–21. https://doi.org/10.1038/s41372-022-01313-9.

26. Edwards EM, Greenberg LT, Profit J, et al. Quality of care in US NICUs by race and ethnicity. Pediatrics 2021;812:1–11, e2020037622.

27. Profit J, et al. Baby-MONITOR: a composite indicator of NICU quality. Pediatrics 2014;134(1):74–82.

28. Montoya-Williams D, Fraiman YS, Pena MM, et al. Antiracism in the field of neonatology: a foundation and concrete approaches. Neoreviews 2022;23:e1–12.

29. Al Maghaireh DF, Abdullah KL, Chan CM, et al. Systematic review of qualitative studies exploring parental experiences in the neonatal intensive care unit. J Clin Nurs 2016;25:45–56.

30. Witt RE, Colvin BN, Lenze SN, et al. Lived experiences of stress of Black and Hispanic mothers during hospitalization of preterm infants in neonatal intensive care units. J Perinatology 2022;42:195–201.

31. Hammonds EM, Reverby SM. Toward a historically informed analysis of racial health disparities since 1619. AJPH 2019;109(10):1348–9.

32. Kindig D. Population health equity: rate and burden, race and class. JAMA 2017; 317(5):467–8.

33. Hardeman RR, Karbeah J, Kozhimannil KB. Applying a critical race lens to relationship-centered care in pregnancy and childbirth: an antidote to structural racism. Birth 2020;47:3–7.

34. Aaron DG, Stanford FC. Medicine, structural racism, and systems. Soc Sci Med 2022;298:114856. https://doi.org/10.1016/j.socscimed.2022.114856.

35. Antoine C, Young BK. Cesarean section one hundred years 1920-2020: the Good, the Bad and the Ugly. J Perinat Med 2020;49(1):5–16. https://doi.org/10. 1515/jpm-2020-0305. Published 2020 Sep 4.

36. Bailey ZD, Krieger N, Agénor M, et al. Structural racism and health inequities in the USA: evidence and interventions. Lancet 2017;389(10077):1453–63. https:// doi.org/10.1016/S0140-6736(17)30569-X.

37. Boakye E, Sharma G, Ogunwole SM, et al. Relationship of preeclampsia with maternal place of birth and duration of residence among non-hispanic black women in the United States. Circ Cardiovasc Qual Outcomes 2021;14(2): e007546. https://doi.org/10.1161/CIRCOUTCOMES.120.007546.

38. Chen A, Oster E, Williams H. Why is infant mortality higher in the United States than in Europe? Am Econ J Econ Policy 2016;8(2):89–124. https://doi.org/10. 1257/pol.20140224. PMID: 27158418; PMCID: PMC4856058.

39. Ely DM, Driscoll AK. Infant Mortality in the United States, 2019: data from the period linked birth/infant death file. Natl Vital Stat Rep 2021;70(14):1–18.

40. Fryer K, Munoz MC, Rahangdale L, et al. Multiparous black and latinx women face more barriers to prenatal care than white women. J Racial Ethn Health Disparities 2021;8(1):80–7.

41. Greenwood BN, Hardeman RR, Huang L, et al. Physician-patient racial concordance and disparities in birthing mortality for newborns. Proc Natl Acad Sci U S A 2020;117(35):21194–200. https://doi.org/10.1073/pnas.1913405117.

42. Hoyert DL. Maternal mortality rates in the United States, 2020. NCHS Health E-Stats; 2022. https://doi.org/10.15620/cdc:113967.

43. Why black women face a high risk of pregnancy complications. News. Published February 25, 2019. Available at: https://www.hsph.harvard.edu/news/hsph-in-the-news/black-women-pregnancy-complications/.

44. PRB. Black women over three times more likely to die in pregnancy, postpartum than white women, new research finds. PRB. Published December 6, 2021. Available at: https://www.prb.org/resources/black-women-over-three-times-more-likely-to-die-in-pregnancy-postpartum-than-white-women-new-research-finds/.

45. U.S.-Born Black women at higher risk of preeclampsia than foreign-born counterparts; race alone does not explain disparity. johns hopkins medicine newsroom. Published December 29, 2021. Available at: https://www.hopkinsmedicine.org/ news/newsroom/news-releases/us-born-black-women-at-higher-risk-of-pre-eclampsia-than-foreign-born-counterparts-race-alone-does-not-explain-dispari-ty#:~:text=Black%20women%20had%20the%20highest.

46. MacDorman MF, Thoma M, Declcerq E, et al. Racial and ethnic disparities in maternal mortality in the United States using enhanced vital records, 2016–2017. Am J Public Health 2021;111(9):1673–81. https://doi.org/10.2105/AJPH.2021.306375.

47. Tahirkheli NN, Cherry AS, Tackett AP, et al. Postpartum depression on the neonatal intensive care unit: current perspectives. Int J Womens Health 2014;6:975–87. https://doi.org/10.2147/IJWH.S54666. Published 2014 Nov 24.

48. Kilgoe A. Available at: https://www.nami.org/Blogs/NAMI-Blog/July-2021/Addressing-the-Increased-Risk-of-Postpartum-Depression-for-Black-Women. NAMI Blog. Published July 25, 2021. Accessed June 30, 2022.

49. Murthy S, Haeusslein L, Bent S, et al. Feasibility of universal screening for postpartum mood and anxiety disorders among caregivers of infants hospitalized in NICUs: a systematic review. J Perinatol 2021;41(8):1811–24. https://doi.org/10.1038/s41372-021-01005-w.

50. Total cesarean deliveries by maternal race: United States, 2018-2020 Average. March of Dimes | PeriStats. Available at: https://www.marchofdimes.org/peristats/data?lev=1&obj=1&=99&slev=1&stop=355&top=8.

51. Howell EA. Reducing disparities in severe maternal morbidity and mortality. Clin Obstet Gynecol 2018;61(2):387–99. https://doi.org/10.1097/GRF.0000000000000349. PMID: 29346121; PMCID: PMC5915910.

52. Barfield WD. Social disadvantage and its effect on maternal and newborn health. Semin Perinatol 2021;45(4):151407. https://doi.org/10.1016/j.semperi.2021.151407.

53. Infant mortality rate by country 2020. worldpopulationreview.com. 2021. Available at: https://worldpopulationreview.com/country-rankings/infant-mortality-rate-by-country.

54. Bailey ZD, Krieger N, Agénor M, et al. Structural racism and health inequities in the USA: evidence and interventions. Lancet 2017;389(8):1453–63. Available at: www.thelancet.com.

55. Sheares KD, et al. Racial disparities in clinical medicine: conversations, perspectives, and research on advancing medical equity. NEJMGroup 2021.

56. Hardeman RR, Hardeman-Jones SL, Medina EM. Fighting for America's paradise: the struggle against structural racism. J Health Polit Policy L 2021;46(4):563–75.

57. David R, Collins JW. Why does racial inequity in health persist? J Perinatology 2021;41:346–50.

58. Pronk N, Kleinman DV, Goekler SF, et al. Promoting health and well-being in Healthy People 2030. J Public Health Manag Pract 2021;27(Suppl 6):S242–8. https://doi.org/10.1097/PHH.0000000000001254.

59. Horbar JD, Edwards EM, Ogbolu Y. Our responsibility to follow through for NICU infants and their families. Pediatrics 2020;146(6):e20200360.

60. Braveman PA, Heck K, Curtis M, et al. The role of socioeconomic factors in black-white disparities in preterm birth. Am J Public Health 2015;105:694–702. https://doi.org/10.2105/AJPH.2014.3022008.

61. DeSisto CL, Hirai AH, Collins JW, et al. Deconstructing a disparity: explaining excess preterm birth among U.S.-born black women. Ann Epidemiol 2018;28:225–30.

62. Matoba N, Collins JW. Racial disparity in infant mortality. Semin Perinatol 2017;41:354–9.

63. MacDorman MF, Matthews TJ, Zeitling J, et al. International comparisons of infant mortality and related factors: United States and Europe, 2010. Natl Vital Stat Rep 2014;63:1–6.

64. Glazer KB, Zeitlin J, Howell EA, et al. Hospital quality of care and racial and ethnic disparities in unexpected newborn complications. Pediatrics 2021;148(3). e2020024091.

65. Karnati S, Kollikonda S, Abu-Shaweesh J. Late preterm infants – changing trends and continuing challenges. Int J Pediatr Adolesc Med 2020;7(1):36–44. https://doi.org/10.1016/j.ijpam.2020.02.006.

66. Matthews TJ, MacDorman MF, Thoma ME. Infant mortality statistics 2013. Natl Vital Stat Rep 2015;64(9):1–30.

67. Anderson JD, Rojas EE, Baer RJ, et al. Racial and ethnic disparities in preterm infant mortality and severe morbidity. Neonatology 2018;113:44–54.

68. Stoll BJ, Hansen NI, Bell EF, et al. Eunice kennedy shriver national institute of child health and human development neonatal research network. trends in care practices, morbidity, and mortality of extremely preterm neonates, 1993-2012. JAMA 2015;314(10):1039–51. https://doi.org/10.1001/jama.2015.10244.

69. Janevic T, Zeitlin J, Howell EA, et al. Association of race/ethnicity with very preterm neonatal morbidities. JAMA Pediatr 2018;172(11):1061–9. https://doi.org/10.1001/jamapediatrics.2018.2029.

70. Travers CP, Carlo WA, Higgins RD, et al. Racial/ethnic disparities among extremely preterm infants in the United States from 2002 to 2016. JAMA Netw Open 2020;3(6):e206757.

71. Burris HH, Parker MG. Racial and ethnic disparities in preterm birth outcomes: a call to action for neonatal providers. J Perinatol 2021;41:365–6.

72. Martin JA, Hamilton BE, Osterman MJR. Births in the United States 2018. Hyattsville MD: National Center for Health Statistics; 2019.

73. Swearingen C, Simpson P, Cabacungan E, et al. Social disparities negatively impact neonatal follow-up clinic attendance of premature infants discharged from the NICU. J Perinatol 2020;40:790–7.

74. Fraiman YS, Stewart Jane E, Litt JS. Race, language and neighborhood predict high risk preterm infant follow-up program participation. J Perinatol 2021;1–6. https://doi.org/10.1038/s41372-021-01188-2.

75. Litt JS, Hintz SR. Quality improvement for NICU graduates: feasible, reliant, impactful. Semin Fetal Neonatal Med 2021;26(1):101205.

76. Litt JS, Edwards EM, Hartman T, et al. Optimizing high-risk infant follow-up in nonresearched-based paradigms: the New England follow-up network. Pediatr Qual Saf 2020;5(3):e287. https://doi.org/10.1097/pq9.0000000000000287.

77. Parker MG, Hwang SS. Quality improvement approaches to reduce racial/ethnic disparities in the neonatal intensive care unit. Semin Perinatology 2021;45:1–8.

78. Patel AL, Meier PP, Canvasser J. Strategies to increase the use of mother's own milk for infants at risk of necrotizing enterocolitis. Pediatr Res 2020;88:21–4. https://doi.org/10.1038/s41390-020-1075-3.

79. Barfield WD. Social disadvantage and its effect on maternal and newborn health. Semin Perinatology 2021;45:1–7.

80. Frieden TR. A Framework for public health action: the health impact pyramid. Am J Public Health 2010;100(4):590–5.

81. Beck AF, Edwards EM, Horbar JD, et al. The color of health: how racism, segregation, and inequality affect the health and well-being of preterm infants and their families. Pediatr Res 2020;87:227–34.

82. Ravi D, Main E, Profit J. Institutional racism: a key contributor to perinatal health inequity. Pediatrics 2021;148(3). e2021050768.

# A Comparison of the Clinical Presentation of Preterm Birth and Autism Spectrum Disorder

## Commonalities and Distinctions in Children Under 3

Adriana I. Mendez, MA[a,b,c,d], Hannah Tokish, BA[b,c,d], Emma McQueen, BS[b,c,d], Shivaang Chawla, BS[b,c,d], Ami Klin, PhD[b,c,d], Nathalie L. Maitre, MD, PhD[c,d], Cheryl Klaiman, PhD[b,c,d],*

### KEYWORDS

- Prematurity • Autism spectrum disorder • Early symptomatology

### KEY POINTS

- Premature infants and infants later diagnosed with autism spectrum disorder (ASD) share many features of clinical presentation in early childhood while also showing unique symptoms.
- Understanding overlapping and distinct symptomatology in these two populations is important for the accurate early detection of ASD and the timely implementation of efficacious interventions.
- We document commonalities and distinctions of clinical presentations in the first 3 years of life in the following domains: social, language and communication, sensory, motor, internalizing/externalizing behaviors, and executive function.
- Given similarities in symptomatology, evidence-based interventions designed specifically for preterm toddlers or toddlers with ASD may ultimately aid both populations.
- Health care disparities affect both populations and contribute to suboptimal outcomes for those in marginalized communities; therefore, policies and programs should be designed to reduce these disparities in both populations.

---

[a] Department of Psychology, Emory University, 36 Eagle Row, Atlanta, GA 30322, USA; [b] Marcus Autism Center, 1920 Briarcliff Road, Atlanta, GA 30329, USA; [c] Department of Pediatrics, Emory University School of Medicine, 2015 Uppergate Drive, Atlanta, GA 30322, USA; [d] Children's Healthcare of Atlanta, 1405 Clifton Road Northeast, Atlanta, GA 30322, USA
* Corresponding author. Marcus Autism Center, 1920 Briarcliff Road Northeast, Atlanta, GA 30329.
E-mail address: Cheryl.klaiman@emory.edu

Clin Perinatol 50 (2023) 81–101
https://doi.org/10.1016/j.clp.2022.11.001
0095-5108/23/© 2022 Elsevier Inc. All rights reserved.
perinatology.theclinics.com

## INTRODUCTION

For the past two decades, there has been increased interest in the overlap of developmental symptomatology between autism spectrum disorder (ASD) and prematurity,[1,2] especially in infancy and toddlerhood.[2,3] This early period is especially important because it corresponds to a time of rapid behavior-brain developmental progression when targeted early interventions are crucial to optimize outcomes.[4] ASD is currently estimated to occur in 2.27% (1 in 44) of 8-year-old children in the United States.[5] Prematurity is estimated to occur in 11.9% of births in the United States and ~10% to 11% of births globally.[6–9] More specifically, of these ~11% of preterm infants, 85% are moderately preterm (32 to 33 weeks' gestation) to late-preterm (34 to 36 weeks' gestations), 10% are very preterm (28 to 31 weeks' gestation), and 5% are extremely preterm (<28 weeks gestation), with lower gestational ages being associated with greater morbidity and higher likelihood of compromised neurodevelopment.[7]

Within the preterm population, studies have reported a range of prevalence rates of ASD of approximately 7% to 12.9%,[10–13] with a recent study by Crump and colleagues[14] reporting prevalence rates of 6.1% for extremely preterm, 2.6% for very to moderately preterm, 1.9% for late preterm, and 2.1% for all preterm. Importantly, recent research suggests that the risk for ASD increases with each additional week of prematurity.[15] Overall, the prevalence of ASD within this population remains notably higher than the prevalence in the general population - regardless of gestation week. Indeed, atypical behavior commonalities exist within these populations and findings from neuroimaging research suggest possibly overlapping brain abnormalities underlying their evolving symptomatology (for example,[16]). Nevertheless, important distinctions also exist, together with highly heterogeneous etiologies underlying both conditions, separately and in cases of co-occurrence. Given the high prevalence of ASD and prematurity separately *and* their co-occurrence for a significant percentage of children, examining differences and similarities in these populations can improve diagnostic accuracy and advance targeted, effective treatment and intervention.

The lack of specificity in current diagnostic tools contributes to confusion in this research area. In early infancy, extremely preterm infants have 13% to 26% of positive screens on the Modified Checklist for Autism in Toddlers (M-CHAT;[17,18]), the most commonly used ASD screener by pediatricians. However, only about 1.8% of preterm children with a positive MCHAT subsequently receive a true diagnosis of ASD, resulting in very high false positive rates.[18] Motor, cognitive, visual, hearing impairments, sensorimotor differences, and emotional and behavioral dysregulation contribute to M-CHAT preterm misclassifications.[19,20] The current, most commonly used ASD screener may not be accurate in the preterm population, with only 52% sensitivity, 84% specificity, a positive predictive value of 20% and a negative predictive value of 96%.[21] This tool was designed to increase specificity at the expense of sensitivity and these trends are also observed in the full-term population.[22] However, given the common presence of developmental abnormalities in prematurity that may be confounded with ASD symptomatology, the MCHAT may have less value for preterm infant screening. Shedding light on potential areas of symptom overlap that are currently misunderstood or mischaracterized is of paramount importance given the danger of false positive screens of preterm children with ASD and, conversely, of false negative screens of preterm children with true comorbid ASD.

More clearly delineating the clinical presentations of prematurity and ASD would directly aid in the accurate diagnosis of ASD within the preterm population *and* the provision of adequate, ASD-specific services. However, this challenge is further compounded by the additional effects on development by health care disparities: for both of these populations, suboptimal outcomes are more likely in families of lower socioeconomic status (SES). For preterm infants, the prevalence of developmental delay is 12.5% in low SES, 7.8% in intermediate SES, and only 5.6% in high SES. Importantly, given that no interaction was found between gestational age and SES, researchers suggest these effects are multiplicative.[23] Children with prematurity *and* low SES are at heightened risk for worse outcomes. Preterm delivery was 2, 9.1, and 13.2 times higher in cases of food insecurity, stress, and inadequate prenatal care, respectively than without these conditions.[24] Pregnant African American mothers were more likely than pregnant White mothers to report living in disadvantaged neighborhoods and experience racial discrimination, psychological stress, and depressive symptoms, all of which contribute to the previously stated risk factors for preterm birth.[25] Similarly, in ASD, factors decreasing the likelihood of early identification or early intervention (low SES; being from underserved racial or ethnic groups) contribute to suboptimal outcomes. A 2020 CDC report revealed that African American toddlers with ASD are significantly less likely than White toddlers with ASD to receive a diagnosis before 36 months and are at increased risk for co-morbid intellectual disability.[26] In addition, families of African American and Latinx children with ASD have more and greater barriers in completing the diagnostic process, including needing to visit more providers to receive a diagnosis than families of White children with ASD.[27,28] Finally, prevalence of intellectual delays in ASD is higher in geographic areas with the most socioeconomic challenges, and after obtaining a diagnosis, higher gross family income is a predictor of service utilization.[29,30] Taken together, these findings suggest that the effects of low SES and/or being from an ethnically or racially underserved community increases the risk for suboptimal outcomes in both prematurity and ASD. Importantly, these effects are likely less apparent within the first 3 years: further studying this impact longitudinally is crucial to mitigate these adverse outcomes.

In our review of ASD and prematurity characteristics, we prioritized domains with past research, and those relevant to understanding of developmental trajectories during this formative period: social behavior, language and communication, sensory processing, motor function, internalizing and externalizing behaviors, and executive function (EF). These domains are neither exhaustive nor completely distinct. They constitute clusters of challenges that are either core symptomatology (in the case of ASD) or major factors influencing outcomes (in both prematurity and ASD), and which should be prioritized for early intervention.

### Developmental Domains

#### Social behavior
Social impairment is a core symptom and part of the ASD definition, irrespective of prematurity. It is present in young preterm children, but whether symptoms are secondary to prematurity or due to the presence of autism is critically important. Both populations show reduced social attention, specifically when measured via eye-tracking. Infants later diagnosed with ASD show trajectories of decreased eye-looking as early as 2 months of age.[31] Similarly, preterm infants fixate to the eye less than the mouths of others on eye-tracking tasks.[32] In eye-tracking comparisons of visual fixation patterns of preterm and full-term toddlers with ASD, no differences were found, suggesting that toddlers with ASD regardless of preterm birth show decreased fixation to facial regions.[33] Within the preterm sample, preterm toddlers with ASD showed decreased fixation to facial regions, whereas preterm children with non-ASD developmental delays or no current delays showed comparable fixation patterns to full-term typically developing (TD) toddlers.[34] In addition, at 6, 12, and

18 months, preterm infants spend less time looking at a dynamic face stimulus and follow another person's gaze directions compared with full-term counterparts.[35] Social withdrawal is also common to both populations, suggesting they attend to social stimuli less frequently and may also avoid them.[36,37] In toddlerhood, both populations also show a decrease in initiation of and response to joint attention, a common measure of social ability.[38,39]

Some important markers of decreased social ability in ASD have not been extensively studied in preterm infants. For example, imitation skills are often reduced in ASD[39] with decreased empathic concern at 22, 28, and 34 months[40]; preterm children at school-age show weaker empathic development than full-term children,[41] but no data at comparable infant ages or on imitation skills is provided.

Social development is consistently diminished in ASD, whereas a systematic review in preterm infants found mixed results. For example, some studies found differences in prosocial behavior, whereas others did not.[42] This is important to note because although social differences may be present in both populations, these seem to be more likely *and* more robustly documented in ASD. Nonetheless, social development may represent a particularly complex domain of differences and commonalities in these populations (**Table 1**).

### Language and Communication

Language development and communication deficits are a hallmark feature of ASD and common in preterm children. In toddlerhood, both preterm and ASD populations show low volubility (ie, number of utterances;[43,44]); they have more pronounced deficits in speech production, or expressive language, than in speech comprehension or receptive language. Their developmental trajectories are altered, with expressive language developing later and slower than receptive language.[45,46] In ASD, more complex discrepancies may exist between expressive and receptive language development.[47] Nonetheless, documented differences in phoneme perception in early infancy in both populations may contribute to later expressive language deficits. Very prematurely born infants do not show perceptual narrowing for non-native phoneme contrasts, which has been associated with later expressive language deficits.[48] Infants later diagnosed with ASD perform significantly worse on phoneme categorization tasks when compared with control stimuli.[49] Both populations show alterations in functional connectivity in areas of the brain associated with language development.[50,51] Young children experiencing delays in language acquisition may use non-verbal communication. Interestingly, both populations show deficits in gesture production: at 18 months, both preterm toddlers and those with ASD show decreased pointing.[52,53]

Although toddlers with ASD do not show deficits in processing speed, preterm 2-year-olds show slower lexical and language processing,[54,55] the populations in this review have more similarities than differences in language and communication.

### Sensory Processing

Both toddlers with ASD and toddlers born preterm show atypicality in sensory processing, including decreased registration and increased sensation avoidance behaviors.[56–63] They both have increased oral sensory behaviors and tactile sensitivity, in addition to impairments in visual and auditory processing[60,64,65]; both have breastfeeding challenges such as altered sucking behaviors and latching difficulties[66–69]; both have altered neural responses to auditory stimuli in both ASD and preterm toddlers.[70–73]

With regards to etiology, preterm infants may be at higher risk for sensory atypicality due to early medical complexities and altered experiences in the context of an

**Table 1**
Commonalities and differences between autism spectrum disorder and prematurity by domain

| | Commonalities | Differences |
|---|---|---|
| Social | <ul><li>Decreased social attention measured via eye-looking in infancy[31,32]</li><li>Decreased initiation and response to joint attention[38,39]</li><li>Weaker empathic development and concern[40,41]</li><li>Increased withdrawal behaviors in infancy[36,167]</li></ul> | <ul><li>ASD: deficits in imitation skills[39]</li><li>ASD: decreased in overall socialization skills[168]</li><li>Preterm: mixed literature, some find weak prosocial behavior, whereas others do not[42]</li></ul> |
| Language/communication | <ul><li>Decreased number and length of utterances[43,44]</li><li>Reduced pointing at 18 mo[52,53]</li><li>Delays in expressive language development are more pronounced than delayed in receptive language development[45,46]</li><li>Differences in phoneme perception[49]</li></ul> | <ul><li>Preterm: at 24 mo, show slower lexical and language processing speeds[55,169]</li></ul> |
| Sensory | <ul><li>Sensory differences/atypicality[56-61]</li><li>Decreased registration[56,60,63]</li><li>Increased sensation avoiding[59,62,65]</li><li>Increased oral sensory behaviors[63,64] and dysregulated breastfeeding[66-69]</li><li>Increased tactile sensitivity[64]</li><li>Differences in visual/auditory processing[60,63,64]</li><li>Altered neural responses to auditory stimuli measured by ERP[70-73]</li></ul> | <ul><li>Preterm: may be at risk for sensory atypicality due to early medical issues and immature CNS[74] vs ASD: may be a core feature, a co-occurring feature, or underlying cause of the disorder[76,77]</li><li>ASD: decreased seeking[59,78,79] or hyperresponsiveness, which is correlated with social disability and RRB severity[61,64,79] vs Preterm: no corresponding research</li><li>Preterm: abnormal reactivity to deep pressure and vestibular stimulation- related to poorer motor outcomes[58,81,82] vs ASD: no corresponding research</li><li>Preterm: altered neural response to predicted visual stimuli, suggesting deficits in top-down sensory prediction[83] vs ASD: no corresponding research</li></ul> |

(continued on next page)

**Table 1**
*(continued)*

| | Commonalities | Differences |
|---|---|---|
| | | • ASD: heightened visual preference for geometric over social images– related to worse cognitive, language and social outcomes[84] vs Preterm: no corresponding research<br>• Preterm: vision and hearing impairments decrease with increased gestational age[170] vs ASD: sensory overreponsivity remains stable over time and predicts later anxiety[80]<br>• Preterm: parenting style related to sensory responsivity[85] vs ASD: related to parental stress and family life impairment[86] |
| Motor | • Motor impairments are common in the first year of life, varying from 8%–38% in both populations[87–90,92–95,97–99,114,171]<br>• Few studies have looked at specific skills in each domain but there are deficits are present in both fine and motor domains<br>• Gross Motor: late walking, sitting, head in midline, poor postural control (prone and supine)[96,105,109–113,115,117–120,172]<br>• Poor postural control and neck/flexor tone is associated with worse outcomes later in development[118,122]<br>• Fine Motor: Delays in visuomotor coordination, reaching, grasping, and grip[89,113,125,127,171,173]<br>• 61%–68% of children have abnormal general movements during the first months of life[102,135]<br>• Increased incidence of Toe-walking and hypotonia contributing to motor impairments[105–107] | • In autism: motor delays predict social impairments[113,115]<br>• In autism: motor stereotypies (banging and unusual sensory exploration is common)[113]<br>• CP is diagnosed in 7%–32% of preterm infants and contributes to some motor impairment,[88,174] of children diagnosed with CP, 7% have co-occurring ASD[175]<br>• In autism, motor difficulties increased with increasing age of diagnosis[99] |

| Internalizing/externalizing behaviors | • Increased internalizing and lower competence scores on ITSEA and CBCL[36,133–136]<br>• Internalizing related to increased regulatory problems and emotional regulation difficulties[134–136,138–140,176]<br>• Increased depression, withdrawal, inattention, anxiety, and risk of ADHD[36,136,140–143]<br>• Increased externalizing behavior problems like aggressive, oppositional behavior[132,144] except one preterm study[135]<br>• Externalizing behaviors predicted by temperament[141,148,150]<br>• Internalizing and externalizing associated with parenting style, parental mental health and stress, and negative affectivity[36,85,138,141,145,146,148–150,176] | • ASD: increased anxiety predicted by sensory overresponsivity and higher receptive and expressive communication skills[80,151] vs Preterm: internalizing predicted by poor infant pain management in hospital[152]<br>• Preterm: more typical ERP processing related to less internalizing[153] vs ASD: no corresponding research<br>• Preterm: increased basal vagal tone predicted decreased externalizing[156] vs ASD: no corresponding research<br>• ASD: presence of stereotypic behavior and self-injurious behavior[154,155] vs Preterm: no corresponding research<br>• ASD: externalizing behaviors related to lower levels of adult/peer interaction[155] vs Preterm: increased externalizing associated with more time spent in neonatal ICU[149] |
| Executive function | • Decreased adaptive skills[37,157–160]<br>• Impairments in working memory[159,161] and other domains of EF[157,159]<br>• Impairments in response inhibition[157,159,162]<br>• Impairments in cognitive flexibility[159,164]<br>• Impairments in communication[37,157,159] | • ASD: associations between EF problems (ie, response inhibition, cognitive flexibility) and stereotyped, self-injurious, ritualistic, restrictive, repetitive, and compulsive behaviors[163] |

immature central nervous systems.[74] In addition, given the development of sensory and perceptual systems, which develop as a function of timing, amount and type of sensory systems, it is clear that development can go awry in these domains in infants born prematurely.[75] In ASD, there is debate about whether sensory differences are a core feature of the disorder, a co-occurring feature, or an underlying cause of core deficits.[76,77] Furthermore, ASD and preterm children show unique behaviors associated with different sensory modalities. Some children with ASD show decreased seeking behaviors, whereas others show hyperresponsiveness to sensory stimuli.[59,61,64,78–80] Longitudinal research suggests that hyperresponsiveness remains stable over time and correlates with social disability and severity of restricted and repetitive behaviors (RRBs).[61,64,79,80] Preterm infants have abnormal reactivity to deep pressure and vestibular stimulation associated with poorer motor skills development[58,81,82] and altered neural responses to visual stimuli (deficits in top-down sensory prediction abilities).[83] In infants with ASD, an increased preference for geometric images over social images is associated with poorer cognitive, language, and social skills.[84] In preterm infants, sensory responsivity has been associated with parenting style, whereas in ASD it has been studied in association with parental stress and family life impairment.[85,86] Overall, atypicality in sensory responsivity and resulting behavioral differences are prevalent in both ASD and preterm children, and ultimately may complicate differential diagnosis between the two populations.

### Motor Function

Motor impairment is frequently associated with both ASD and prematurity, typically emerging within the first 3 to 6 months of life with many overlapping features.[87–99] Prevalence of motor delays in these populations ranges from 8% to 37% depending on exact inclusion criteria and motor assessments (eg, Movement Assessment Battery for Children – 2nd Edition [MABC-2], Bayley Scales of Infant and Toddler Development – 2nd and 3rd Edition [BSID-2 & 3], Vineland Adaptive Behavior Scales –2nd Edition [Vineland-II], and Alberta Infant Motor Scale [AIMS]).[100,101] Abnormalities in general movements in infancy, specifically cramped synchronized or poor repertoire patterns in the writhing phase and absent fidgety movements at 3 to 4 months post term, later predict atypical neurodevelopmental outcomes. These patterns are reported in up to 61% to 68% of children later diagnosed with ASD and those preterm infants with neuromotor delays and impairments.[100,102–104]

Neurologic findings common in prematurity and ASD can contribute to delays in motor skills. Hypotonia occurs in 51% of children with ASD and is common in preterm infants.[105,106] Idiopathic toe-walking occurs in 19% of children with ASD and is also more common in preterm infants than in term-born children.[107] When cerebral palsy (CP) is diagnosed in conjunction with both ASD and prematurity, motor impairments tend to be more prevalent than when diagnosed with prematurity alone.[19,88,108]

Gross and fine motor impairments are characteristic of both children with ASD and those born preterm. Both show significantly delayed gross motor skills as early as 6 to 8 months[109] (van Haastert and colleagues, 2006; Ming and colleagues, 2007; Estes and colleagues, 2015; Pusponegoro and colleagues, 2016; Haaster and colleagues, 2006; Bos and colleagues, 2013). Gross motor deficits are reported in 9% to 20% of ASD cases, whereas up to 40% of preterm infants have a mild-to-moderate impairment and 20% moderate impairment. Specifically, late walking, delayed unsupported sitting, head support in the midline position, balance, ball skills and poor postural control (prone and supine) are all common to both populations.[105,109–121] In addition, head lag in coordination with postural control during pull-to-sit was associated with an ASD diagnosis at 36 months.[118] Similarly, in preterm infants, poor neck extensor and flexor tone is associated with worse developmental outcomes at later ages.[122] Fine motor delays are similarly common to both ASD and preterm infants for object exploratory behavior, reaching, grasping, and visuomotor coordination within the first year of life.[89,91,113,116,117,123–127]

Despite the many similarities in motor impairments shared between ASD and prematurity, some are unique to each phenotype. In ASD, motor delays within the first few years of life are related to communication skills and later predict social impairments, whereas no corresponding literature was found for preterm children.[95,113,115,128] Early fine motor delays may be predictive of social disability and increased ASD symptomatology at 36 months[129] and motor impairments are amplified with increasing age of diagnosis.[95,99]

### Internalizing and Externalizing Behaviors

Preterm infants and infants diagnosed with ASD show many similarities in the prevalence of both internalizing and externalizing behaviors. Defined as mood and emotional reactivity problems, internalizing behaviors often include social-emotional dysfunction, anxiety, depression, and avoidance.[23,130] Externalizing behaviors, defined as oppositional and conduct problems, encompass aggressive and oppositional behaviors, tantrums, and hyperactivity.[130–132] On the Infant Toddler Social Emotional Assessment (ITSEA) and the Child Behavior Checklist (CBCL), measures of early psychopathology and behavior challenges, both groups have shown increased internalizing traits and lower competence scores.[36,133–136] Internalizing behaviors were associated with increased emotional and self-regulation difficulties.[134–140] Both preterm infants and infants later diagnosed with ASD show increased depression and withdrawal symptoms, as well as increased attention, anxiety, and risk of ADHD.[36,136,140–143] Furthermore, both show increased externalizing problems such as aggressive and oppositional behaviors.[132,144] However, the preterm literature is somewhat mixed, with one study by Spittle and colleagues[135] finding no significant differences in externalizing symptoms. Studies suggest that temperament is a significant predictor of externalizing behavior in both populations, and both internalizing and externalizing behaviors are associated with parenting style, parental mental health and stress, and heightened negative affectivity.[36,85,137,138,145–150]

Studies of children with ASD show increased anxiety is associated with sensory overresponsivity and higher receptive and expressive language abilities.[80,151] In preterm populations, internalizing symptoms are associated with exposure to painful procedures.[152] More typical cortical multiprocessing at term equivalent age is predictive of fewer internalizing tendencies.[153] Uniquely, children with ASD show stereotypic and self-injurious behavior, not a characteristic of preterm externalizing tendencies.[154,155] In ASD, aggression and destructive, stereotypic, and self-injurious behaviors have been associated with lower levels of interactions with peers and adults.[155] In prematurity, the association is less clear but some research is indicating that if mothers show depressive symptomatology, there is increased risk of opposition to maternal requests and increased health problems.[149,156] Although differences exist in the factors that impact internalizing and externalizing behaviors, both preterm and ASD populations nonetheless face challenges in both behavioral domains, with ASD distinguished by the presence of RRBs and self-injury.

### Executive Function

Though the existing literature on EF in children under 36 months (about 3 years) is limited, there are similarities between prematurity and ASD in adaptive behavior, working memory, response inhibition, cognitive flexibility, and verbal fluency during the first 3 years of life.

In studies using the Behavior Assessment for Children (BASC), both preterm toddlers and toddlers with ASD showed lower overall adaptive skill scores when compared with full term, TD children.[37,157] Preterm toddlers also had decreased scores in the adaptive behavior scales of the Vineland-II, and on the adaptive behavior scale of the parent-reported Bayley Scales of Infant Development, particularly within the social and practical domains.[158,159] Similarly, toddlers with ASD have poor social adaptive skills indicative of early emerging social deficits, which typically increase in severity throughout life.[160]

Impairments in working memory are seen at 8 to 10 months in preterm infants[161] and within the first 2 years in children with autism.[162] In addition, preterm children are more impaired than full-term children as measured using the parent-reported Behavior Rating Inventory of Executive Function (BRIEF-P), in domains of inhibition, shifting, emotional control, working memory, and planning/organization.[159] Deficits are also noted on performance-based EF tasks for working memory, response inhibition, cognitive flexibility, and verbal fluency. Similarly, children with ASD have increased scores on the BRIEF-P[163,164] and significant impairments on performance-based EF tasks of working memory and response inhibition. Furthermore, children with ASD have problems with mental shifting[164] and functional communication[37] when compared with their TD counterparts.

Overall, preterm children and those with ASD have similar patterns of EF impairments.[159,164] However, many of the stereotypical, self-injurious, ritualistic, restrictive, repetitive, and compulsive behaviors seen in ASD are significantly correlated with problems in EF,[163] which may serve to distinguish them.

## DISCUSSION

Although published research on early development in prematurity and ASD shows commonalities and distinctions, there are also profound research gaps requiring further study. The development of social adaptation, speech-language, and communication in infancy occurs within the context of early infant-caregiver interaction, beginning with behavior and brain mechanisms involved in preferential orientation toward, and interaction with, other people. These early predispositions lead to canalized development via ever more complex cycles of contingent behavior, with achievements in one cycle becoming the initial task for the next cycle and so on.[165] This normative process may be disrupted by initial vulnerabilities originating from multiple causes, including obstetric or genetic as is the case in prematurity and ASD, respectively. The question is whether such disruptions in development can be mitigated via similar means irrespective of the etiology that caused the disruption in the first place.

For example, early intervention efforts in ASD focus on promoting social communication. Could this equally benefit the disorders of preterm infants? Conversely, scaffolding early infant-caregiver contact through skin-to-skin care is recommended from birth in preterm infants, potentially promoting social contingency across all modalities of interaction (including early-emerging tactile, vocal, and motor functions). Could infants at elevated likelihood of autism (eg, infant siblings of children with autism) benefit from neonatal and early-infancy interventions that are more common-place in preterm infants? Such research could also promote better standards of care for both groups of vulnerable children and families.

Similarly, health care disparity factors contribute to increased prevalence of preterm birth, reduced and delayed diagnosis in ASD, and overall, worsened outcomes.[23,24,26]

It is possible that the full impact of these disparities will not be apparent in the first 3 years of life. Therefore, policies, programs and practices designed to reduce health care disparities are necessary, as are interventions developed to mitigate the impact of adverse environments and experiences on child development.[166]

Overall, given the similarities in trajectories and developmental manifestations of children with ASD and preterm birth, there are major advantages for researchers and clinicians alike to collaborate, with the ultimate goal of not only elucidating commonalities and distinctions between the two conditions—in etiology and neurodevelopment—but to also join forces in advancing better standards of care, services, and outcomes.

---

**Best practices**

■ Children born prematurely should be screened for autism spectrum disorder and may need a more comprehensive assessment as the screening tools in current practice may not be sensitive enough for children born premature. (REF 15)

---

## CLINICS CARE POINTS

---

- Symptoms can overlap between children born premature and those with autism spectrum disorder.
- There is increased prevalence of autism in those born prematurely, and the prevalence increases with each additional week of prematurity.
- Delaying detection of autism in those born premature increases delays in appropriate interventions.

---

## DISCLOSURE

The authors have nothing to disclose.

## REFERENCES

1. Hernandez-Fabian A, Canal-Bedia R, Magan-Maganto M, et al. [Autism spectrum disorder and prematurity: towards a prospective screening program]. Rev Neurol 2018;66(S01):S25–9.
2. Limperopoulos C. Autism spectrum disorders in survivors of extreme prematurity. Clin Perinatology 2009;36(4):791–805.
3. Wallace KS, Rogers SJ. Intervening in infancy: implications for autism spectrum disorders. J Child Psychol Psychiatry 2010;51(12):1300–20.
4. Shultz S, Klin A, Jones W. Early infant transitions in social adaptive action and implications thereof for autism. Trends Cogn Sci 2018;22:452–69.
5. Maenner MJ, Shaw KA, Bakian AV, et al. Prevalence and characteristics of autism spectrum disorder among children aged 8 Years - autism and developmental disabilities monitoring network, 11 sites, United States, 2018. MMWR Surveill Summ 2021;70(11):1–16.
6. McCabe ER, Carrino GE, Russell RB, et al. Fighting for the next generation: US Prematurity in 2030. Pediatrics 2014;134(6):1193–9.
7. Torchin H, Ancel PY, Jarreau PH, et al. [Epidemiology of preterm birth: prevalence, recent trends, short- and long-term outcomes]. J Gynecol Obstet Biol Reprod (Paris) 2015;44(8):723–31.

8. Ferré C, Callaghan W, Olson C, et al. Effects of maternal age and age-specific preterm birth rates on overall preterm birth rates — United States, 2007 and 2014. MMWR Morbidity Mortality Weekly Rep 2016;65:1181–4.

9. Purisch SE, Gyamfi-Bannerman C. Epidemiology of preterm birth. Semin Perinatol 2017;41(7):387–91.

10. Agrawal S, Rao SC, Bulsara MK, et al. Prevalence of autism spectrum disorder in preterm infants: a meta-Analysis. Pediatrics 2018;142(3):1–14.

11. Soul JS, Spence SJ. Predicting autism spectrum disorder in very preterm infants. Pediatrics 2020;146(4):1–2.

12. Hirschberger RG, Kuban KCK, O'Shea TM, et al. Co-occurrence and severity of neurodevelopmental burden (cognitive impairment, cerebral palsy, autism spectrum disorder, and epilepsy) at age ten years in children born extremely preterm. Pediatr Neurol 2018;79:45–52.

13. Joseph RM, O'Shea TM, Allred EN, et al. Prevalence and associated features of autism spectrum disorder in extremely low gestational age newborns at age 10 years. Autism Res : official J Int Soc Autism Res 2017;10(2):224–32.

14. Crump C, Sundquist J, Sundquist K. Preterm or early term birth and risk of autism. Pediatrics 2021;148(3):1–12.

15. Allen L, Leon-Attia O, Shaham M, et al. Autism risk linked to prematurity is more accentuated in girls. PLoS One 2020;15(8):1–12.

16. Fleiss B, Gressens P, Stolp HB. Cortical gray matter injury in encephalopathy of prematurity: link to neurodevelopmental disorders. Front Neurol 2020;11:575.

17. Limperopoulos C, Bassan H, Sullivan NR, et al. Positive screening for autism in ex-preterm infants: prevalence and risk factors. Pediatrics 2008;121(4):758–65.

18. Pritchard MA, de Dassel T, Beller E, et al. Autism in toddlers born very preterm. Pediatrics 2016;137(2):e20151949.

19. Kuban KCK, O'Shea TM, Allred EN, et al. Positive screening on the modified checklist for autism in toddlers (M-CHAT) in extremely low gestational age newborns. J Pediatr 2009;154(4):535–40.e1.

20. Luyster RJ, Kuban KCK, O'Shea TM, et al. The Modified Checklist for Autism in Toddlers in extremely low gestational age newborns: individual items associated with motor, cognitive, vision and hearing limitations. Paediatric Perinatal Epidemiol 2011;25(4):366–76.

21. Kim SH, Joseph RM, Frazier JA, et al. Predictive validity of the modified checklist for autism in toddlers (M-CHAT) born very preterm. J Pediatr 2016;178:101–7.e2.

22. Guthrie W, Wallis K, Bennett A, et al. Accuracy of autism screening in a large pediatric network. Pediatrics 2019;144(4):1–12.

23. Potijk MR, Kerstjens JM, Bos AF, et al. Developmental delay in moderately preterm-born children with low socioeconomic status: risks multiply. J Pediatr 2013;163(5):1289–95.

24. Dolatian M, Sharifi N, Mahmoodi Z. Relationship of socioeconomic status, psychosocial factors, and food insecurity with preterm labor: a longitudinal study. Int J Reprod Biomed 2018;16(9):563–70.

25. Giurgescu C, Misra DP. Psychosocial factors and preterm birth among black mothers and fathers. MCN Am J Matern Child Nurs 2018;43(5):245–51.

26. Maenner MJ. Prevalence of autism spectrum disorder among children aged 8 Years — autism and developmental disabilities monitoring network, 11 sites, United States, 2016. MMWR Surveill Summ 2020;69(4):1–12.

27. Constantino JN, Abbacchi AM, Saulnier C, et al. Timing of the diagnosis of autism in african American children. Pediatrics 2020;146(3):1–9.

28. Zuckerman KE, Sinche B, Mejia A, et al. Latino parents' perspectives on barriers to autism diagnosis. Acad Pediatr 2014;14(3):301–8.
29. Delobel-Ayoub M, Ehlinger V, Klapouszczak D, et al. Socioeconomic disparities and prevalence of autism spectrum disorders and intellectual disability. PLoS One 2015;10(11):e0141964.
30. Nguyen CT, Krakowiak P, Hansen R, et al. Sociodemographic disparities in intervention service utilization in families of children with autism spectrum disorder. J Autism Dev Disord 2016;46(12):3729–38.
31. Jones W, Klin A. Attention to eyes is present but in decline in 2-6-month-old infants later diagnosed with autism. Nature 2013;504(7480):427–31.
32. Telford EJ, Fletcher-Watson S, Gillespie-Smith K, et al. Preterm birth is associated with atypical social orienting in infancy detected using eye tracking. J Child Psychol Psychiatry 2016;57(7):861–8.
33. McQueen E, Tokish H, Rudrabhatla A, et al, editors. Early patterns of social visual engagement in preterm and full-term toddlers with autism spectrum disorder. Austin, TX: International Society for Autism Research; 2021.
34. Tokish H, McQueen E, Rudrabhatla A, et al, editors. Quantifying social visual engagement in preterm toddlers with and without autism spectrum disorder. Austin, TX: International Society for Autism Research; 2021.
35. Imafuku M, Kawai M, Niwa F, et al. Preference for dynamic human images and gaze-following abilities in preterm infants at 6 and 12 months of age: an eye-tracking study. Infancy 2017;22:223–39.
36. Moe V, Braarud C, Wentzel-Larsen T, et al. Precursors of social emotional functioning among full-term and preterm infants at 12 months: early infant withdrawal behavior and symptoms of maternal depression. Infant Behav Dev 2016;44:159–68.
37. Bradstreet LE, Juechter JI, Kamphaus RW, et al. Using the BASC-2 parent rating scales to screen for autism spectrum disorder in toddlers and preschool-aged children. J Abnorm Child Psychol 2017;45(2):359–70.
38. Zmyj N, Witt S, Weitkämper A, et al. Social cognition in children born preterm: a perspective on future research directions. Front Psychol 2017;8:1–7.
39. Colombi C, Liebal K, Tomasello M, et al. Examining correlates of cooperation in autism: imitation, joint attention, and understanding intentions. Autism 2009;13(2):143–63.
40. Campbell SB, Moore EL, Northrup J, et al. Developmental changes in empathic concern and self-understanding in toddlers at genetic risk for autism spectrum disorder. J autism Dev Disord 2017;47(9):2690–702.
41. Campbell C, Horlin C, Reid C, et al. How do you think she feels? Vulnerability in empathy and the role of attention in school-aged children born extremely preterm. Br J Dev Psychol 2015;33(3):312–23.
42. Ritchie K, Bora S, Woodward LJ. Social development of children born very preterm: a systematic review. Dev Med Child Neurol 2015;57(10):899–918.
43. Sanchez K, Spittle AJ, Boyce JO, et al. Conversational language in 3-year-old children born very preterm and at term. J speech, Lang hearing Res : JSLHR 2019;63(1):206–15.
44. Patten E, Belardi K, Baranek GT, et al. Vocal patterns in infants with autism spectrum disorder: canonical babbling status and vocalization frequency. J autism Dev Disord 2014;44(10):2413–28.
45. Bühler KE, Limongi SC, Diniz EM. Language and cognition in very low birth weight preterm infants with PELCDO application. Arquivos de neuro-psiquiatria 2009;67(2A):242–9.

46. Davidson MM, Ellis Weismer S. A discrepancy in comprehension and production in early language development in ASD: is it clinically relevant? J autism Dev Disord 2017;47(7):2163–75.
47. Kjelgaard MM, Tager-Flusberg H. An investigation of language impairment in autism: implications for genetic subgroups. Lang Cogn Process 2001;16(2–3): 287–308.
48. Jansson-Verkasalo E, Ruusuvirta T, Huotilainen M, et al. Atypical perceptual narrowing in prematurely born infants is associated with compromised language acquisition at 2 years of age. BMC Neurosci 2010;11:1–7.
49. Bestelmeyer P, Davis NJ, Poliva O, et al. Neuromodulation of right auditory cortex selectively increases activation in speech-related brain areas in brainstem auditory agnosia. Cogn Behav Neurol 2018;31(3):151–5.
50. Kwon SH, Scheinost D, Vohr B, et al. Functional magnetic resonance connectivity studies in infants born preterm: suggestions of proximate and long-lasting changes in language organization. Dev Med Child Neurol 2016;58(Suppl 4): 28–34.
51. Righi G, Tenenbaum EJ, McCormick C, et al. Sensitivity to audio-visual synchrony and its relation to language abilities in children with and without ASD. Autism Res 2018;11(4):645–53.
52. Sansavini A, Guarini A, Zuccarini M, et al. Low rates of pointing in 18-month-olds at risk for autism spectrum disorder and extremely preterm infants: a common index of language delay? Front Psychol 2019;10:1–12.
53. Barbaro J, Dissanayake C. Developmental profiles of infants and toddlers with autism spectrum disorders identified prospectively in a community-based setting. J autism Dev Disord 2012;2(9):1939–48.
54. Chita-Tegmark M, Arunachalam S, Nelson CA, et al. Eye-tracking measurements of language processing: developmental differences in children at high risk for ASD. J Autism Developmental Disord 2015;45:3327–38.
55. Marchman VA, Ashland MD, Loi EC, et al. Predictors of early vocabulary growth in children born preterm and full term: a study of processing speed and medical complications. Child Neuropsychol 2019;25(7):943–63.
56. Rahkonen P, Lano A, Pesonen AK, et al. Atypical sensory processing is common in extremely low gestational age children. Acta Paediatr (Oslo, Norway 1992) 2015;104(5):522–8.
57. Boone KM, Gracious B, Klebanoff MA, et al. Omega-3 and -6 fatty acid supplementation and sensory processing in toddlers with ASD symptomology born preterm: a randomized controlled trial. Early Hum Dev 2017;115:64–70.
58. Chorna O, Solomon JE, Slaughter JC, et al. Abnormal sensory reactivity in preterm infants during the first year correlates with adverse neurodevelopmental outcomes at 2 years of age. Arch Dis Child Fetal neonatal edition 2014;99(6): F475–9.
59. Ben-Sasson A, Cermak SA, Orsmond GI, et al. Extreme sensory modulation behaviors in toddlers with autism spectrum disorders. Am J Occup Ther 2007; 61(5):584–92.
60. Germani T, Zwaigenbaum L, Bryson S, et al. Brief report: assessment of early sensory processing in infants at high-risk of autism spectrum disorder. J autism Dev Disord 2014;44(12):3264–70.
61. Wolff JJ, Dimian AF, Botteron KN, et al. A longitudinal study of parent-reported sensory responsiveness in toddlers at-risk for autism. J Child Psychol Psychiatry 2019;60(3):314–24.

62. Niedźwiecka A, Domasiewicz Z, Kawa R, et al. Sensory processing in toddlers with autism spectrum disorders. Eur J Dev Psychol 2019;17(4):527–55.
63. Eeles AL, Anderson PJ, Brown NC, et al. Sensory profiles obtained from parental reports correlate with independent assessments of development in very preterm children at 2 years of age. Early Hum Dev 2013;89(12):1075–80.
64. Wiggins LD, Robins DL, Bakeman R, et al. Brief report: sensory abnormalities as distinguishing symptoms of autism spectrum disorders in young children. J autism Dev Disord 2009;39(7):1087–91.
65. Eeles AL, Spittle AJ, Anderson PJ, et al. Assessments of sensory processing in infants: a systematic review. Developmental Med child Neurol 2013;55(4):314–26.
66. Lucas RF, Cutler A. Dysregulated breastfeeding behaviors in children later diagnosed with autism. J Perinat Educ 2015;24(3):171–80.
67. Lau C. Breastfeeding challenges and the preterm mother-infant dyad: a conceptual model. Breastfeed Med 2018;13(1):8–17.
68. Lau C. Development of infant oral feeding skills: what do we know? Am J Clin Nutr 2016;103(2):616s–21s.
69. Mizuno K, Fujimaki K, Sawada M. Sucking behavior at breast during the early newborn period affects later breast-feeding rate and duration of breast-feeding. Pediatr Int 2004;46(1):15–20.
70. Riva V, Cantiani C, Mornati G, et al. Distinct ERP profiles for auditory processing in infants at-risk for autism and language impairment. Scientific Rep 2018;8(1):715.
71. Antinmaa J, Lapinleimu H, Salonen J, et al. Neonatal brainstem auditory function associates with early receptive language development in preterm children. Acta Paediatr 2020;109(7):1387–93.
72. Key AP, Lambert EW, Aschner JL, et al. Influence of gestational age and postnatal age on speech sound processing in NICU infants. Psychophysiology 2012;49(5):720–31.
73. Maitre NL, Slaughter JC, Aschner JL, et al. Hemisphere differences in speech-sound event-related potentials in intensive care neonates: associations and predictive value for development in infancy. J child Neurol 2014;29(7):903.
74. Lecuona E, Van Jaarsveld A, Raubenheimer J, et al. Sensory integration intervention and the development of the premature infant: a controlled trial. S Afr Med J 2017;107(11):976–82.
75. Lickliter R. The influence of prenatal experience on behavioral and social development: the benefits and limitations of an animal model. Dev Psychopathol 2018;30(3):871–80.
76. Ben-Sasson A, Hen L, Fluss R, et al. A meta-analysis of sensory modulation symptoms in individuals with autism spectrum disorders. J Autism Dev Disord 2009;39(1):1–11.
77. Marco EJ, Hinkley LBN, Hill SS, et al. Sensory processing in autism: a review of neurophysiologic findings. Pediatr Res 2011;69(8):48–54.
78. Ben-Sasson A, Cermak SA, Orsmond GI, et al. Sensory clusters of toddlers with autism spectrum disorders: differences in affective symptoms. J child Psychol Psychiatry allied disciplines 2008;49(8):817–25.
79. Boyd BA, Baranek GT, Sideris J, et al. Sensory features and repetitive behaviors in children with autism and developmental delays. Autism researchh 2010;3(2):78–87.

80. Green SA, Ben-Sasson A, Soto TW, et al. Anxiety and sensory over-responsivity in toddlers with autism spectrum disorders: bidirectional effects across time. J autism Dev Disord 2012;42(6):1112–9.

81. Cabral TI, da Silva LG, Martinez CM, et al. Analysis of sensory processing in preterm infants. Early Hum Dev 2016;103:77–81.

82. Cabral TI, Pereira da Silva LG, Tudella E, et al. Motor development and sensory processing: a comparative study between preterm and term infants. Res Dev disabilities 2015;36C:102–7.

83. Emberson LL, Boldin AM, Riccio JE, et al. Deficits in top-down sensory prediction in infants at risk due to premature birth. Curr Biol 2017;27(3):431–6.

84. Pierce K, Marinero S, Hazin R, et al. Eye tracking reveals abnormal visual preference for geometric images as an early biomarker of an autism spectrum disorder subtype Associated with increased symptom severity. Biol Psychiatry 2016;79(8):657–66.

85. Neel MLM, Stark AR, Maitre NL. Parenting style impacts cognitive and behavioural outcomes of former preterm infants: a systematic review. Child Care Health Dev 2018;44(4):507–15.

86. Ben-Sasson A, Soto TW, Martínez-Pedraza F, et al. Early sensory over-responsivity in toddlers with autism spectrum disorders as a predictor of family impairment and parenting stress. J Child Psychol Psychiatry 2013;54(8):846–53.

87. Evensen KAI, Ustad T, Tikanmäki M, et al. Long-term motor outcomes of very preterm and/or very low birth weight individuals without cerebral palsy: a review of the current evidence. Semin Fetal Neonatal Med 2020;25(3):101116.

88. Lenke MC. Motor outcomes in premature infants. Newborn Infant Nurs Rev 2003;3(3):104–9.

89. Bos AF, Van Braeckel KN, Hitzert MM, et al. Development of fine motor skills in preterm infants. Developmental Med child Neurol 2013;55(SUPPL.4):1–4.

90. Williams J, Lee KJ, Anderson PJ. Prevalence of motor-skill impairment in preterm children who do not develop cerebral palsy: a systematic review. Dev Med Child Neurol 2010;52(3):232–7.

91. Van Hus JW, Potharst ES, Jeukens-Visser M, et al. Motor impairment in very preterm-born children: links with other developmental deficits at 5 years of age. Dev Med Child Neurol 2014;56(6):587–94.

92. Pascal AG, Govaert P, Oostra A, et al. Neurodevelopmental outcome in very preterm and very-low-birthweight infants born over the past decade: a meta-analytic review. Developmental Med child Neurol 2018;60(4):342–55.

93. Wolf MJ, Koldewijn K, Beelen A, et al. Neurobehavioral and developmental profile of very low birthweight preterm infants in early infancy. Acta Paediatr 2002; 91(8):930–8.

94. Di Rosa G, Cavallaro T, Alibrandi A, et al. Predictive role of early milestones-related psychomotor profiles and long-term neurodevelopmental pitfalls in preterm infants. Early Hum Dev 2016;101:49–55.

95. West KL. Infant motor development in autism spectrum disorder: a synthesis and meta-analysis. Child Dev 2019;90(6):2053–70.

96. Estes A, Munson J, Rogers SJ, et al. Long-term outcomes of early intervention in 6-year-old children with autism spectrum disorder. J Am Acad Child Adolesc Psychiatry 2015;54(7):580–7.

97. McPhillips M, Finlay J, Bejerot S, et al. Motor deficits in children with autism spectrum disorder: a cross-syndrome study. Autism Res 2014;7(6):664–76.

98. Heathcock JC, Tanner K, Robson D, et al. Retrospective analysis of motor development in infants at high and low risk for autism spectrum disorder. Am J Occup Ther 2015;69(5):6905185070.

99. Licari MK, Alvares GA, Varcin K, et al. Prevalence of motor difficulties in autism spectrum disorder: analysis of a population-based cohort. Autism Res 2020; 13(2):298–306.

100. Spittle AJ, Brown NC, Doyle LW, et al. Quality of general movements is related to white matter pathology in very preterm infants. Pediatrics 2008;121(5):e1184–9.

101. Spittle AJ, Cameron K, Doyle LW, et al. Motor impairment trends in extremely preterm children: 1991-2005. Pediatrics 2018;141(4):1–8.

102. Einspieler C, Sigafoos J, Bölte S, et al. Highlighting the first 5 months of life: general movements in infants later diagnosed with autism spectrum disorder or Rett Syndrome. Res autism Spectr Disord 2014;8(3):286–91.

103. Skiöld B, Eriksson C, Eliasson AC, et al. General movements and magnetic resonance imaging in the prediction of neuromotor outcome in children born extremely preterm. Early Hum Dev 2013;89(7):467–72.

104. Dimitrijević L, Bjelaković B, Čolović H, et al. Assessment of general movements and heart rate variability in prediction of neurodevelopmental outcome in preterm infants. Early Hum Dev 2016;99:7–12.

105. Ming X, Brimacombe M, Wagner GC. Prevalence of motor impairment in autism spectrum disorders. Brain Dev 2007;29(9):565–70.

106. Stephens BE, Liu J, Lester B, et al. Neurobehavioral assessment predicts motor outcome in preterm infants. J Pediatr 2010;156(3):366–71.

107. Baber S, Michalitsis J, Fahey M, et al. A Comparison of the birth characteristics of idiopathic toe walking and toe walking gait due to medical reasons. J Pediatr 2016;171:290–3.

108. Pan PY, Bölte S, Kaur P, et al. Neurological disorders in autism: a systematic review and meta-analysis. Autism 2021;25(3):812–30.

109. van Haastert IC, de Vries LS, Helders PJ, et al. Early gross motor development of preterm infants according to the Alberta Infant Motor Scale. J Pediatr 2006; 149(5):617–22.

110. Jeng S-F, Chen L-C, Tsou K-I, et al. Relationship between spontaneous kicking and age of walking attainment in preterm infants with very low birth weight and full-term infants. Phys Ther 2004;84(2):159–72.

111. Lemcke S, Juul S, Parner ET, et al. Early signs of autism in toddlers: a follow-up study in the Danish National Birth Cohort. J autism Dev Disord 2013;43(10): 2366–75.

112. Ozonoff S, Young GS, Goldring S, et al. Gross motor development, movement abnormalities, and early identification of autism. J autism Dev Disord 2008; 38(4):644–56.

113. Bhat AN, Landa RJ, Galloway JC. Current perspectives on motor functioning in infants, children, and adults with autism spectrum disorders. Phys Ther 2011; 91(7):1116–29.

114. Estes A, Zwaigenbaum L, Gu H, et al. Behavioral, cognitive, and adaptive development in infants with autism spectrum disorder in the first 2 years of life. J neurodevelopmental Disord 2015;7(1):24–34.

115. Pusponegoro HD, Efar P, Soedjatmiko, et al. Gross motor profile and its association with socialization skills in children with autism spectrum disorders. Pediatr Neonatal 2016;57(6):501–7.

116. van der Fits IG, Klip AW, van Eykern LA, et al. Postural adjustments during spontaneous and goal-directed arm movements in the first half year of life. Behav Brain Res 1999;106(1–2):75–90.

117. Babik I, Galloway JC, Lobo MA. Infants born preterm demonstrate impaired exploration of their bodies and surfaces throughout the first 2 years of life. Phys Ther 2017;97(9):915–25.

118. Flanagan JE, Landa R, Bhat A, et al. Head lag in infants at risk for autism: a preliminary study. Am J Occup Ther 2012;66(5):577–85.

119. Lidstone DE, Miah FZ, Poston B, et al. Children with autism spectrum disorder show impairments during dynamic versus static grip-force tracking. Autism Res 2020;13(12):2177–89.

120. Gima H, Kihara H, Watanabe H, et al. Early motor signs of autism spectrum disorder in spontaneous position and movement of the head. Exp Brain Res 2018; 236(4):1139–48.

121. Jeng S-F, Lau T-W, Hsieh W-S, et al. Development of walking in preterm and term infants: age of onset, qualitative features and sensitivity to resonance. Gait Posture 2008;27(2):340–6.

122. Ross G, Lipper E, Auld PA. Early predictors of neurodevelopmental outcome of very low-birthweight infants at three years. Dev Med Child Neurol 1986;28(2): 171–9.

123. Lobo MA, Kokkoni E, Cunha AB, et al. Infants born preterm demonstrate impaired object exploration behaviors throughout infancy and toddlerhood. Phys Ther 2015;95(1):51–64.

124. LeBarton ES, Iverson JM. Fine motor skill predicts expressive language in infant siblings of children with autism. Dev Sci 2013;16(6):815–27.

125. Stoit AMB, van Schie HT, Slaats-Willemse DIE, et al. Grasping motor impairments in autism: not action planning but movement execution is deficient. J Autism Developmental Disord 2013;43(12):2793–806.

126. Sacrey LAR, Bennett JA, Zwaigenbaum L. Early infant development and intervention for autism spectrum disorder. J Child Neurol 2015;30(14):1921–9.

127. FitzGerald TL, Cameron KL, Albesher RA, et al. Strength, motor skills, and physical activity in preschool-aged children born either at less than 30 Weeks of gestation or at term. Phys Ther 2021;101(5):pzab037.

128. Bradshaw J, Bearss K, McCracken C, et al. Parent education for young children with autism and disruptive behavior: response to active control treatment. J Clin Child Adolesc Psychol 2018;47(sup1):S445–55.

129. Iverson JM, Shic F, Wall CA, et al. Early motor abilities in infants at heightened versus low risk for ASD: a Baby Siblings Research Consortium (BSRC) study. J Abnormal Psychol 2019;128(1):69–80.

130. Ding N, Gao H, Jiang J, et al. The characteristics and factors of the internalizing and externalizing behaviours of children at high risk for autism spectrum disorder. BMC Psychiatry 2021;21(1):523.

131. de la Osa N, Granero R, Trepat E, et al. The discriminative capacity of CBCL/1½-5-DSM5 scales to identify disruptive and internalizing disorders in preschool children. Eur Child Adolesc Psychiatry 2016;25:17–23.

132. Cibralic S, Kohlhoff J, Wallace N, et al. Treating externalizing behaviors in toddlers with ASD traits using parent-child interaction therapy for toddlers: a case study. Clin Case Stud 2021;20(2):165–84.

133. Månsson J, Stjernqvist K, Bäckström M. Behavioral outcomes at corrected age 2.5 years in children born extremely preterm. J Dev Behav Pediatr : JDBP. 2014; 35(7):435–42.

134. Raza S, Sacrey LR, Zwaigenbaum L, et al. Relationship between early social-emotional behavior and autism spectrum disorder: a high-risk sibling study. J autism Dev Disord 2020;50(7):2527–39.
135. Spittle AJ, Treyvaud K, Doyle LW, et al. Early emergence of behavior and social-emotional problems in very preterm infants. J Am Acad Child Adolesc Psychiatry 2009;48(9):909–18.
136. Rogers EE, Hintz SR. Early neurodevelopmental outcomes of extremely preterm infants. Semin perinatology 2016;40(8):497–509.
137. Montirosso R, Giusti L, De Carli P, et al. Developmental care, neonatal behavior and postnatal maternal depressive symptomatology predict internalizing problems at 18 months for very preterm children. J Perinatol 2018;38(2):191–5.
138. Smith CG, Jones EJH, Wass SV, et al. Infant effortful control mediates relations between nondirective parenting and internalising-related child behaviours in an autism-enriched infant cohort. J autism Dev Disord 2021;52(8):3496–511.
139. Laurent AC, Gorman K. Development of Emotion self-regulation among young children with autism spectrum disorders: the role of parents. J Autism Developmental Disord 2018;48(4):1249–60.
140. Arpi E, Ferrari F. Preterm birth and behaviour problems in infants and preschool-age children: a review of the recent literature. Developmental Med Child Neurol 2013;55(9):788–96.
141. Chetcuti L, Uljarević M, Varcin KJ, et al. Subgroups of temperament associated with social-emotional difficulties in infants with early signs of autism. Autism Res 2020;13(12):2094–101.
142. Ross GS, Rescorla LA, Perlman J M. Patterns and prediction of behavior problems during the toddler and preschool periods in preterm children. Int J Behav Dev 2020;44(5):404–11.
143. Tureck K, Matson JL, Cervantes P, et al. Autism severity as a predictor of inattention and impulsivity in toddlers. Developmental Neurorehabil 2015;18(5): 285–9.
144. Shah PE, Robbins N, Coelho RB, et al. The paradox of prematurity: the behavioral vulnerability of late preterm infants and the cognitive susceptibility of very preterm infants at 36 months post-term. Infant Behav Dev 2013;36(1):50–62.
145. Davis AS. Children with down syndrome: implications for assessment and intervention in the school. Sch Psychol Q 2008;23(2):271–81.
146. Huhtala M, Korja R, Lehtonen L, et al. Parental psychological well-being and behavioral outcome of very low birth weight infants at 3 years. Pediatrics 2012;129(4):937–44.
147. Chetcuti L, Uljarević M, Varcin KJ, et al. The role of negative affectivity in concurrent relations between caregiver psychological distress and social-emotional difficulties in infants with early signs of autism. Autism Res 2020;13(8):1349–57.
148. Martins CBS, Cassiano RGM, Linhares MBM. Negative affectivity moderated by preterm birth predicted toddlers' behavior problems. Infant Behav Dev 2021;63: 101544.
149. Gracioli SMA, Linhares MBM. Neonatal and temperament variables predict behavior problems of preterm children at toddlerhood. J Hum Growth Development 2019;29(3):313–24.
150. Guilherme Monte Cassiano R, Gaspardo CM, Cordaro Bucker Furini G, et al. Impact of neonatal risk and temperament on behavioral problems in toddlers born preterm. Early Hum Dev 2016;103:175–81.
151. Davis TE Iii. Where to from here for ASD and anxiety? Lessons learned from child anxiety and the issue of DSM-5. Clin Psychol Sci Pract 2012;19:358–63.

152. Montirosso R, Casini E, Prete AD, et al. Neonatal developmental care in infant pain management and internalizing behaviours at 18 months in prematurely born children. Eur J Pain 2016;20(6):1010–21.

153. Maitre NL, Key AP, Slaughter JC, et al. Neonatal multisensory processing in preterm and term infants predicts sensory reactivity and internalizing tendencies in early childhood. Brain topography 2020;33(5):586–99.

154. Matson JL, Boisjoli J, Rojahn J, et al. A factor analysis of challenging behaviors assessed with the Baby and Infant Screen for Children with aUtism Traits (BIS-CUIT-Part 3). Res Autism Spectr Disord 2009;3(3):714–22.

155. Matson JL, Mahan S, Hess JA, et al. Progression of challenging behaviors in children and adolescents with autism spectrum disorders as measured by the Autism Spectrum Disorders-Problem Behaviors for Children (ASD-PBC). Res Autism Spectr Disord 2010;4:400–4.

156. Poehlmann J, Miller Schwichtenberg AJ, Hahn E, et al. Compliance, opposition, and behavior problems in toddlers born preterm or low birthweight. Infant Ment Health J 2012;33(1):34–44.

157. Baron IS, Kerns KA, Müller U, et al. Executive functions in extremely low birth weight and late-preterm preschoolers: effects on working memory and response inhibition. Child Neuropsychol 2012;18(6):586–99.

158. Nagy BE, Kenyhercz F. Adaptive behavioral, social-emotional, and neurodevelopmental outcomes at 2 Years of age in Hungarian preterm infants based on Bayley III. Developmental Neurorehabil 2021;24(1):18–24.

159. Alduncin N, Huffman LC, Feldman HM, et al. Executive function is associated with social competence in preschool-aged children born preterm or full term. Early Hum Dev 2014;90(6):299–306.

160. Ventola PE, Saulnier CA, Steinberg E, et al. Early-emerging social adaptive skills in toddlers with autism spectrum disorders: an item analysis. J Autism Developmental Disord 2014;44(2):283–93.

161. Sun J, Buys N. Early executive function deficit in preterm children and its association with neurodevelopmental disorders in childhood: a literature review. Int J Adolesc Med Health 2012;24(4):291–9.

162. St. John T, Estes AM, Dager SR, et al. Emerging executive functioning and motor development in infants at high and low risk for autism spectrum disorder. Front Psychol 2016;7:1–12.

163. Sadeghi S, Pouretemad HR, Badv RS. Impaired executive functions predict repetitive behaviors in toddlers under 36 months old with autism spectrum disorder symptoms. Res Square 2021;67:101721.

164. Carotenuto M, Ruberto MG, Fontana ML, et al. Executive functioning in autism spectrum disorders: a case-control study in preschool children. Curr Pediatr Res 2019;23:112–6.

165. Klin A, Micheletti M, Klaiman C, et al. Affording autism an early brain development re-definition. Development Psychopathology 2020;32(4):1175–89.

166. Shonkoff JP, Bales SN. Science does not speak for itself: translating child development research for the public and its policymakers. Child Dev 2011;82(1):17–32.

167. Narzisi A, Calderoni S, Maestro S, et al. Child behavior check list 1½–5 as a tool to identify toddlers with autism spectrum disorders: a case-control study. Res Developmental Disabilities 2013;34(4):1179–89.

168. Yang S, Paynter JM, Gilmore L. Vineland adaptive behavior scales: II profile of young children with autism spectrum disorder. J autism Dev Disord 2016;46(1):64–73.

169. Casas M, Chatzi L, Carsin AE, et al. Maternal pre-pregnancy overweight and obesity, and child neuropsychological development: two Southern European birth cohort studies. Int J Epidemiol 2013;42(2):506–17.
170. Hirvonen M, Ojala R, Korhonen P, et al. Visual and hearing impairments after preterm birth. Pediatrics 2018;142(2):1–10.
171. Van Hus JW, Jeukens-Visser M, Koldewijn K, et al. Comparing two motor assessment tools to evaluate neurobehavioral intervention effects in infants with very low birth weight at 1 year. Phys Ther 2013;93(11):1475–83.
172. de Groot L, de Groot CJ, Hopkins B. An instrument to measure independent walking: are there differences between preterm and fullterm infants? J child Neurol 1997;12(1):37–41.
173. Sacrey LR, Zwaigenbaum L, Bryson S, et al. The reach-to-grasp movement in infants later diagnosed with autism spectrum disorder: a high-risk sibling cohort study. J neurodevelopmental Disord 2018;10(1):41–52.
174. Baghdadli A, Picot MC, Pascal CI, et al. Relationship between age of recognition of first disturbances and severity in young children with autism. Eur Child Adolesc Psychiatry 2003;12(3):122–7.
175. Baio J. Prevalence of autism spectrum disorders: autism and developmental disabilities monitoring network, 14 sites, United States 2008. Morbidity Mortality Weekly Rep 2012;61(3):1–24.
176. Montirosso R, Tronick E, Borgatti R. Promoting neuroprotective care in neonatal intensive care units and preterm infant development: insights from the neonatal adequate care for quality of life study. Child Development Perspect 2017;11(1):9–15.

# Interventions for Executive Function in High-Risk Infants and Toddlers

Andrea F. Duncan, MD, MSClinRes[a,b,*]

## KEYWORDS

- Executive function • Intervention • High-risk • Self-regulation

## KEY POINTS

- Executive functioning (EF) development during infancy and toddlerhood provides a critical foundation for later academic success, health, and wealth.
- Very few EF interventions exist for children aged younger than 3 years, and intervention targets and dosages are highly variable.
- Self-regulation is the most studied EF construct in intervention trials for young children, followed by general executive behaviors.
- Positive results for EF interventions were often skewed toward participants with the lowest gestational ages or the most medical complexity.

## BACKGROUND

Children born preterm are at high risk for long-term neurodevelopmental deficits, including deficits in executive functioning (EF).[1] Executive function denotes higher order cognitive capabilities involved in goal-making, mapping out how to achieve those goals, and carrying out the plans that were made.[2] Multiple aspects of EF must synergistically interact for optimal function: anticipation and attentional control, impulse control and self-regulation, activity initiation, working memory, cognitive flexibility, planning and organization, problem solving, and self-performance monitoring.[2–4] Foundations of EF emerge during the first year of life, and the development of these early skills provides the basis for higher order EF skills in later childhood.[5] Early social-emotional ability, EF, and related self-regulation skills during infancy and toddlerhood are necessary for later academic achievement, health, and wealth.[6,7]

Disclosure Statement: The author has nothing to disclose.
[a] Division of Neonatology, Children's Hospital of Philadelphia, 3401 Civic Center Boulevard, 2nd Floor Main, Philadelphia, PA 19104, USA; [b] Department of Pediatrics, Perelman School of Medicine, University of Pennsylvania, Philadelphia, PA, USA
* Division of Neonatology, Children's Hospital of Philadelphia, 3401 Civic Center Boulevard, 2nd Floor Main, Philadelphia, PA 19104.
E-mail address: duncana2@chop.edu

Clin Perinatol 50 (2023) 103–119
https://doi.org/10.1016/j.clp.2022.10.003        perinatology.theclinics.com
0095-5108/23/© 2022 Elsevier Inc. All rights reserved.

Children born at high risk for neurodevelopmental concerns who demonstrate EF deficits are at much higher risk for school failure, special education needs, and teacher reports of behavioral and general academic delays.[8,9] Up to 50% of children born extremely preterm (EPT; <28 weeks gestation) exhibit such deficits, and they are largely linked to morbidities associated with preterm birth, including brain injury[9,10] and track into adulthood.[1]

More than 70% of EPT children have microstructural white matter abnormalities, with 20% exhibiting moderate-to-severe abnormalities.[11] Disruption of early white matter development resulting from EP birth may, in part, be responsible for the EF deficits in this population.[11,12] Evidence suggests that concepts vital for EF and self-regulatory functioning are shaped during infancy, and emergence of these skills is intimately linked to the development of the prefrontal limbic system (PrLS) in the first year of life.[13] The PrLS system has one of the longest developmental periods, with major developmental shifts in the structural integrity of white matter; functional connectivity between brain regions largely occurring late in gestation and postnatally.[13] Postnatal myelination of PrLS white matter develops rapidly throughout the first 3 postnatal years.[13] Due to its protracted developmental course, PrLS maturation and organization is heavily influenced by experience.[13] For example, numerous animal studies indicate that the quality of maternal care in early life results in experience-driven synaptic reorganization in the PrLS.[14–16] Given that experiences in the first days to months of life result in experience-related PrLS development, and early PrLS development is related to emergence of foundational EF skills, interventions targeted at EF in very early life may have far-reaching benefits. To date, however, there have been few interventions developed for EPT children.

## EARLY EXECUTIVE FUNCTION DEVELOPMENT IS SEQUENTIAL

The development of EF is sequential and extremely complex. In addition to the interactions between EF development and experience, interactions with higher order neural systems are integral to establishment of the varied functions that are categorized as EF. In infancy, focused attention is believed to signal the emergence of EF.[17,18] The somewhat dissociable EF components of inhibitory control, working memory, and cognitive flexibility begin to appear during infancy and the toddler years.[19] Inhibitory control and working memory rapidly develop from ages 2 to 5 years, setting the foundation for the development of cognitive flexibility.[18,20] These constituents are foundational for the higher order EF, including goal setting, planning, and problem solving.[5] Given the dynamic nature of EF in the early years, it is little wonder that determining feasible, accurate, and predictive early EF tasks has proven difficult; there is very little validation of EF assessment methodology for infants and toddlers.[21,22]

## EXECUTIVE FUNCTION INTERVENTIONS FOR CHILDREN AGED 0 TO 3 YEARS

Numerous intervention trials have demonstrated benefit to EF in older children and adolescents born preterm, high-risk, and with other disease states. Interventions such as mindfulness courses,[1] exercise programs,[23–25] music instruction,[26] and Judo training[27] have all been shown to improve EF in 4 to 18-year-old children who were born preterm, were overweight, had attention deficit hyperactivity disorder (ADHD), or traumatic brain injury, as well as typically developing children. However, compared with the number of EF-focused interventions for older children, very few EF interventions exist for children aged younger than 3 years. The interventions are heterogenous in methodology, outcome measures, timing, frequency and intensity of treatment, and intervention targets (**Table 1**). The length of the interventions, for example, varies from

**Table 1**
**Executive function interventions for children aged 0 to 3 y**

| Age Range Studied (Y) | Intervention and Description | Target |
|---|---|---|
| 3–9 | *Internet-Based Interacting Together Everyday: Recovery After Childhood TBI [I-InTERACT])*[49]: A self-guided and live online intervention with psychoeducational modules and synchronous videoconferencing meetings with a trained therapist. Sessions provided information about effects of early TBI, effective parenting skills, stress/anger management, and communication methods. 14 sessions *I-InTERACT Express:*[49] Abbreviated 7-session self-guided and live intervention focusing exclusively on effective parenting skills with a trained therapist | *Parents* of children with TBI |
| 2–3 | *Mediational Intervention for Sensitizing Caregivers:*[31] Caregiver–child dyad interactions videotaped monthly and how to focus and direct their child; provide meaning (name experiences/things/people and convey emotional excitement and affection, expand and regulate. Trainings in home and laboratory for 1 y | *Parents* of children exposed to HIV but uninfected |
| 3–5 | *Circle of Security-Parenting:*[50] A 10-wk program emphasizing responsive parenting using child distress stock video footage to encourage parental reflective dialog, emotion regulation, empathy toward the child, and sensitivity to child distress to create secure base | *Parents* of children in Head Start |
| 3–7 | *Parental Occupation Executive Training*[51]: An 8-session parent-training program promoting the use of cognitive strategies to support daily functioning of children with ADHD | *Parents* of children with ADHD |
| 24–35 mo | *FCU:*[33,35] A home-delivered parenting intervention targeting parenting skills for families identified to be at risk for problem behavior. Uses motivational interviewing to provide parents with direct feedback about their child's and family's behavior FCU aims to motivate parents to modify their behavior in service of their child's welfare, engaging in postfeedback treatment sessions aimed at learning new skills based on evidence-based practices derived from social learning principles | *Parents* of children with social and behavioral risks |

(continued on next page)

| Table 1 (continued) | | |
| --- | --- | --- |
| **Age Range Studied (Y)** | **Intervention and Description** | **Target** |
| <6 mo | *IBAIP*:[36–38] Assists parents and interventionists to adjust their interaction style to match the neurobehavioral needs of the infant. Uses the Infant Behavioral Assessment (IBA), which provides a 2-min "observation window" of the infant's behavioral repertoire during interaction. Based on the IBA, facilitation strategies are used to support the infant's self-regulation including environmental facilitation, handling/positioning, and cue-matched facilitation. After each intervention session, parents receive a report that describes the infant's neurobehavioral and developmental progress and gives suggestions to support the infant's explorations and self-regulation | *Parents* of <6-mo-old children born preterm |
| 0–4 | *Early responsive stimulation (RS)*[29,30]: A 2-y program focused on enhancing caregiver (1) Sensitivity—the capacity of the caregiver to observe and understand the infant and young child's needs and wants) and (2) Responsiveness—the capacity of the caregiver to respond in a timely and developmentally appropriate manner to the infant and young child's signals. Occurs via individualized coaching, support, and feedback during monthly home visits and community group meetings | *Parents* of rural disadvantaged children |
| 3–5 | *Hitkashrut*[52]: Master's degree–level educational psychologists provide 14 manual-based meetings with groups of 5 to 11 couples to provide a "common elements" coparent training program to teach behavior management skills | *Couples* parenting children at risk for conduct problems |
| 0–2 | *Psychosocial stimulation*[39]: Home visits by community health workers for 19 mo focused on maternal responsiveness to the infant's cues, talking to the infant, play, and praise/positive reinforcement of desired behaviors | *Parents* of children born LBW |
| 3–4 | *Group Positive Parenting Program (Triple P)*:[53] This 5-wk parenting program aims to improve child self-regulation via multiple avenues. For example, by giving clear and logical consequences to guide behavior and using techniques | *Parents* |

(continued on next page)

| Table 1 | | |
| --- | --- | --- |
| (*continued*) | | |
| **Age Range Studied (Y)** | **Intervention and Description** | **Target** |
| | such as quiet time and time out to allow children space and time to self-soothe | |
| 1–2 | *CBIP or HBIP:*[40] 8 identical in-clinic or in-home child-focused, parent-focused, and dyad-focused sessions incorporating modulation of the neonatal intensive care unit and home environment, teaching of child developmental skills, instructions on health and feeding, massage, parental support and education, and parent–infant interaction activities | *Parents, dyads,* and *children* born preterm |
| 2 wk–11 mo | *Preventative Care Program:*[32] Home-based intervention delivered during 9 home visits by a physiotherapist and psychologist together to improve infant cognitive, motor, and language development by working with the family to understand their infant's behavioral cues, enrich the environment by encouraging positive play and interactions, positioning and handling, problem-solving difficult tasks, providing information on milestones specific to preterm infants, and optimizing parent mental health | Maternal-infant *dyads* of 2 wk to 11-mo-old born preterm |
| 3–4 | *Generating Attention, Inhibition, and Memory Intervention*[54]: Children meet in small groups for 8 wk with 2 interventionists and participate in activities to practice EF and related skills, including attention, inhibition, memory, hand–eye coordination, balance, sensory awareness, listening skills, and visual focusing. While children are in small groups, parents meet in a group with a psychologist who explains and models implementing the activities at home with emphases on skill building and on how to use specific and labeled praise | *Parents* of *children* at risk for ADHD |
| 3–5 | *Head Start* Research-Based, Developmentally Informed[55]: Teacher-delivered 1-y intervention integrated into Head Start classrooms that are using the High/Scope or Creative Curriculum. The intervention is delivered by classroom teachers and integrated into their ongoing classroom programs. It includes curriculum-based lessons, center-based extension activities, and | *Children* in Head Start primarily (parents receive information for home) |
| | | (*continued on next page*) |

| Table 1 (continued) | | |
|---|---|---|
| **Age Range Studied (Y)** | **Intervention and Description** | **Target** |
| | training and weekly classroom coaching in "teaching strategies" to use throughout the day. It is focused primarily on social-emotional skill enrichment using the PATHS Preschool curriculum and language/emergent literacy skill enrichment. Parents also receive take-home materials describing the importance of positive support, emotion coaching, and interactive reading, with parenting tips and learning activities to use at home | |
| 3–4 | *Enhancing Neurobehavioral Gains with the Aid of Games and Exercise*[53,56]: This 8-wk intervention involves parents playing several well-known games with their children in a structured manner daily for half an hour a day (eg, puzzles, ball games, musical statues, blocks, skip rope). Each game parents play requires self-regulation (eg, waiting your turn, inhibiting a response, regulating emotion). | *Children* with hyperactivity |
| 3–5 | *Yoga*[57]: using a manualized curriculum from If I Was a Bird Yoga led by a trained children's yoga instructors and 1–2 assistants | *Children* with ADHD symptoms |
| 0–6 mo | *Supporting Play Exploration, and Early Developmental Intervention:*[41] Phase 1 in takes place in the Neonatal Intensive Care Unit (NICU): provided by the parent and therapist jointly and in response to the infant's behavioral cues based on the synactive theory of development. 33 Videos of positive and negative interaction available to parents throughout phase 1. Coaching on behavioral states, self-calming, environmental modification, and choosing times for feeding-based and play-based interactions using dolls or video clips if the infant was not alert or fatigued. Phase 2 starts at end of phase 1. An activity booklet used to encourage parents to provide motor and cognitive opportunities daily in a variety of play positions, environments, and with objects. Intervention lasts roughly 15 wk | Very preterm *children* |
| EF assessed at 5–10 | *Kangaroo Care:*[34] Skin-to-skin contact in the NICU for an hour per day for 2 wk in the NICU | *Children* born preterm after kangaroo care in the NICU |
| | | *(continued on next page)* |

| Table 1 (continued) | | |
|---|---|---|
| **Age Range Studied (Y)** | **Intervention and Description** | **Target** |
| 3–4 | *Let's Play in Tandem:*[58] A 40-wk, parent-delivered school readiness intervention intended to bolster prereading skills, basic numerical skills, and general knowledge. Activities are in the form of games designed to elicit sustained one-on-one verbal interactions, joint attention, and maternal scaffolding of the children's learning. The mother's role is to provide children with prompts, demonstrations, instructions, and encouragement. Project workers taught parents new activities in home once per week | *Children* with social and economic deprivation |
| 7–16 mo | *START-Play:*[42] Physical therapy intervention based on the theory that the mind and body are inextricably linked. Infants learn performing movements and experiencing consequences related to cognitive constructs such as means-end relations, object permanence, object affordances, and joint attention. Key components are cognitive constructs embedded within motor activities; motor and cognitive skills advanced together at "just-right" level; parent and therapist brainstorming cognitive motor interaction; movement flexibility allowed without rigid adherence to "normal patterns"; and all therapy provided within a social, engaging context guided by degrees of joint attention | *Children* with motor delays |
| 24 mo | *Music Intervention*[43]: 3 tracks were created to help infant awaken, support calm awake, and to help infant fall asleep. Music was by Andreas Vollenweider, consisted of background, bells, harp, and punji and was 30–65 dBA. Occurred roughly 5 times per week from gestational age of 33 wk until hospital discharge or term-equivalent age | *Children* born preterm |
| 3 | *Extra experience learning:*[28] Children practiced a card memory game with an experimenter. The experimenter familiarized the child with each matching pair of cards, then flipped over and scrambled them. The child was shown how to play the game by turning over 2 nonmatching cards and said, | Typically developing *children* |

*(continued on next page)*

| Age Range Studied (Y) | Intervention and Description | Target |
|---|---|---|
| | "These 2 are not the same shape." and the child and experimenter took turns looking for matches. If the pair matched, the cards were removed from the game. If the pair was not a match, the experimenter said, "These are not the same shape" and flipped the cards back over. Children were required to make 4 of 5 matches. After that, the game was repeated one more time. Immediately following the second memory game, the experimenter administered the Dimensional Change Card Sort task to test cognitive flexibility. This was repeated for color—both matching and dissimilar | |
| 3–6 | Early Intensive Behavioral Training[59]: Each child's training was delivered for 15 mo by a team of trained preschool teachers, teaching assistants, and parents. Areas including as compliance skills, joint attention, language and communication skills, play and social skills, self-help skills, and preschool skills are targeted. Within these areas, more specific training is individually tailored to teach the children skills such as planning, sequencing, initiating, flexibility, organizing, and self-regulation | *Children* with autism spectrum disorder (ASD) |
| 3–4 | *Tools of the Mind* [60]: A 15-mo play-based, preschool and kindergarten curriculum that emphasizes self-control, language, and literacy skills. Children are taught by teachers to use a variety of cognitive tools, including language (to self and to others), to help regulate their behavior | *Children* in urban day cares |
| 2–4 | *Program Intensified habilitation:*[44] Group sessions take place in the rehabilitation unit in the hospital, where the children are given an individual training to strengthen motor, communication, and executive functions based on developmentally appropriate play-oriented interventions. Children and their parents live at the hospital for 1–2 wk and local professionals also participate for one or more days. During periods in between, although children are in their home settings, parents, and local professionals arrange the training | *Children* with cerebral palsy (CP) |

(continued on next page)

| Table 1 *(continued)* | | |
|---|---|---|
| **Age Range Studied (Y)** | **Intervention and Description** | **Target** |
| | based on the interventions agreed on in the group sessions. Executive functions are stimulated through role play, activities of daily life, and structured activities both in the child's preschool and at home. Lasts 1 y | |
| 2–5 (int) 9 (assess) | *Choline supplementation*[48] at 500 mg daily for 9 mo | *Children* exposed to alcohol in utero |
| 3–5 | Complete extracapsular tonsillectomy and adenoidectomy[61] | *Children* with mild or moderate obstructive sleep apnea |
| 2–6 | *CSRP:*[45–47] A 30-wk early childhood intervention to improve children's self-regulation and executive function through changing the classroom quality of Head Start centers by providing: (1) professional development to improve teacher behavior management strategies; (2) mental health consultant (MHC) classroom visits to assist teachers in implementing the behavioral management program; (3) MHC provision of stress reduction workshops for teachers; (4) MHC services targeted at 3–4 children per classroom identified as having especially severe emotional and behavioral issues | *Teachers* and *children* in Head Start |

1 session[28] to 2 years.[29,30] In some cases, EF is assessed immediately after the intervention[31]; in others EF is assessed 8[32,33] or even 10 years[34] following the intervention, which may have occurred in the neonatal period.[34]

Although 3-year-old children were included in the studies of these interventions, 3-year olds were most often the youngest study participants. Very few interventions have focused mostly on children aged younger than 3 years. Those include the Mediational Intervention for Sensitizing Caregivers,[31] Family Check-Up (FCU),[33,35] Infant Behavioral Assessment and Intervention Program (IBAIP),[36–38] Early responsive stimulation (RS),[29,30] Psychosocial stimulation,[39] Clinic-Based Intervention (CBIP) and Home-Based Intervention Programs (HBIP),[40] Preventative Care Program,[32] Supporting Play Exploration, and Early Developmental Intervention,[41] In-hospital Kangaroo Care,[34] START-Play,[42] In-hospital Music Intervention,[43] Program Intensified habilitation,[44] and the Chicago School Readiness Project (CSRP).[45–47] Most of these interventions target the parent or the parent–child dyad. A single pharmaceutical intervention trialed for EF in children exposed to alcohol in utero was choline supplementation.[48]

Although many of the children included in the trials were at high risk for developmental concerns, they were not necessarily NICU graduates, although many of them suffered neurodevelopmental and behavioral disorders more common in children with a history of prematurity such as ADHD, ASD, CP, and motor delay. Lejeune (2019),[43] Feldman (2014),[34] Dusing (2018),[62] Spittle (2016),[32] Koldewijn (2005,

**Table 2**
Outcomes of executive functioning interventions in children aged 0 to 3 y

| EF Construct | Studies Demonstrating Improvement with Intervention | Intervention | Studies Demonstrating Negative or no Difference after Intervention | Intervention |
|---|---|---|---|---|
| Attentional Control | Bierman et al,[55] 2008<br>Cohen et al,[57] 2018c<br>Feldman et al,[34] 2014 | Head Start Research-Based, Developmentally Informed (REDI)<br>Yoga<br>Kangaroo Care in the NICU | Boivin et al,[31] 2017<br>Walker et al,[39] 2010<br>Verkerk et al,[38] 2012<br>Tamm et al,[54] 2019<br>Spittle et al,[32] 2016 | Mediational Intervention for Sensitizing Caregivers<br>Psychosocial stimulation<br>IBAIP<br>Generating Attention, Inhibition, and Memory Intervention<br>Preventative Care Program |
| Impulse Control/Self-Regulation | Cassidy et al,[50] 2017<br>Hentges et al,[33] 2020<br>Koldewijn et al,[36,37] 2005, 2009<br>Obradović et al,[29,30] 2016, 2019<br>Somech et al,[52] 2012<br>Wu et al,[40] 2016<br>Healey et al,[53] 2019<br>Feldman et al,[34] 2014<br>Ford et al,[58] 2009<br>Raver et al,[45] 2011 | Circle of Security -Parenting<br>FCU<br>IBAIP<br>Early RS<br>Hitkashrut<br>CBIP and HBIP<br>Enhancing Neurobehavioral Gains with the Aid of Games and Exercise and Positive Parenting Program (Triple P)<br>Kangaroo Care in the NICU<br>Let's Play in Tandem<br>CSRP | Meijssen et al,[64] 2010<br>Verkerk et al,[38] 2012<br>Spittle et al,[32] 2016<br>Bierman et al,[55] 2008<br>Cohen et al,[57] 2018<br>Healey et al,[56] 2015<br>Lejeune et al,[43] 2019<br>Solomon et al,[60] 2018e<br>Wozniak et al,[48] 2020<br>Watts et al,[46] 2018<br>McCoy et al,[47] 2019 | IBAIP<br>IBAIP<br>Preventative Care Program<br>Head Start REDI<br>Yoga<br>Enhancing Neurobehavioral Gains with the Aid of Games and Exercise<br>Music Intervention in NICU<br>Tools of the Mind<br>Choline Supplementation<br>CSRP<br>CSRP |
| Working Memory | Obradović et al, 2019[30]<br>Wozniak et al, 2020[48] | Early RS<br>Choline Supplementation | Walker et al,[39] 2010<br>Spittle et al,[32] 2016<br>Bierman et al,[55] 2008<br>Healey et al,[56] 2015 | Psychosocial stimulation<br>Preventative Care Program<br>Head Start REDI<br>Enhancing Neurobehavioral Gains with the Aid of Games and Exercise |

| Domain | | | | |
|---|---|---|---|---|
| Cognitive Flexibility | Obradović et al, 2019[30]<br>Perone et al, 2019[28] | Early RS<br>Extra experience learning | Cassidy et al,[50] 2017<br>Bierman et al,[55] 2008<br>Cohen et al,[57] 2018 | Circle of Security -Parenting<br>Head Start REDI<br>Yoga |
| General Executive Behaviors | Tamm et al, 2019[54]<br>Skogli et al, 2020[59]<br>Sørensen et al, 2016[44]<br>Raver et al, 2011[45]<br>McCoy et al, 2019[47] | Generating Attention, Inhibition, and Memory Intervention<br>Early Intensive Behavioral Training<br>Program Intensified Habilitation<br>CSRP<br>CSRP | Boivin et al,[31] 2017<br>Aguilar et al, 2019[49]<br>Frisch et al,[51] 2020<br>Lunkenheimer et al,[35] 2008<br>Verkerk et al,[38] 2012[b]<br>Wozniak et al,[48] 2020<br>Waters et al,[61] 2020<br>Watts et al,[46] 2018 | Mediational Intervention for Sensitizing Caregivers<br>Internet-Based Interacting Together Every day: Recovery After Childhood TBI [I-InTERACT]) and I-InTERACT Express[a]<br>Parental Occupation Executive Training<br>FCU<br>IBAIP<br>Choline Supplementation<br>Complete extracapsular tonsillectomy and adenoidectomy<br>CSRP |
| Planning/Organization | Feldman et al,[34] 2014 | Kangaroo Care in the NICU | Spittle et al,[32] 2016 | Preventative Care Program |
| Problem Solving | Dusing et al,[62] 2018<br>Feldman et al,[34] 2014<br>Harbourne et al,[42] 2021[d] | Supporting Play Exploration, and Early Developmental Intervention<br>Kangaroo Care in the NICU<br>START-Play | – | |
| Initiation | – | – | – | – |
| Monitoring of Performance | – | – | – | – |

[a] No difference for either versus control group, but I-InTERACT Express significantly better than I-InTERACT.
[b] Positive interaction effect between extreme prematurity and EB.
[c] No significant difference after controlling for ADHD symptoms.
[d] Improvement only seen for children with severe motor deficits.
[e] Improvements only seen for children with baseline high levels of hyperactivity.

2009),[36,37] Verkerk (2012),[38] Walker(2010),[39] and Wu (2016)[40] studied the effects various interventions on preterm children.

## EFFECTS OF EXECUTIVE FUNCTIONING INTERVENTIONS ON CHILDREN 0 TO 3

Self-regulation was the EF construct most often studied in intervention trials in young children, followed by general executive behaviors. Executive behaviors are behaviors that require a range of EFs and are measured by questionnaires, rather than direct assessment.[63] The Circle of Security-Parenting, Let's Play in Tandem, Positive Parenting Program (Triple P), CBIP and HBIP, Hitkashrut, Early RS, and FCU interventions all demonstrated improvements in infant self-regulation. The IBAIP, Enhancing Neurobehavioral Gains with the Aid of Games and Exercise, and CSRP showed mixed results for child self-regulation. Although Kangaroo Care for 2 weeks in the NICU has been associated with better self-regulation, this was assessed roughly a decade after the neonatal intervention. Attentional control, working memory, mental/cognitive flexibility, and executive behaviors were rare targets of studied interventions, with very few interventions demonstrating benefit (**Table 2**). No studies assessed initiation or monitoring; few studies assessed problem solving and all demonstrated benefit; 2 studies assessed planning/organization, with mixed results (see **Table 2**).

Some populations at risk for EF deficits demonstrated improvements in various EF domains—particularly self-regulation—after the intervention. Positive results were often limited to those who were born at the earliest gestation and who had the most severe medical problems.

In a systematic review and meta-analysis of interventions for ADHD, Shephard and colleagues (2021)[65] found no evidence for improvements EF after interventions before age 5 in children diagnosed with ADHD, with the exception of working memory. Development of successful EF interventions for children 0 to 3 is of paramount importance because EF is critical to school performance and participation. Beginning interventions at this early age may allow early neuroplasticity to be leveraged to the benefit of high-risk children. Currently, there are few studies of EF interventions in this age range—the current interventions are highly variable. However, current studies do demonstrate some encouraging results. Further research is needed to develop feasible interventions that can be used in high-risk children. Should interventions prove efficacious in this age group, the consideration of context will be critical. Given that these intervention(s) should occur during the preschool years to maximize EF development by school age, integration of EF interventions into preschool/day-care programs could be considered so as not to unduly burden parents or create disparities between working parents and those who are at home and able to provide interventions. Consideration of various intervention environments should be a component of future research in this area.

## SUMMARY

Early EF skills are critical to the development of higher order cognitive skills and are developing when neuroplasticity peaks during the first 3 years of life.[66,67] Therefore, EF interventions should be designed for children aged younger than 3 years because the positive developmental effects could be far-reaching.

**Best practices**

*What is the current practice for executive function interventions in high-risk children from 0 to 3 years of age?*

Although high-risk children are at increased risk for EF deficits, currently there are no recommendations for targeted EF interventions before the age of 3. Currently, studied interventions are extremely heterogenous.

*What changes in current practice are likely to improve outcomes?*

- Creation of novel, feasible EF interventions for children at the youngest ages
- Longitudinal assessment of EF following the interventions with studies powered to assess those outcomes a priori
- Further assessment of the neuroanatomical and functional mechanisms that underlie EF development in high-risk children and intervention effects
- New EF targets for interventions

Bibliographic Source(s):

See article references

## CLINICS CARE POINTS

- Executive function can be assessed prior to the age of 3.
- Executive function formation is sequential and synergistic. Assessments and interventions must take this into account.
- The context wherein executive function interventions are provided should be considered when designing new interventions to ensure feasibility and equity.

## REFERENCES

1. Siffredi V, Liverani MC, Hüppi PS, et al. The effect of a mindfulness-based intervention on executive, behavioural and socio-emotional competencies in very preterm young adolescents. Sci Rep 2021;11(1):19876.
2. Anderson PJ, Reidy N. Assessing executive function in preschoolers. Neuropsychol Rev 2012;22(4):345–60.
3. Anderson PJ, Doyle LW. Cognitive and educational deficits in children born extremely preterm. Semin perinatology 2008;32(1):51–8.
4. Anderson P. Assessment and development of executive function (EF) during childhood. Child Neuropsychology 2002;8(2):71–82.
5. Diamond A. Executive functions. Annu Rev Psychol 2013;64:135.
6. Woodward LJ, Clark CAC, Pritchard VE, et al. Neonatal white matter abnormalities predict global executive function impairment in children born very preterm. Developmental Neuropsychol 2011;36(1):22.
7. Inder TE, Wells SJ, Mogridge NB, et al. Defining the nature of the cerebral abnormalities in the premature infant: a qualitative magnetic resonance imaging study. J Pediatr 2003;143(2):171–9.
8. Bock J, Rether K, Gröger N, et al. Perinatal programming of emotional brain circuits: an integrative view from systems to molecules. Front Neurosci 2014;8:11.
9. Bock J, Braun K. The impact of perinatal stress on the functional maturation of prefronto-cortical synaptic circuits: implications for the pathophysiology of ADHD? Prog Brain Res 2011;189:155–69.
10. Mayes LC. Arousal regulation, emotional flexibility, medial amygdala function, and the impact of early experience: comments on the paper of Lewis et al. Ann New York Acad Sci 2006;1094(1):178–92.

11. Blair C, Diamond A. Biological processes in prevention and intervention: the promotion of self-regulation as a means of preventing school failure. Development psychopathology 2008;20(3):899–911.
12. Goldsmith DF, Rogoff B. Mothers' and toddlers' coordinated joint focus of attention: variations with maternal dysphoric symptoms. Developmental Psychol 1997; 33(1):113.
13. Kochanska G, Murray K, Jacques TY, et al. Inhibitory control in young children and its role in emerging internalization. Child Development 1996;67(2): 490–507.
14. Kochanska G, Knaack A. Effortful control as a personality characteristic of young children: Antecedents, correlates, and consequences. J Personal 2003;71(6): 1087–112.
15. Lengua LJ, Honorado E, Bush NR. Contextual risk and parenting as predictors of effortful control and social competence in preschool children. J Appl Dev Psychol 2007;28(1):40–55.
16. Forcada-Guex M, Pierrehumbert B, Borghini A, et al. Early dyadic patterns of mother–infant interactions and outcomes of prematurity at 18 months. Pediatrics 2006;118(1):e107–14.
17. Blankenship TL, Slough MA, Calkins SD, et al. Attention and executive functioning in infancy: Links to childhood executive function and reading achievement. Developmental Sci 2019;22(6):e12824.
18. Garon N, Bryson SE, Smith IM. Executive function in preschoolers: a review using an integrative framework. Psychol Bull 2008;134(1):31–60.
19. Miyake A, Friedman NP, Emerson MJ, et al. The unity and diversity of executive functions and their contributions to complex "frontal lobe" tasks: a latent variable analysis. Cogn Psychol 2000;41(1):49–100.
20. Best JR, Miller PH. A developmental perspective on executive function. Child Development 2010;81(6):1641–60.
21. Mehsen V, Morag L, Chesta S, et al. Hot executive function assessment Instruments in preschool children: a systematic review. Int J Environ Res Public Health 2021;19(1):95.
22. Silva C, Sousa-Gomes V, Fávero M, et al. Assessment of preschool-age executive functions: a systematic review. Clin Psychol Psychotherapy 2022;29(4):1374–91.
23. Ortega FB, Mora-Gonzalez J, Cadenas-Sanchez C, et al. Effects of an exercise program on brain health outcomes for children with overweight or Obesity: the ActiveBrains randomized clinical trial. JAMA Netw open 2022;5(8):e2227893.
24. Li L, Zhang J, Cao M, et al. The effects of chronic physical activity interventions on executive functions in children aged 3-7 years: a meta-analysis. J Sci Med Sport 2020;23(10):949–54.
25. Liang X, Li R, Wong SHS, et al. The impact of exercise interventions concerning executive functions of children and adolescents with attention-deficit/hyperactive disorder: a systematic review and meta-analysis. Int J Behav Nutr Phys activity 2021;18(1):68.
26. Rodriguez-Gomez DA, Talero-Gutiérrez C. Effects of music training in executive function performance in children: a systematic review. Front Psychol 2022;13: 968144.
27. Ludyga S, Mücke M, Leuenberger R, et al. Behavioral and neurocognitive effects of judo training on working memory capacity in children with ADHD: a randomized controlled trial. NeuroImage Clin 2022;36:103156.
28. Perone S, Plebanek DJ, Lorenz MG, et al. Empirical tests of a brain-based model of executive function development. Child Development 2019;90(1):210–26.

29. Obradović J, Portilla XA, Ballard PJ. Biological Sensitivity to family income: Differential effects on early executive functioning. Child Development 2016;87(2): 374–84.

30. Obradović J, Finch JE, Portilla XA, et al. Early executive functioning in a global context: developmental continuity and family protective factors. Developmental Sci 2019;22(5):e12795.

31. Boivin MJ, Nakasujja N, Familiar I, et al. Effect of caregiver training on neurodevelopment of HIV-exposed uninfected children and caregiver mental health: a Ugandan cluster randomized controlled trial. J Dev Behav Pediatr JDBP 2017; 38(9):753.

32. Spittle AJ, Barton S, Treyvaud K, et al. School-age outcomes of early intervention for preterm infants and their parents: a randomized trial. Pediatrics 2016;138(6).

33. Hentges RF, Krug CMW, Shaw DS, et al. The long-term indirect effect of the early Family Check-Up intervention on adolescent internalizing and externalizing symptoms via inhibitory control. Development psychopathology 2020;32(4):1544–54.

34. Feldman R, Rosenthal Z, Eidelman AI. Maternal-preterm skin-to-skin contact enhances child physiologic organization and cognitive control across the first 10 years of life. Biol Psychiatry 2014;75(1):56–64.

35. Lunkenheimer ES, Dishion TJ, Shaw DS, et al. Collateral benefits of the Family Check-Up on early childhood school readiness: indirect effects of parents' positive behavior support. Developmental Psychol 2008;44(6):1737.

36. Koldewijn K, Wolf M-J, Van Wassenaer A, et al. The Infant Behavioral Assessment and Intervention Program to support preterm infants after hospital discharge: a pilot study. Developmental Med child Neurol 2005;47(2):105–12.

37. Koldewijn K, Wolf M-J, van Wassenaer A, et al. The infant behavioral assessment and intervention program for very low birth weight infants at 6 months corrected age. J Pediatr 2009;154(1):33–8, e32.

38. Verkerk G, Jeukens-Visser M, Houtzager B, et al. The infant behavioral assessment and intervention program in very low birth weight infants; outcome on executive functioning, behaviour and cognition at preschool age. Early Hum Dev 2012;88(8):699–705.

39. Walker SP, Chang SM, Younger N, et al. The effect of psychosocial stimulation on cognition and behaviour at 6 years in a cohort of term, low-birthweight Jamaican children. Dev Med Child Neurol 2010;52(7):e148–54.

40. Wu YC, Hsieh WS, Hsu CH, et al. Intervention effects on emotion regulation in preterm infants with very low birth weight: a randomize controlled trial. Res Dev disabilities 2016;48:1–12.

41. Dusing SC. Postural variability and sensorimotor development in infancy. Dev Med Child Neurol 2016;58(Suppl 4):17–21.

42. Harbourne RT, Dusing SC, Lobo MA, et al. START-play physical therapy intervention impacts motor and cognitive outcomes in infants with neuromotor disorders: a multisite randomized clinical trial. Phys Ther 2021;101(2):pzaa232.

43. Lejeune F, Lordier L, Pittet MP, et al. Effects of an early postnatal music intervention on cognitive and emotional development in preterm children at 12 and 24 months: preliminary findings. Front Psychol 2019;10:494.

44. Sørensen K, Liverød JR, Lerdal B, et al. Executive functions in preschool children with cerebral palsy–Assessment and early intervention–A pilot study. Developmental Neurorehabil 2016;19(2):111–6.

45. Raver CC, Jones SM, Li-Grining C, et al. CSRP's impact on low-income preschoolers' preacademic skills: self-regulation as a mediating mechanism. Child Development 2011;82(1):362–78.

46. Watts TW, Gandhi J, Ibrahim DA, et al. The Chicago School Readiness Project: Examining the long-term impacts of an early childhood intervention. PloS one 2018;13(7):e0200144.

47. McCoy DC, Gonzalez K, Jones S. Preschool self-regulation and preacademic skills as Mediators of the long-term impacts of an early intervention. Child Development 2019;90(5):1544–58.

48. Wozniak JR, Fink BA, Fuglestad AJ, et al. Four-year follow-up of a randomized controlled trial of choline for neurodevelopment in fetal alcohol spectrum disorder. J Neurodev Disord 2020;12(1):9.

49. Aguilar JM, Cassedy AE, Shultz EL, et al. A Comparison of 2 online parent skills training interventions for early childhood brain injury: improvements in internalizing and executive function behaviors. J head Trauma Rehabil 2019;34(2): 65–76.

50. Cassidy J, Brett BE, Gross JT, et al. Circle of Security-parenting: a randomized controlled trial in Head Start. Development psychopathology 2017;29(2):651–73.

51. Frisch C, Tirosh E, Rosenblum S. Parental occupation executive training (POET): an efficient innovative intervention for young children with attention deficit hyperactive disorder. Phys Occup Ther In Pediatr 2020;40(1):47–61.

52. Somech LY, Elizur Y. Promoting self-regulation and cooperation in prekindergarten children with conduct problems: a randomized controlled trial. J Am Acad Child Adolesc Psychiatry 2012;51(4):412–22.

53. Healey D, Healey M. Randomized controlled trial comparing the effectiveness of structured-play (ENGAGE) and behavior management (TRIPLE P) in reducing problem behaviors in preschoolers. Scientific Rep 2019;9(1):1–9.

54. Tamm L, Epstein JN, Loren REA, et al. Generating attention, inhibition, and memory: a pilot randomized trial for preschoolers with executive functioning deficits. J Clin child Adolesc Psychol 2019;48(sup1):S131–45.

55. Bierman KL, Nix RL, Greenberg MT, et al. Executive functions and school readiness intervention: impact, moderation, and mediation in the Head Start REDI program. Development psychopathology 2008;20(3):821–43.

56. Healey DM, Halperin JM. Enhancing Neurobehavioral Gains with the Aid of Games and Exercise (ENGAGE): Initial open trial of a novel early intervention fostering the development of preschoolers' self-regulation. Child Neuropsychol 2015;21(4):465–80.

57. Cohen SCL, Harvey DJ, Shields RH, et al. Effects of Yoga on attention, Impulsivity, and hyperactivity in preschool-aged children with attention-deficit hyperactivity disorder symptoms. J Dev Behav Pediatr 2018;39(3):200–9.

58. Ford RM, McDougall SJ, Evans D. Parent-delivered compensatory education for children at risk of educational failure: Improving the academic and self-regulatory skills of a Sure Start preschool sample. Br J Psychol 2009;100(4):773–97.

59. Skogli EW, Andersen PN, Isaksen J. An exploratory study of executive function development in children with autism, after receiving early intensive behavioral training. Developmental Neurorehabil 2020;23(7):439–47.

60. Solomon T, Plamondon A, O'Hara A, et al. A cluster randomized-controlled trial of the impact of the Tools of the Mind curriculum on self-regulation in Canadian preschoolers. Front Psychol 2018;8:2366.

61. Waters KA, Chawla J, Harris MA, et al. Cognition after early Tonsillectomy for Mild OSA. Pediatrics 2020;145(2).

62. Dusing SC, Tripathi T, Marcinowski EC, et al. Supporting play exploration and early developmental intervention versus usual care to enhance development

outcomes during the transition from the neonatal intensive care unit to home: a pilot randomized controlled trial. BMC Pediatr 2018;18(1):1–12.
63. Vugs B, Hendriks M, Cuperus J, et al. Working memory performance and executive function behaviors in young children with SLI. Res Dev disabilities 2014; 35(1):62–74.
64. Meijssen D, Wolf MJ, Koldewijn K, et al. The effect of the Infant Behavioral Assessment and Intervention Program on mother–infant interaction after very preterm birth. J Child Psychol Psychiatry 2010;51(11):1287–95.
65. Shephard E, Zuccolo PF, Idrees I, et al. Systematic review and meta-analysis: the science of early-life precursors and interventions for attention-deficit/hyperactivity disorder. J Am Acad Child Adolesc Psychiatry 2021;61(2):187–226.
66. Heckman JJ. Skill formation and the economics of investing in disadvantaged children. Science 2006;312(5782):1900–2.
67. DeMaster D, Bick J, Johnson U, et al. Nurturing the preterm infant brain: leveraging neuroplasticity to improve neurobehavioral outcomes. Pediatr Res 2019;85(2):166–75.

# Interventions for Motor Disorders in High-Risk Neonates

Lynda McNamara, BPhty (Hons)[a],
Catherine Morgan, PhD, BAppSc (Phty)[b],
Iona Novak, PhD, MSc (Hons), BAppSc OT[b,*]

## KEYWORDS

- High-risk infants • Motor interventions • Preterm • Cerebral palsy • Degenerative
- Physical therapy • Occupational therapy

## KEY POINTS

- Infants at high risk of motor impairments constitute three different subpopulations: (1) motor delay, (2) nondegenerative motor impairment, and (3) degenerative.
- For infants with motor delay consider coaching; developmental care; NIDCAP; generic or specific motor training; hydrotherapy; treadmill training for improving motor skills.
- For infants with motor impairment (cerebral palsy) consider bimanual training, CIMT, environmental enrichment, and task-specific motor training (eg, GAME); standing frames, exoskeletons, and powered mobility are appropriate for non-weightbearing infants.
- For infants with a degenerative physical disability, balance motor skills advancement (such as treadmill training for walking) versus preparation for degeneration, with accommodations (eg, powered wheelchairs).

## INTRODUCTION

The brain undergoes substantial changes in childhood, both in anatomic structure and connectivity[1]. Brain development arises from complex interactions between physiologic conditions and social and physical environments, all modulated by gene transcription and expression[2]. Infants exposed to genetic, environmental, inflammatory, metabolic, and psychosocial risk factors during either pregnancy, delivery, or immediately after birth are known as high-risk infants[3,4]. Prematurity, asphyxia, and metabolic pathways pose some of the greatest risks for brain injury

[a] The Children's Hospital Westmead Clinical School, The University of Sydney, Locked Bag 4001, Westmead, Sydney, NSW 2145, Australia; [b] Cerebral Palsy Alliance Research Institute, Specialty of Child and Adolescent Health, Sydney Medical School, The University of Sydney, PO Box 171, Forestville, Sydney, NSW 2006, Australia
* Corresponding author. PO Box 171, Forestville NSW 2087.
*E-mail addresses:* iona.novak@sydney.edu.au; inovak@cerebralpalsy.org.au

Clin Perinatol 50 (2023) 121–155
https://doi.org/10.1016/j.clp.2022.11.002
0095-5108/23/© 2022 Elsevier Inc. All rights reserved.
**perinatology.theclinics.com**

and resultant life-long motor disability[5,6]. Survival following preterm birth or high-risk term born sequalae today exceeds 95% in high-income contexts, following intense research, clinical, and public health efforts[5]. These are the infants cared for in High-Risk Infant Follow-Up programs (HRIF). Their mission is increasingly focused on the reduction of morbidity associated with childhood disabilities including autism spectrum disorder (ASD), congenital heart disease (CHD), cerebral palsy (CP), developmental coordination disorder (DCD), epilepsy, intellectual disability, and stroke. The range and severity of disability consequences depends on the intensity, duration, location, size, and maturity of the brain malformations or brain region damaged affecting connectivity[5]. The developing brain is extremely vulnerable to injury because of periods of unique susceptibility; the complexity of motor ontogenesis, and the adaptive responses to genetic and environmental processes[1,2]. Inequity also has a profound impact on infant's health and development[4,7]. Thus, early detection of disability is a major priority of HRIF to harness and direct plasticity through early intervention and environmental enrichment[6,8]. In addition, many adult diseases have their origins in early childhood[5]. Lifelong motor disabilities have a major effect on surviving infants, their families, and societal costs[5,9].

## CONSIDERATIONS

Early intervention aims to prevent, lessen, or enrich motor, cognitive, sensory, and social impairments in high-risk infants disadvantaged by biological, social, or environmental risk factors[2,4,10]. In this review, we take a special focus on evidence-based early interventions that treat motor abnormalities in high-risk infants. In a broad sense, three populations of high-risk infants may benefit from early motor interventions, and the interventions for these three populations differ in purpose, specificity, type, and dose (**Fig. 1**).

Interventions to advance the functioning of the motor system, for infants with delayed or non-degenerative motor impairments, seek to harness neuroplasticity and adaptation to the environment during the "critical periods" of motor development[1]. Neuroplasticity directs the excitation generated by responses to experiences, and modifies neuronal circuitry so as to fine-tune the infant's actions, thoughts, and behaviors[1]. Whereas accommodations, also known as compensations, seek to fully

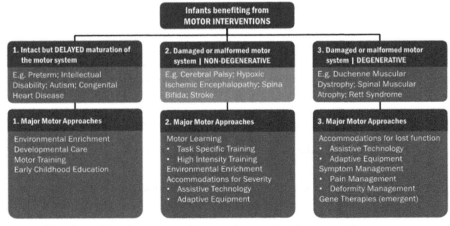

**Fig. 1.** Infants benefiting from motor interventions and major approaches.

include the infant with a physical disability, without treating the infant, but instead by adapting the task or environment, usually through technology or adaptive equipment. Accommodations (such as powered wheelchairs) are appropriate for infants with degenerative conditions, but also for infants with severe non-degenerative physical disabilities not predicted to walk.

## NATURE OF THE PROBLEM

Health care professionals are faced with challenges in answering important parent questions about the risk of disability in high-risk infants and providing timely evidence-based care. Parents want honest and open communication about their child's risk profile, including prognosis and diagnosis-specific interventions and support. The historical "wait and see" approach can delay or deny opportunities during the most critical neuroplastic window[8]. A fundamental change in practice is required to determine exactly "what an infant is at risk of?" rather than an infant is "at risk."

Advances in genetic testing, sensitive biomarkers, and improvements in neuroimaging have paved the way for a fundamental shift toward a new era of evidence-informed early prognostication to differentiate between delayed or non-degenerative motor impairments and degenerative conditions. Although the specification of risk profiles early in life is a complex process, complicated by rapid changes in development, low motor repertoire, and emerging cognitive and preverbal skills, accurate tests exist with predictive validity to enable early prediction of disability. Examples of delayed maturation of the early motor system can be seen in infants with ASD from 0 to 6 months corrected age[11]. Further discussion of the similarity of ASD and preterm infant motor delays can be found in this issue (Mendez and colleagues). Clinical guidelines for early detection of ASD recommend the most accurate ASD-specific tools to predict the risk of ASD[12,13]. Using CP as an example of non-degenerative motor impairment, an accurate clinical diagnosis of CP can be made before 6-month corrected age using a combination of (1) medical history; (2) term-age MRI indicating abnormality in motor pathways; (3) Prechtl's General Movement Assessment indicating "absent fidgety" or reduced quality of spontaneous movements; and (4) a standardized Hammersmith Infant Neurologic Examination score <57 indicating neurologic damage to motor domains[8].

Early prediction of subpopulation or diagnosis may support parents and clinicians on a pathway toward evidence-based diagnostic-specific interventions as opposed to the historical generic "early intervention" referral to state services. Parents may benefit from individualized support for their infant and family, and education on their fundamental role in their child's development. Early engagement of parents is key to achieving the repetition and intensity of child-active training in infancy required to drive neuroplasticity, in particular as infants' have developmental endurance limitations and high sleep requirements[10,14].

## AIMS

This review aimed to (1) clarify key concepts in the literature; (2) identify and map the best-available evidence for effective motor interventions for infants at high-risk of a motor impairment across three different populations of delayed motor maturation; non-degenerative motor impairment; and degenerative motor impairment; (3) examine current research in the topic area; and (4) to identify and analyze knowledge gaps.

## METHODOLOGY

A scoping review was conducted to address the study's aims[15]. An explicit, transparent, peer-reviewed search strategy was used using the following PICOs search terms: Population = High-risk infants OR at-risk infants OR cerebral palsy OR preterm OR encephalopathy OR Down syndrome OR autism spectrum disorder OR spinal muscular atrophy OR Rett syndrome; Intervention = Motor intervention OR motor training OR physiotherapy/physical therapy OR occupational therapy; Comparison = not specified, all accepted; Outcome = motor; Study Design = Systematic Review OR Randomized Controlled Trial (RCT) (if published after the systematic review) OR Clinical Practice Guidelines. The search was limited to humans aged 0 to 2 years and published from 2013 onwards (ie, in the last decade given the substantive changes in intervention approaches over time). Databases searched included MEDLINE, Cochrane, CINAHL, supplemented by hand searching. The search yield is summarized in a flow diagram (**Fig. 2**). Forty-one studies were included in this review. Excluded studies are summarized in Supplemental Table S1.

Data were extracted to a standardized extraction form. Quality and strength of recommendations were assessed using Grading of Recommendations Assessment, Development, and Evaluation (GRADE) evidence to decision framework[16]. We used GRADE terminology to make recommendations. "We recommend" denotes strong recommendations supported by moderate-high quality evidence, and "we suggest" denotes conditional recommendations supported by very low-low quality evidence or moderate quality evidence with small sample sizes. We also applied the Evidence Alert Traffic Light System[17] to color-code the evidence, where green means effective (correlating to strong for recommendations), red means ineffective (correlating to strong against recommendations), and yellow means more research is needed to

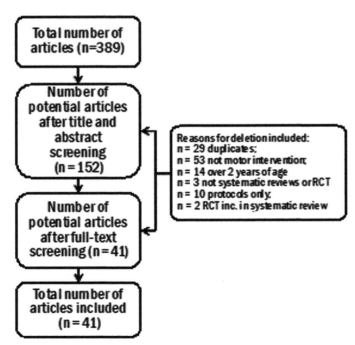

**Fig. 2.** Flow diagram.

increase our confidence in the estimate of effect and could be either for or against the intervention (correlating to conditional for or against recommendations).

## KEY CONCEPTS ABOUT THERAPEUTIC OPTIONS

Parent education and parent coaching are an essential component of care for infants at high-risk of motor impairment. Parent education can assist parents to learn knowledge about their child's condition and self-management techniques. Parent coaching can be used to assist parent to solve problems, and to practice new ways of interacting with and supporting their child. Both approaches seek to empower parents and are supported by evidence[18,19]. Health professionals must draw on a range of evidence-based knowledge to facilitate parental understanding of the "what, why, how, and when" of therapeutic options[18,19].

### What?

Motor learning approaches using active infant-initiated training of skills and are superior for improving motor function compared with passive hands-on therapy[20,21]. An understanding of this essential catalyst of experience-dependent activity is fundamental for effective motor interventions. In addition, repetition of task-specific practice induces neuroplasticity more than generic therapy techniques[22]. For infants, this means real-life practice of meaningful skills such as active reaching for a desired toy rather than passively mobilizing an infant to guide a movement pattern desired by a therapist.

### Why?

Information-seeking behavior on the part of parents is a necessary process on the pathway to acceptance responses after receiving news of a diagnosis of disability[18]. Parents are challenged with choosing therapy options for their infant, in particular when searching through web-based information sources. Knowledge of these key concepts of child-generated movements, task-specific practice, and repetition that induce neuroplasticity and drive motor function can shine a light on effective training approaches and enhance decision-making skills of parents. In addition, early classification of subpopulation and prediction of future outcomes further guides parents to seek the most beneficial tailored interventions to focus on early in their child's life. For example, multiple markers with high accuracy for detecting CP motor severity, type, and topography are available for infants under 12 months of age to answer parent questions regarding the spectrum of CP[8]. An early understanding of severity (ambulant vs nonambulant CP) can assist parents with developing a plan specific for their child, in particular for more severe forms of CP where early accommodations are necessary for mobility and to avoid secondary complications. Understanding of type and topography can guide targeted task-specific interventions specific for brain injury (for example, unilateral or asymmetrical brain injury) rather than generic or umbrella approaches to normalize movement patterns[21]. Parents play a crucial role in the enrichment of their child's motor learning environment and early goal setting and coaching to enhance engagement is essential. This also involves providing parents with high-quality information sources outlining when there is strong evidence against an intervention, for example, passive movement[20,21].

### How?

Intrinsic motivation is key to practicing a new task as infants gain enjoyment through active repetitive practice[22] further driving neuroplastic change. In older children, high intensity of practice is a significant factor in inducing functional change, with recommendations of 90-h of child-active training within a 6-week period[23]. In infants, lower doses are used to accommodate sleep routines, endurance, and optimize bonding, but the paradigm is toward high intensity by creating regular short bursts of practice throughout the day at the right challenge level to the infant's arousal level. Optimizing parent-infant interactions, daily routines and awake play environments contextualized for their individual infant and family is, therefore, critical for infants with motor impairment[10]. Therapeutic options should aim to harness these drivers of neuroplasticity in addition to coaching parents toward environmental enrichment specific to their infant's goals[10].

## When to Adapt?

Targeted interventions are indicated for severe forms of motor impairment or for degenerative conditions. An early understanding of assistive technologies such as early switch use, powered mobility, and accommodations through equipment can offer pathways of independent self-mobility, learning, and play. Assistive devices (such as for walking and communication) and equipment can assist with conserving energy and time and improve safety (such as for feeding activities). In addition, early accommodations and equipment can reduce caregiver burden for activities of daily living and manual handling.

## CURRENT BEST-AVAILABLE EVIDENCE

Current best-avialable evidence is summarised in **Table 1**.

## CURRENT GUIDELINES AND RECOMMENDATIONS

Comprehensive clinical guidelines regarding motor interventions in the majority of high-risk subpopulations are limited. Although rehabilitation interventions are for the most part regarded as low risk from a safety perspective, there are almost no investigations into safety or the impact on the family and their health. An example of an exception is CIMT for infants, where it has been shown that short-duration, low-dose intervention wearing a soft constraint has no negative effects on the dominant hand[21]. In addition, the GRADE methodology integrally involves consumers on the expert panel to determine the strength of the recommendations. Some of the systematic reviews and clinical practice guidelines cited within this review had included consumers during the GRADE panel process, but not all. Given this was an academic paper not a clinical practice guideline, we also did not have consumers on the panel. Therefore, all conclusions must be interpreted with this limitation in mind.

Systematic reviews in preterm groups variably demonstrate positive effects of early intervention strategies on motor outcomes; however, the size of the effect varies significantly between reviews[30,39]. The interventions described vary markedly in content and age of initiation. Consequently, no strong recommendations for practice have been made in terms of the content of early motor-focused intervention to address delays. Similarly, best practice recommendations for early intervention in ASD focus on cognition, communication, behavior, and social skills but are yet to identify key ingredients to minimize motor delays in these children[13]. Guidelines for infants with CHD focus on monitoring standards but lack specific guidance on early intervention content to optimize motor skill acquisition[28]. Programs have been developed but not rigorously tested[57]. For infants with Down syndrome, treadmill training has a strong recommendation for improving mobility outcomes including age at the onset of walking.

**Table 1**
Best available evidence results

| Citation | Method | Population | n | Intervention | Results | Grade |
|---|---|---|---|---|---|---|
| Subpopulation 1: intact but delayed maturation of the motor system | | | | | | |
| Aita et al.[24] 2021 | Systematic review of 12 studies | Preterm | 901 | NIDCAP Physical therapy | NIDCAP conferred superior results to usual care for improvements in the motor system short-term [−1.04; 95%CI −1.58 to −0.50] No difference between hydrotherapy and passive range of motion or a combination of both (Moyer-Mileur protocol). Note: Low statistical power | ○○⊕⊕ Low–very low quality for NIDCAP |
| Anderson et al.[25] 2020 | Review, included 2 motor studies | Preterm | N/A | Developmental care NIDCAP | Most interventions targeted general development, only two trials targeted advancing motor skills. Note: Low statistical power  NIDCAP conferred small short-term superior results to usual care for improvements in the motor system short-term [0.79SD better off]. | ○○⊕⊕ Low quality for developmental care ○○⊕⊕ Low quality for NIDCAP |
| Angulo-Barroso et al.[26] 2013 | RCT | Preterm | 28 | Treadmill training | Treadmill training conferred superior results to usual care for improvements in stepping, but there were no differences between groups for onset of walking. Note: Low statistical power | ○○⊕⊕ Low quality for treadmill training |

(continued on next page)

**Table 1**
*(continued)*

| Citation | Method | Population | n | Intervention | Results | Grade |
|---|---|---|---|---|---|---|
| Cabrera-Martos et al.[27] 2021 | Systematic review of 6 studies | Non-synostotic positional head deformities | 364 | Stretching Motor stimulation Manual therapy BabyDorm pillow | Physical therapy (including stretching, motor stimulation, and manual therapy) and helmets conferred equal improvements in cranial asymmetry and motor development. Pillows conferred superior gains. Note: Low statistical power. Although pillows appeared effective, they are contraindicated for preventing SIDS. | ○○⊕⊕ Low quality for stretching, motor stimulation, manual therapy, and BabyDorm Pillow |
| Cassidy et al.[28] 2021 | Clinical practice guideline | Congenital heart disease | N/A | Developmental care | No data existed specific to the congenital heart disease population and thus no recommendations were made. | ○○○⊕ Very low quality |
| Harbourne et al.[29] 2021 | RCT | Motor delay | 134 | START-play (includes motor-based problem solving; dynamic low support in sitting; cognitive and social input) | For infants with significant motor delay, START-Play conferred superior short-term results compared with usual care, for improvements in reaching, problem-solving, cognitive, and fine motor skills No difference between START-Play and usual care for improving motor skills in infants with mild motor delay | ○○⊕⊕ Low quality for START-Play |
| Hughes et al.[30] 2016 | Systematic review of 36 studies | Preterm | 3484 | Motor interventions (including interactions; | Motor intervention conferred superior gains to usual care at 3 mo [1.37; 95%CI 0.48–2.27], | ○○○⊕ Moderate quality for |

| Study | Design | Population | N | Intervention | Findings | Quality |
|---|---|---|---|---|---|---|
| | | | | handling and positioning; fine and gross motor activities) | 6 mo [0.34; 95%CI 0.11–0.57], 12 mo [0.73; 95%CI 0.20–1.26], and 24 mo [0.28; 95%CI 0.07–0.49], for improving motor skills but the size of the benefits declined over time. At 3 mo, there were large effects from motor-specific interventions [2.00; 95%CI 0.28–3.72] but not from generic interventions [0.33; 95%CI −0.03 to −0.69]. | motor specific interventions |
| Kaplan et al.[31] 2018 | Clinical practice guideline | Torticollis | N/A | PROM & AROM Symmetric movement | Passive and active range of motion of the neck, plus training in symmetric movement produces superior gains to usual care for improving neck symmetry. | ◯◯◯⊕ Moderate quality for PROM, AROM, and Symmetric Movement |
| Khurana et al.[32] 2020 | Systematic review of 15 studies | Preterm | 1268 | Parent-delivered motor intervention Postural control intervention Developmental care | Parent-delivered motor intervention conferred superior gains to usual care for improvements is motor skills short-term and possibly long-term. Therapist delivered postural control intervention conferred superior gains to usual care for improvements is motor skills short-term. | ◯◯◯⊕ Moderate quality for Parent delivered motor interventions ◯◯◯⊕ Moderate quality for postural control interventions |
| McCarty et al.[33] 2019 | Clinical practice guideline | Neonatal abstinence syndrome | N/A | Developmental care Swaddling hydrotherapy | Hydrotherapy, swaddling and developmental care appeared to reduce stress and withdrawal pain and may contribute to motor skills | ◯◯◯⊕ Very low quality for developmental care, hydrotherapy, swaddling |

(continued on next page)

**Table 1**
*(continued)*

| Citation | Method | Population | n | Intervention | Results | Grade |
|---|---|---|---|---|---|---|
| Novak et al.[34] 2019 | Systematic review of 129 studies | Preterm | N/A | Developmental care | Developmental Care with a focus on motor intervention conferred superior gains to usual care for improving motor skills short-term | ○○○⊕ Moderate quality for developmental care |
| Ohlsson et al.[35] 2013 | Systematic review of 18 studies | High-risk infants | 627 | NIDCAP | NIDCAP did not reduce rates of death or major disability [RR0.89; 95%CI 0.61–1.29], nor disability-free survival [0.97; 95%CI 0.69–1.35] | ○○○⊕ Moderate quality for NIDCAP |
| Paleg et al.[36] 2018 | Systematic review of 31 studies | Hypotonia (Down syndrome, noonan syndrome, rett syndrome) | 585 | Orthotics Treadmill training | Treadmill training appeared to accelerate the development of walking skills for infants with Down syndrome Orthoses appear to improve foot alignment in ambulatory children with hypotonia | ○○○⊕ Moderate quality in Down syndrome for treadmill training ○⊕⊕⊕ Very low quality in other syndromes for treadmill training & orthotics |
| Poole et al.[37] 2019 | Systematic review of 7 studies | Torticollis | 464 | Stretching | Stretching conferred superior gains to usual care for head ROM | ○○⊕⊕ Low quality for stretching |
| Soleimani et al.[38] 2020 | Systematic review of 21 studies | Preterm | 1200 | Developmental care | Developmental care conferred superior gains to usual care at 12 mo in psychomotor development [0.33; 95%CI 0.07–0.58] | ⊕⊕⊕⊕ High quality for developmental care |

| | | | | | | |
|---|---|---|---|---|---|---|
| Spittle et al.[39] 2015 | Systematic review of n = 16 studies | Preterm | 2379 | Motor intervention + parent education | There was little evidence of an effect of early intervention on motor outcomes in the short, medium or long-term [Superseded by Hughes & Soleimani]NOTE: Interventions that target the infant and parent dyad produce superior outcomes to treating just the infant or parent alone | ○○⊕⊕ Low quality for motor for motor intervention developmental care |
| Tanner et al.[40] 2020 | Systematic review of 56 studies (19 in EI) | At-risk | N/A | General EI NIDCAP coaching | General EI conferred superior gains to usual care for improvement in motor skills. NIDCAP intervention conferred superior gains to usual care for improvement in motor skills short-term. Coaching conferred superior gains to usual care for improvement in motor skills. | ○○○⊕ Moderate quality for EI & NIDCAP ○○⊕⊕ Low quality for coaching |
| Valentin-Gudiol et al.[41] 2017 | Systematic Review of 7 studies | At-risk (including Down syndrome, develop-mental delay) | 175 | Treadmill training | In infants with Down syndrome, treadmill training conferred superior gains to usual care for accelerating walking onset [MD -4.00, 95% CI -6.96 to − 1.04] In infants with developmental delay, treadmill training did not confer superior gains to usual care for walking onset [MD 0.60; 95%CI -2.34–1.14] | ⊕⊕⊕⊕ High quality for treadmill training in Down syndrome |
| Zwaigen-baum et al.[13] 2015 | Clinical practice guideline | Autism spectrum disorder | N/A | No motor recommendations made | | |

Subpopulation 2: damaged or malformed motor system non-degenerative

(continued on next page)

**Table 1**
*(continued)*

| Citation | Method | Population | n | Intervention | Results | Grade |
|---|---|---|---|---|---|---|
| Baker et al.[42] 2022 | Systematic review of 11 studies | Cerebral palsy | 363 | Task-specific motor training CIMT | Task-specific motor training conferred superior gains to usual care for improving motor function [0.41; 95%CI 0.05–0.78] CIMT may be more effective than bimanual play or massage for improving hand function in the hemiplegic hand [0.59; 95% CI −0.18–1.37] Note: CI crosses line of no effect, thus this is not likely to be an accurate interpretation of study findings High-intensity treadmill training was no more effective than low-intensity for improving walking | ⊘⊕⊕⊕ Very low quality for task-specific training |
| Basu et al.[43] 2018 | Feasibility trial | Stroke | 13 | eTIPS motor training | Early motor training in infants with stroke is feasible to conduct and acceptable to parents. NOTE: More research needed to determine efficacy | ⊘⊕⊕⊕ Very low quality for eTIPS |
| Bunge et al.[44] 2021 | Systematic review of 13 studies | Cerebral palsy | 82 | Powered lower limb exoskeletons | Exoskeletons may promote walking skills and walking speed, but the effects on energy expenditure are unclear | ⊘⊘⊕⊕ Low quality for walking |
| Case Smith et al.[45] 2013 | Systematic review of 24 studies | Cerebral palsy | | Superseded by Damiano et al 2021; Morgan et al. 2016; and Novak et al 2019 | | |
| Damiano et al.[46] 2021 | Systematic review of 3 systematic | Cerebral palsy | N/A | Environmental enrichment | Environmental enrichment and activity-based approaches appeared to produce gains in | ⊘⊘⊘⊕ Moderate quality for environmental |

| | | | | Intervention | Findings | Quality |
|---|---|---|---|---|---|---|
| | reviews of 46 studies | | | CIMT GAME | motor development with moderate effect sizes. CIMT appeared to confer large effect sizes, but was not superior to intense bimanual training or occupational therapy. GAME intervention initiated before 5 mo of age was superior to equally intense standard care | enrichment ◯◯⊕⊕ Low quality for CIMT ◯◯⊕⊕ Low quality for GAME |
| Dionisio et al.[47] 2022 | Scoping review of 8 studies | Cerebral palsy | 148 | CIMT | CIMT appeared to confer improved hand use of the hemiplegic hand | ◯◯◯⊕ Low quality for CIMT |
| Inamdar et al.[48] 2022 | Systematic review of 12 studies | Cerebral palsy | 460 | Physical therapy (including developmental care; COPCA; task-orientated; context focused; NDT; kinesio-tape) | Physical Therapy appeared to confer improvements in sitting skills [0.78; 95%CI -.51, 2.07] Note: CI crosses line of no effect. Kinesio-taping may be an effective adjunct to physical therapy to improve sitting skills. Task-specific, intensive, and child-initiated intervention components may be effective for improving sitting skills | ◯◯◯⊕ Low quality for physical therapy inclusive of kinesio-taping or task-specific training |
| Khamis et al.[49] 2020 | Systematic review of 5 studies | Cerebral palsy | 208 | Motor learning feeding interventions | Motor learning feeding interventions may improve feeding skills. Note: Most studies also included some compensatory strategies, which are not compatible with a training approach | ◯◯◯⊕ Very low quality for motor learning feeding interventions |
| Mailleux et al.[50] 2021 | Systematic review of 3 studies | Cerebral palsy, unilateral | 88 | CIMT Bimanual training | CIMT is effective and safe for improving upper limb function. Bimanual Training was found to be equally effective to CIMT in one study | ◯◯◯⊕ Low quality for CIMT |

(continued on next page)

**Table 1**
(*continued*)

| Citation | Method | Population | n | Intervention | Results | Grade |
|---|---|---|---|---|---|---|
| Maitre et al 2020 [51] | RCT | Cerebral palsy, unilateral or asymmet-rical | 73 | Bimanual Training + CIMT + motor training + sensory-motor training + parent education | A multi-component approach conferred superior gains to bimanual training alone for improvements in smoothness of reach and unimanual fine motor skills | ○○⊕⊕ Low quality for multi-component |
| Morgan et al.[10] 2013 | Systematic review of 7 studies | Cerebral palsy | 150 | Environmental enrichment | Environmental Enrichment intervention conferred superior gains to usual care for improvement in motor skills [0.39; 95%CI 0.05–0.72] | ○○○⊕ Moderate quality for Environmental Enrichment |
| Morgan et al.[21] 2021 | Clinical practice guideline based on systematic review | Cerebral palsy | N/A | Early intervention Task-specific motor training Environmental enrichment NDT CIMT Bimanual training | Early intervention that includes child-initiated movement, targeted motor training activities, and task-specific and context-specific exercises confers superior gains to NDT for producing improvements in motor skills  CIMT and Bimanual Training confer equal results for improving upper limb function in unilateral cerebral palsy | ○○○⊕ Moderate quality for early intervention  ○○○⊕ Moderate quality for task-specific and environment enrichment  ○○○⊕ Moderate quality against NDT  ○○⊕⊕ Low quality for CIMT or Bimanual |

| Source | Study type | Population | N | Interventions | Findings | Quality |
|---|---|---|---|---|---|---|
| Morgan et al.[14] 2016 | Systematic review of 34 studies | Cerebral palsy | 509 | NDT; Task-specific training; environmental enrichment | The body of literature evaluating motor interventions was sparse. NDT was the most common intervention studied. Most studies showed no benefit over usual care for improving motor skills. Child-initiated movement, environment modification/enrichment, and task-specific training were the only interventions to confer gains in motor skills compared with usual care [Effect size >0.7] | ○○○⊕ Low quality for task-specific training |
| Novak et al.[8] 2017 | Clinical practice guideline based on systematic review | Cerebral palsy | Superseded by Morgan et al 2021 | | | |
| Novak et al.[34] 2013 | Systematic review | Cerebral palsy | Superseded by Novak et al 2020 | | | |
| Novak et al.[52] 2020 | Systematic review of systematic reviews of 247 studies | Cerebral palsy | N/A | CIMT; Bimanual training; Motor training GAME; General stimulation; COPCA; Conductive education; Vojta; NDT | Baby-CIMT; Baby-Bimanual Training; GAME; "small steps" a motor training intervention conferred superior gains to usual care for improvement in motor skills | ○○○⊕ Low quality for CIMT; bimanual; motor training; GAME; general stimulation; COPCA; ○○○⊕ Low quality against conductive education; Vojta; NDT |
| Paleg et al.[53] 2013 | Systematic review of 30 studies | Cerebral palsy, non-weight bearing | 122+ | Standing | A standing program in a standing device at 45–60 min daily conferred improvements to ROM, especially for the knee from the hamstring stretching | ○○○⊕ Moderate–low quality for standing devices |

*(continued on next page)*

**Table 1**
*(continued)*

| Citation | Method | Population | n | Intervention | Results | Grade |
|---|---|---|---|---|---|---|
| te Velde et al.[20] 2022 | Systematic review of 34 studies | Cerebral palsy | 1332 | NDT | No difference between NDT and no intervention for improving motor skills [0.13; 95%CI 0.20–0.46]<br><br>Activity-Based intervention conferred superior gains to NDT for improving motor skills [0.76; 95%CI 0.12–1.40]<br><br>Body function and structures intervention conferred superior gains to NDT for improving motor skills [0.77; 95%CI 0.19–1.35]<br><br>No difference between higher- and lower-dose NDT [0.32; 95% CI 0.11–0.75] | ◯◯◯⊕ Moderate quality against NDT |
| Subpopulation 3: damaged or malformed motor system degenerative | | | | | | |
| Fonzo et al.[54] 2020 | Systematic review of 22 studies | Rett syndrome | 77 | Environmental enrichment<br>Hydrotherapy<br>Treadmill training | Environmental enrichment appeared to improve and protect motor skills<br><br>Hydrotherapy appeared to improve walking skills and reduce stereotypic movements<br><br>Treadmill training appeared to improve walking skills | ◯⊕⊕⊕ Very low quality for Environmental Enrichment Hydrotherapy Treadmill training |

| Livingstone et al.[55] 2014 | Systematic review of 28 studies | Physical disability affecting mobility | 559 | Powered mobility | Powered mobility appeared to improve overall development, independent mobility, and self-initiated movement<br>NOTE: Findings also relevant to infants with a severe physical disability that is non-degenerative motor impairment such as cerebral palsy | ○○⊕⊕<br>Low–very low quality for powered mobility |
| Mercuri et al.[56] 2018 | Clinical practice guideline | Spinal muscular atrophy | N/A | Exercise<br>Gait training<br>Positioning and bracing<br>stretching<br>powered mobility | Stretching contractures, positioning and bracing to provide respiratory support, and powered mobility are recommended for those unable to sit independently.<br>Positioning and bracing to provide respiratory support, and wheeled or powered mobility or gait training, plus exercise are recommended for those who can sit.<br>Exercise and braces are recommended for those who can walk. | ○○⊕⊕<br>Low–very low quality |

*Abbreviations*: AROM, active range of motion; CIMT, constraint-induced movement therapy; COPCA, coping with and caring for infants with special needs; Development, and Evaluation; eTIPS, early Therapy In Perinatal Stroke; GAME, Goals-Activity-Motor Enrichment; GRADE, Grading of Recommendations Assessment; N/A, Not applicable; NDT, Neurodevelopmental Therapy; NIDCAP, Newborn Individualized Developmental Care and Assessment Program; NOTE, When a systematic review reported on multiple domains of development; only, the motor data was reported in this table; PROM, Passive Range Of Motion; RCT, Randomized Controlled Trial; ROM, Range of Motion; SIDS, Sudden Infant Death Syndrome.; EI, Early Intervention.

A recent clinical practice guideline found moderate quality evidence for effective motor interventions for infants with CP[21]. It is strongly recommended that motor interventions should start as early as possible and be task and context-specific, with an emphasis on creating optimal environments to invite practice and repetition. Both baby-friendly constraint-induced movement therapy (CIMT) and bimanual therapy are recommended for infants with or at high risk of unilateral CP[21]. A strong recommendation is made against passive approaches to early motor interventions including the range of motion exercises and interventions that rely on facilitation techniques including NDT or Bobath. Conditional recommendations against Conductive Education and Vojta[20,21] are made for the same reason and thus these interventions are deemed to be below the worth-it line.

Nearly all early intervention approaches seeking to improve motor skills have a focus on parent coaching and education, as it is known children learn best in natural environments and parents and carers are crucial for providing enriching and responsive environments. Adequate opportunities for repetition and intensity of practice can only be realized in the context of a clinician-parent partnership where parents are coached and empowered to create targeted play opportunities for their child.

Clinical guidelines for infants with degenerative disorders focus on symptom management and optimization of function through judicial use of adaptive equipment, targeted exercise, and environmental enrichment.

## CURRENT STUDIES/TRIALS OR PRECLINICAL STUDIES

Whereas new studies in degenerative disorders focus on pharmacologic or gene therapies aiming to halt or slow progression[4], the last 8 to 10 years have seen a significant increase in published protocols and registered randomized trials in clinical trial registries in both CP and preterm infants. Many of these protocols importantly adopt evidence-based motor learning strategies in line with contemporary neuroscience and theoretical frameworks about how children learn. Modes of delivery of early intervention are the subject of multiple new studies[58] with a renewed focus on telehealth, for example, the TEDI-PREM trial (https://www.tediprem.org/login; ACTRN12621000364875. https://trialsearch.who.int/Trial2.aspx?; APPLES-tele (https://clinicaltrials.gov/ct2/show/NCT04997109) amongst others[59,60]. A number of these studies focus on a clinician-parent partnership in achieving an adequate dose of practice.

Studies comparing the dose or intensity of intervention are underway for infants with asymmetrical brain injury (I-ACQUIRE https://www.nihstrokenet.org/i-acquire/home) and diplegia (https://clinicaltrials.gov/ct2/show/NCT03672877). HABIT-ILE (intensive 2 weeks) is being trialed in infants with unilateral CP compared with usual care (https://clinicaltrials.gov/ct2/show/NCT04698395). Outcomes of these important studies will provide clinicians and policy makers with better evidence to assist in clinical decision-making around dose and intensity of therapy required in these early years.

## CONTROVERSIES

The historical "wait and see" approach to diagnosing life-long disability after a motor impairment is evident and has negatively impacted the evidence base for early intervention during infancy. The absence of early diagnostic labels has precluded the recruitment of alike samples to clinical trials. Resultant underpowered studies and participants with heterogeneous outcomes have led to a paucity of high-quality early intervention trials for infants with motor impairment (eg, clinical trials in infants born preterm that attempt to examine the outcomes for cerebral palsy while also including

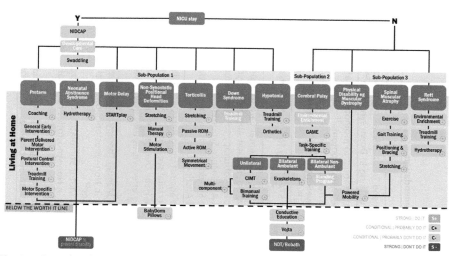

**Fig. 3.** Algorithm for decision-making.

some participants with normal outcomes). Implementation of evidence-based clinical indicators and clinical consensus statements[61] to accurately detect the risk of motor impairment specific to a subpopulation[8] opens up the field for targeted intervention studies for delayed, damaged, malformed, and degenerative motor systems.

De-implementation of ineffective interventions warrants attention in the field of motor impairment[20]. For example, in cerebral palsy subpopulations, passive interventions (facilitation, passive stretching, sensory support, or positioning to normalize movement) at any dose do not improve motor function[20,21]. In contrast, cumulative evidence supports active interventions adopting neuroplasticity principles (active self-generated movements, repetitive, varied specific task practice, real-life problem solving) to improve motor outcomes in CP infants[20,21].

The intensity of active training is another important neuroplasticity criterion to consider when comparing generic versus diagnosis specific-interventions for motor impairment in infants. Maximizing the windows of active play opportunities around required sleep times is important to consider when achieving required doses in infancy. Parents can be empowered with the knowledge that the dosage of therapy can be achieved in their own home environment through evidence-based coaching models. This is significant as many parents feel compelled to try multiple therapy approaches, often traveling long distances for appointments which can impact carer burden and burnout. In addition, as parents develop a greater understanding of how specific practice can induce the greatest neoplastic change[22], they are better able to make their own decisions about generic versus specific interventions for their child's goals.

## FUTURE DIRECTIONS

Early intervention has been studied for many decades and there is now evidence that not providing early intervention for high-risk infants is harmful. This lack of equipoise makes designing and recruiting for future high-quality RCTs challenging. Researchers have moved away from a "one size fits all" approach to EI and these more tailored studies of specific interventions for specific neurodevelopmental disorders are likely to advance the field. The heterogeneity in presentation and severity among children

**Table 2**
Recommendations for clinical practice

| Population | Intervention | Quality | Strength | Direction | Key Recommendation |
|---|---|---|---|---|---|
| Subpopulation 1: intact but delayed maturation of the motor system | | | | | |
| Down syndrome | Treadmill training | ○○○⊕ Moderate | Strong | For | We recommend Treadmill Training to accelerate the onset of walking in Down syndrome[34,36,41] |
| Hypotonia | Orthotics | ○○⊕⊕ Low | Conditional | For | We suggest Orthotics to promote foot alignment in Syndromes with hypotonia[36] |
| | Treadmill training | ○○○⊕ Low | Conditional | For | We suggest Treadmill Training to accelerate the onset of walking in syndromes with hypotonia[36,41] |
| Motor delay | START-play | ○○⊕⊕ Low | Conditional | For | We suggest START-play for infants with significant motor delay[29] |
| Neonatal abstinence syndrome | Developmental care | ○⊕⊕⊕ Very low | Conditional | For | We suggest Developmental Care to improve movement in Neonatal Abstinence Syndrome[33] |
| | Hydrotherapy | ○○⊕⊕ Very low | Conditional | For | We suggest Hydrotherapy to improve movement in Neonatal Abstinence Syndrome[33] |
| | Swaddling | ○⊕⊕⊕ Very low | Conditional | For | We suggest Swaddling to improve movement in Neonatal Abstinence Syndrome[33] |
| Non-synostotic positional head deformities | BabyDorm pillow | ○○⊕⊕ Low | Conditional | Against | We suggest against using BabyDorm Pillow to improve cranial symmetry in Non-synostotic Positional Head Deformities despite pillows appearing effective, as they may elevate the risk for SIDS[27] |
| | Manual therapy | ○○⊕⊕ Low | Conditional | For | We suggest Manual Therapy to improve cranial symmetry in Non-synostotic Positional Head Deformities[27] |
| | Motor stimulation | ○○⊕⊕ Low | Conditional | For | We suggest Motor Stimulation to improve cranial symmetry in Non-synostotic Positional Head Deformities[27] |
| | Stretching | ○○⊕⊕ Low | Conditional | For | We suggest Stretching to improve cranial symmetry in Non-synostotic Positional Head Deformities[27] |

| | Intervention | Quality | Certainty | For/Against | Recommendation |
|---|---|---|---|---|---|
| **Preterm** | Coaching | ◯⊕⊕⊕ Low | Conditional | For | We recommend Coaching to improve motor skills short-term in infants born preterm[40] |
| | Developmental care | ◯◯◯⊕ Moderate–high | Strong | For | We recommend Developmental Care to improve motor skills short-term in infants born preterm[25,32,34,38] |
| | General early intervention | ◯◯◯⊕ Moderate | Conditional | For | We suggest general early intervention to improve motor skills short-term in infants born preterm[40] |
| | Motor-specific interventions | ◯◯◯⊕ Moderate | Conditional | For | We suggest Motor-Specific Interventions to improve motor skills short-term in infants born preterm[30,39] |
| | NIDCAP | ◯◯◯⊕ Moderate | Conditional | For | We suggest NIDCAP to improve motor skills short-term in infants born preterm[24,25,40] |
| | | ◯◯◯⊕ Moderate | Conditional | Against | We suggest against using NIDCAP to prevent disability in infants born preterm[35] |
| | Parent delivered motor interventions | ◯◯◯⊕ Moderate | Conditional | For | We suggest Parent Delivered Motor Interventions to improve motor skills in infants born preterm[32] |
| | Postural control intervention | ◯◯◯⊕ Moderate | Conditional | For | We suggest Therapist Delivered Postural Control Intervention to improve motor skills in infants born preterm[32] |
| | Treadmill training | ◯⊕⊕⊕ Low | Conditional | For | We suggest Treadmill Training to improve stepping in infants born preterm[26] |
| **Torticollis** | Stretching | ◯◯◯⊕ Low | Conditional | For | We suggest Stretching to improve ROM in torticollis[37] |
| **Subpopulation 2: damaged or malformed motor system non-degenerative** | | | | | |
| **Cerebral palsy** | Bimanual training | ◯⊕⊕⊕ Low | Conditional | For | We suggest Bimanual Training to improve motor skills in infants with unilateral cerebral palsy[21,50,52] |
| | CIMT | ◯◯◯⊕ Low | Conditional | For | We suggest CIMT to improve motor skills in infants with unilateral cerebral palsy[21,46,47,50,52] |
| | Conductive education | ◯◯◯⊕ Low | Conditional | Against | We suggest against Conductive Education in infants with cerebral palsy for improving motor skills; however, this intervention may be helpful for social and academic skills[52] |
| | Environmental enrichment | ◯◯◯⊕ Moderate | Strong | For | We suggest Environmental Enrichment to improve motor skills in infants with cerebral palsy[10,14,20,46,52] |
| | Exoskeletons | ◯◯◯⊕ Low | Conditional | For | We suggest Exoskeletons to promote walking skills and walking speed in infants with cerebral palsy[44] |

*(continued on next page)*

**Table 2**
*(continued)*

| Population | Intervention | Quality | Strength | Direction | Key Recommendation |
|---|---|---|---|---|---|
| | Feeding interventions | ⊖⊕⊕⊕ Very low | Conditional | For | We suggest Motor Learning Feeding Interventions to improve feeding skills in infants with cerebral palsy[49] |
| | GAME | ⊖⊕⊕⊕ Low | Conditional | For | We suggest GAME Intervention to improve motor skills in infants with cerebral palsy[46,52] |
| | Kinesio-taping | ⊖⊕⊕⊕ Low | Conditional | For | We suggest Kinesio-taping as an adjunct to Task-Specific Training to improve sitting skills in infants with cerebral palsy[48] |
| | Multicomponent | ⊖⊕⊕⊕ Low | Conditional | For | We suggest a multi-component intervention that includes bimanual, CIMT, motor training, sensory-motor training, and parent education in infants with asymmetrical cerebral palsy to improve upper limb motor skills[51] |
| | NDT | ⊖⊕⊕⊕ Moderate | Strong | Against | We recommend against NDT at any dose for improving motor skills[20,21,52] |
| | Powered mobility | ⊖⊕⊕⊕ Low–very low | Conditional | For | We suggest powered mobility to improve independent mobility and self-initiated movement for infants with a severe physical disability who are predicted to be non-ambulant[55] |
| | Standing devices | ⊖⊕⊕⊕ Moderate–low | Strong | For | We recommend a standing program in a standing device at 45–60 min daily to maintain ROM for non-weightbearing infants with cerebral palsy[53] |
| | Task-specific training | ⊖⊕⊕⊕ Low | Conditional | For | We suggest Task-Specific Training to improve motor skills in infants with cerebral palsy[14,21,42,48,52] |
| | Task-specific training vs NDT | ⊖⊕⊕⊕ Moderate | Strong | For | We recommend Activity-Based Task-Specific Training intervention over NDT for improving motor skills[20] |
| | Vojta | ⊖⊕⊕⊕ Low | Conditional | Against | We suggest against Vojta in infants with cerebral palsy for improving motor skills[52] |

| Subpopulation 3: damaged or malformed motor system degenerative | | | | | |
|---|---|---|---|---|---|
| Physical disability affecting mobility for example, muscular dystrophy | Powered mobility | ○○⊕⊕ Low–very low | Conditional | For | We suggest powered mobility to improve independent mobility and self-initiated movement[55] |
| Rett syndrome | Environmental enrichment | ○⊕⊕⊕ Very low | Conditional | For | We suggest Environmental Enrichment to improve and protect motor skills[54] |
| | Hydrotherapy | ○⊕⊕⊕ Very low | Conditional | For | We suggest Hydrotherapy to improve and protect motor skills[54] |
| | Treadmill training | ○⊕⊕⊕ Very low | Conditional | For | We suggest Treadmill Training to improve and protect motor skills[54] |
| Spinal muscular atrophy | Exercise | ○○⊕⊕ Low–very low | Conditional | For | We suggest exercise to improve endurance, strength, and balance for children who sit or walk[56] |
| | Gait training | ○○⊕⊕ Low–very low | Conditional | For | We suggest gait training for children who can sit to promote walking skills[56] |
| | Positioning and bracing | ○○⊕⊕ Low–very low | Conditional | For | We suggest adaptive seating, positioning, and bracing to optimize inclusion in the seated position for children unable to sit[56] |
| | Powered mobility | ○○⊕⊕ Low–very low | Conditional | For | We suggest powered mobility in children able to sit and unable to sit to promote independent mobility[56] |
| | Stretching | ○○⊕⊕ Low–very low | Conditional | For | We suggest stretching to maintain range of movement and manage contractures in all severities[56] |

The best available positive evidence has been summarised into an algorithm to assist with clinical decision-making. The color codes for the interventions refer to the Evidence Alert Traffic Light System codes.

with CP, for example, has often meant high levels of variability in responsiveness to intervention, dissolving between-group differences. Future research should focus on similar groups of children within the CP population to properly tease out what works and for whom. Another important area to address is about the dose of therapy required and how this can be achieved within funding constraints. Adaptive trial designs have many advantages for these situations and if well thought out can be more efficient and ethical[62].

## DISCUSSION AND CONCLUSION

In the last decade, there have been substantial shifts in thinking about how to identify and treat motor impairments in infants at high-risk of disability. Historically the total population was described as "at-risk or high-risk" and identification of actual disability was made late[8,12,13], hampering the conduct and methodological quality of early intervention clinical trials. With earlier specifications in the risk profile and detection of disability, there is an upsurge in the number of clinical trials being conducted, which will continue to bring new knowledge and enhancements of clinical interventions. Of great consequence, the field now clearly differentiates the high-risk population into three subpopulations and the motor interventions for these subpopulations differ. No longer is the sole provision of generic early intervention considered best-practice for all subpopulations. For infants with delayed motor skills, anticipated to eventually catch up, such as infants born preterm without cerebral palsy, developmental care, NIDCAP, and motor training (either generic or specific) are recommended. Now, for infants on a trajectory to motor impairment (such as cerebral palsy), task-specific, child-active, goal-based, high-intensity motor training using the principles of motor learning and environment enrichment to harness neuroplasticity are strongly recommended for use[21]. In addition, for these infants, former popularized approaches that include child-passive therapist-led movements, (such as Neurodevelopmental Therapy, Vojta, handling, and positioning) are recommended against as clinical trials indicate they produce equal gains to no therapy and effective alternatives exist[20]. For infants with degenerative conditions, gene therapies are emerging, which can transform the treatment paradigm from palliative care to functional training, similar to those with non-degenerative motor impairments. For those without gene therapies, the art and science of selecting interventions involves weighing up how much of the infant's time and childhood should be spent on training skills they will eventually lose, versus, training them on compensatory approaches (such as single-switch technology or powered mobility) to build skills and advance readiness for a deteriorating motor repertoire and fatiguability. Given the state of the evidence and the potential of ongoing and future research studies for motor interventions, HRIF should more than ever emphasize early and accurate detection of motor concerns.

---

**Best Practices**

*What is the current practice for infants at high-risk of motor impairment?*

Up until recently, it was not possible to diagnose most motor impairments early, and therefore usual care for-the-most-part was generic "one-size fits all" early intervention. With the advancement of genetic diagnostics and early identification of cerebral palsy and autism spectrum disorder, infants might now receive the right treatment at the right time.

*What changes in current practice are likely to improve outcomes?*

Early diagnosis of specific disabilities will enable earlier and more relevant interventions. Infants with permanent motor impairment (such as cerebral palsy) require task-specific training; general approaches will be insufficient in dose and specificity. Infants with degenerative conditions (eg, Rett syndrome and spinal muscular atrophy) require training approaches for mild presentations and compensatory adaptations to promote inclusion for severe presentations.

*Is there a Clinical Algorithm?*

Refer to **Fig. 3**.

*Pearls/Pitfalls at the point-of-care*

Early diagnosis of motor impairment versus motor delay requires the use of instruments with high sensitivity and specificity in addition to clinical examination. but is important because "wait and see" monitoring might now be considered harmful as it underutilizes plasticity when specific interventions are safe and effective.

*Major Recommendations:*

Refer to **Table 2**.

## DISCLOSURE

The authors have nothing to disclose.

## REFERENCES

1. Kalia M. Brain development: anatomy, connectivity, adaptive plasticity, and toxicity. Metab 2008;57:S2–5.
2. Cioni G, Inguaggiato E, Sgandurra G. Early intervention in neurodevelopmental disorders: underlying neural mechanisms. Dev Med Child Neurol 2016;58:61–6.
3. Shrestha M. High-risk babies and neurodevelopmental outcome. In: Martin C, Preedy V, Rajendram R, editors. Diagnosis, management and modeling of neurodevelopmental disorders. Academic Press; 2021. p. 39–45, chapter 4.
4. Woolfenden S, Farrar MA, Eapen V, et al. Delivering paediatric precision medicine: genomic and environmental considerations along the causal pathway of childhood neurodevelopmental disorders. DMCN 2022;64(9):1077–84.
5. Ferriero DM. Neonatal brain injury. NEJM 2004;351(19):1985–95.
6. Rizzi R, Menici V, Cioni ML, et al. Concurrent and predictive validity of the infant motor profile in infants at risk of neurodevelopmental disorders. BMC Ped 2021; 21(1):1.
7. Spencer N, Raman S, O'Hare B, et al. Addressing inequities in child health and development: towards social justice. BMJ Paed Open 2019;3(1):e000503.
8. Novak I, Morgan C, Adde L, et al. Early, accurate diagnosis and early intervention in cerebral palsy: advances in diagnosis and treatment. JAMA Pediatr 2017; 171(9):897–907.
9. Stoll BJ, Hansen NI, Bell EF, et al. Neonatal outcomes of extremely preterm infants from the NICHD neonatal research network. Ped 2010;126:443–56.
10. Morgan C, Novak I, Badawi N. Enriched environments and motor outcomes in cerebral palsy: systematic review and meta-analysis. Ped 2013;132(3):e735–46.
11. Lim YH, Licari M, Spittle AJ, et al. Early motor function of children with autism spectrum disorder: a systematic review. Pediatr 2021;147(2). e2020011270.
12. Volkmar F, Siegel M, Woodbury-Smith M, et al. Practice parameter for the assessment and treatment of children and adolescents with autism spectrum disorder. J Amer Acad Child Adoles Psych 2014;53(2):237–57.
13. Zwaigenbaum L, Bauman ML, Fein D, et al. Early screening of autism spectrum disorder: recommendations for practice and research. Pediatr 2015;136(S1): S41–59.

14. Morgan C, Darrah J, Gordon AM, et al. Effectiveness of motor interventions in infants with cerebral palsy: a systematic review. Dev Med Child Neurol 2016;58(9): 900–9.

15. Munn Z, Peters MDJ, Stern C, et al. Systematic review or scoping review? Guidance for authors when choosing between a systematic or scoping review approach. BMC Med Res Method 2018;18:143.

16. Alonso-Coello P, Schuunemann HJ, Moberg J, et al. GRADE Evidence to Decision (EtD) frameworks: a systematic and transparent approach to making well informed healthcare choices. 1: Introduction. BMJ 2016;353:i2016.

17. Novak I, McIntyre S. The effect of education with workplace supports on practitioners' evidence-based practice knowledge and implementation behaviours. Aust Occup Ther J 2010;57(6):386–93.

18. Novak I, Morgan C, McNamara L, et al. Best practice guidelines for communicating to parents the diagnosis of disability. Early Hum Dev 2019;139:104841.

19. Novak I. Evidence to practice commentary new evidence in coaching interventions. Phys Occup Ther Ped 2014;34(2):132–7.

20. Te Velde A, Morgan C, Finch-Edmondson M, et al. Neurodevelopmental therapy for cerebral palsy: a meta-analysis. Ped 2022;149(6). e2021055061.

21. Morgan C, Fetters L, Adde L, et al. Early intervention for children aged 0 to 2 years with or at high risk of cerebral palsy: international clinical practice guideline based on systematic reviews. JAMA Ped 2021;175(8):846–58.

22. Kleim JA, Jones TA. Principles of experience-dependent neural plasticity: implications for rehabilitation after brain damage. J Speech Lang Hear Res 2008; 51(1):S225–39.

23. Sakzewski L, Gordon A, Eliasson AC, et al. The state of the evidence for intensive upper limb therapy approaches for children with unilateral cerebral palsy. J Child Neuro 2014;29(8):1077–90.

24. Aita M, De Clifford Faugère G, Lavallée A, et al. Effectiveness of interventions on early neurodevelopment of preterm infants: a systematic review and meta-analysis. BMC Pediatr 2021;21(1):1–7.

25. Anderson PJ, Treyvaud K, Spittle AJ. Early developmental interventions for infants born very preterm–what works? Sem Fetal Neonatal Med 2020;25(3):101119. WB Saunders.

26. Angulo-Barroso RM, Tiernan C, Chen LC, et al. Treadmill training in moderate risk preterm infants promotes stepping quality–results of a small randomised controlled trial. Res Dev Disabil 2013;34(11):3629–38.

27. Cabrera-Martos I, Ortigosa-Gómez SJ, López-López L, et al. Physical therapist interventions for infants with nonsynostotic positional head deformities: a systematic review. Phys Ther 2021;101(8):pzab106.

28. Cassidy AR, Butler SC, Briend J, et al. Neurodevelopmental and psychosocial interventions for individuals with CHD: a research agenda and recommendations from the Cardiac Neurodevelopmental Outcome Collaborative. Cardiol Young 2021;31(6):888–99.

29. Harbourne RT, Dusing SC, Lobo MA, et al. START-play physical therapy intervention impacts motor and cognitive outcomes in infants with neuromotor disorders: a multisite randomized clinical trial. Phys Ther 2021;101(2):pzaa232.

30. Hughes AJ, Redsell SA, Glazebrook C. Motor development interventions for preterm infants: a systematic review and meta-analysis. Pediatrics 2016;138(4). e20160147.

31. Kaplan SL, Coulter C, Sargent B. Physical therapy management of congenital muscular torticollis: a 2018 evidence-based clinical practice guideline from the APTA academy of pediatric physical therapy. Pediatr Phys Ther 2018;30:240–90.
32. Khurana S, Kane AE, Brown SE, et al. Effect of neonatal therapy on the motor, cognitive, and behavioral development of infants born preterm: a systematic review. Dev Med Child Neurol 2020;62(6):684–92.
33. McCarty DB, Peat JR, O'Donnell S, et al. "Choose physical therapy" for neonatal abstinence syndrome: clinical management for infants affected by the opioid crisis. Phys Ther 2019;99(6):771–85.
34. Novak I, McIntyre S, Morgan C, et al. A systematic review of interventions for children with cerebral palsy: state of the evidence. Dev Med Child Neurol 2013; 55(10):885–910.
35. Ohlsson A, Jacobs SE. NIDCAP: a systematic review and meta-analyses of randomized controlled trials. Ped 2013;131(3):e881–93.
36. Paleg G, Romness M, Livingstone R. Interventions to improve sensory and motor outcomes for young children with central hypotonia: a systematic review. J Pediatr Rehabil Med 2018;11(1):57–70.
37. Poole B, Kale S. The effectiveness of stretching for infants with congenital muscular torticollis. Phys Ther Rev 2019;24(1–2):2–11.
38. Soleimani F, Azari N, Ghiasvand H, et al. Do NICU developmental care improve cognitive and motor outcomes for preterm infants? A systematic review and meta-analysis. BMC Ped 2020;20(1):1–6.
39. Spittle A, Orton J, Anderson PJ, et al. Early developmental intervention programmes provided post hospital discharge to prevent motor and cognitive impairment in preterm infants. Cochrane Database Syst Rev 2015;11:CD005495.
40. Tanner K, Schmidt E, Martin K, et al. Interventions within the scope of occupational therapy practice to improve motor performance for children ages 0-5 Years: a systematic review. Am J Occup Ther 2020;74(2). 7402180060p1-7402180060p40.
41. Valentin-Gudiol M, Mattern-Baxter K, Girabent-Farres M, et al. Treadmill interventions in children under six years of age at risk of neuromotor delay. Cochrane Database Syst Rev 2017;7:CD009242.
42. Baker A, Niles N, Kysh L, et al. Effect of motor intervention for infants and toddlers with cerebral palsy: a systematic review and meta-analysis. Ped Phys Ther 2022; 34(3):297–307.
43. Basu AP, Pearse J, Watson R, et al. Feasibility trial of an early therapy in perinatal stroke (eTIPS). BMC Neurol 2018;18(1):102.
44. Bunge LR, Davidson AJ, Helmore BR, et al. Effectiveness of powered exoskeleton use on gait in individuals with cerebral palsy: a systematic review. PLoS ONE 2021;16(5):e0252193.
45. Case-Smith J, Frolek Clark GJ, Schlabach TL, et al. Systematic review of interventions used in occupational therapy to promote motor performance for children ages birth-5 years. Am J Occup Ther 2013;67(4):413–24.
46. Damiano DL, Longo E. Early intervention evidence for infants with or at risk for cerebral palsy: an overview of systematic reviews. Dev Med Child Neurol 2021; 63(7):771–84.
47. Dionisio MC, Terrill AL. Constraint-induced movement therapy for infants with or at risk for cerebral palsy: a scoping review. Am J Occup Ther 2022;76(2). 7602205120.

48. Inamdar K, Molinini RM, Panibatla ST, et al. Physical therapy interventions to improve sitting ability in children with or at-risk for cerebral palsy: a systematic review and meta-analysis. Dev Med Child Neurol 2021;63(4):396–406.

49. Khamis A, Novak I, Morgan C, et al. Motor learning feeding interventions for infants at risk of cerebral palsy: a systematic review. Dysphagia 2020;35(1):1–17.

50. Mailleux L, De Beukelaer N, Carbone MB, et al. Early interventions in infants with unilateral cerebral palsy: a systematic review and narrative synthesis. Res Dev Disabil 2021;117:104058.

51. Maitre NL, Jeanvoine A, Yoder PJ, et al. Kinematic and somatosensory gains in infants with cerebral palsy after a multi-component upper-extremity intervention: a randomized controlled trial. Brain Topogr 2020;33(6):751–66.

52. Novak I, Morgan C, Fahey M, et al. State of the evidence traffic lights 2019: systematic review of interventions for preventing and treating children with cerebral palsy. Curr Neurol Neurosci Rep 2020;20(2):1–21.

53. Paleg GS, Smith BA, Glickman LB. Systematic review and evidence-based clinical recommendations for dosing of pediatric supported standing programs. Ped Phys Ther 2013;25(3):232–47.

54. Fonzo M, Sirico F, Corrado B. Evidence-Based physical therapy for individuals with Rett syndrome: a systematic review. Brain Sci 2020;10(7):410.

55. Livingstone R, Field D. Systematic review of power mobility outcomes for infants, children and adolescents with mobility limitations. Clin Rehab 2014;28(10):954–64.

56. Mercuri E, Finkel RS, Muntoni F, et al. Diagnosis and management of spinal muscular atrophy: Part 1: recommendations for diagnosis, rehabilitation, orthopedic and nutritional care. Neuromus Dis 2018;28(2):103–15.

57. Doherty N, McCusker C. Chapter 9 - the congenital heart disease intervention program (CHIP) and interventions in infancy. In: McCusker C, Casey F, editors. Congenital heart disease and neurodevelopment. Academic Press; 2016. p. 133–48.

58. Pietruszewski L, Burkhardt S, Yoder PJ, et al. Protocol and feasibility-randomized trial of telehealth delivery for a multicomponent upper extremity intervention in infants with asymmetric cerebral palsy. Child Neurol Open 2020;7. 2329048X20946214.

59. Lima CRG, Dos Santos AN, Dos Santos MM, et al. Tele-care intervention performed by parents involving specific task-environment-participation (STEP protocol) for infants at risk for developmental delay: protocol of randomized controlled clinical trial. BMC Pediatr 2022;22(1):1–13.

60. Mobbs CA, Spittle AJ, Johnston LM. PreEMPT (preterm infant early intervention for movement and participation trial): the feasibility of a novel, participation-focused early physiotherapy intervention supported by telehealth in regional Australia—a protocol. Open J Pediatr 2020;10(04):707.

61. Maitre NL, Byrne R, Duncan A, et al. High-risk for cerebral palsy" designation: a clinical consensus statement. J Ped Rehabil Med 2022;15(1):165–74.

62. Pallmann P, Bedding AW, Choodari-Oskooei B, et al. Adaptive designs in clinical trials: why use them, and how to run and report them. BMC Med 2018;16(1):1–15.

**Supplemental Table S1**
**Excluded citations and rationale**

| Citation | Exclusion Rationale |
|---|---|
| Acton BV, Biggs WS, Creighton DE, Penner KA, Switzer HN, Thomas JH, Joffe AR, Robertson CM. Overestimating neurodevelopment using the Bayley-III after early complex cardiac surgery. Pediatrics. 2011 Oct;128(4):e794–800. | Not motor intervention |
| Abdelhaleem N, Taher S, Mahmoud M, et al. Effect of action observation therapy on motor function in children with cerebral palsy: a systematic review of randomized controlled trials with meta-analysis. Clin Rehabil. 2021;35(1):51–63. | Over 2 y of age |
| Acton BV, Biggs WS, Creighton DE, Penner KA, Switzer HN, Thomas JH, Joffe AR, Robertson CM. Overestimating neurodevelopment using the Bayley-III after early complex cardiac surgery. Pediatrics. 2011 Oct;128(4):e794–800. | Not motor intervention |
| Ammann-Reiffer C, Bastiaenen CH, de Bie RA, van Hedel HJ. Measurement properties of gait-related outcomes in youth with neuromuscular diagnoses: a systematic review. Phys Ther. 2014;94(8):1067–82. | Over 2 y of age |
| Amichai T, Katz-Leurer M. Heart rate variability in children with cerebral palsy: review of the literature and meta-analysis. NeuroRehabilitation. 2014;35(1):113–22. | Not motor intervention |
| Ayala L, Winter S, Byrne R, et al. Assessments and Interventions for Spasticity in Infants With or at High Risk for Cerebral Palsy: A Systematic Review. Pediatr Neurol. 2021;118:72–90. | Not motor intervention |
| Benfer KA, Novak I, Morgan C, et al. Community-based parent-delivered early detection and intervention programme for infants at high risk of cerebral palsy in a low-resource country (Learning through Everyday Activities with Parents (LEAP-CP): protocol for a randomised controlled trial. BMJ Open. 2018;8(6):e021186. | Protocol only |
| Benzies KM, Magill-Evans JE, Hayden KA, Ballantyne M. Key components of early intervention programs for preterm infants and their parents: a systematic review and meta-analysis. BMC pregnancy and childbirth. 2013 Jan;13(1):1–5. | Not motor intervention |
| Bourseul JS, Molina A, Lintanf M, et al. Early Botulinum Toxin Injections in Infants With Musculoskeletal Disorders: A Systematic Review of Safety and Effectiveness. Arch Phys Med Rehabil. 2018;99(6):1160–1176.e5. | Not motor intervention |
| Brady JM, Pouppirt N, Bernbaum J, D'Agostino JA, Gerdes M, Hoffman C, Cook N, Hurt H, Kirpalani H, DeMauro SB. Why do children with severe bronchopulmonary dysplasia not attend neonatal follow-up care? Parental views of barriers. Acta paediatrica. 2018 Jun;107(6):996–1002. | Not motor intervention |
| Brodie N, Keim JL, Silberholz EA, Spector ND, Pattishall AE. Promoting resilience in vulnerable populations: focus on opioid-exposed children, siblings of children with special healthcare needs and support for children through school-based interventions. Current Opinion in Pediatrics. 2019 Feb 1;31(1):157–65. | Over 2 y of age |
| Byers JF. Components of developmental care and the evidence for their use in the NICU. MCN: The American Journal of Maternal/Child Nursing. 2003 May 1;28(3):174–80. | Not motor intervention |

(continued on next page)

| Supplemental Table S1 (*continued*) | |
|---|---|
| **Citation** | **Exclusion Rationale** |
| Charpak N, Gabriel Ruiz J. KMC, concepts, definitions and praxis: what elements are applicable in what settings in which local circumstances? Current Women's Health Reviews. 2011 Aug 1;7(3):232–42. | Not motor intervention |
| Chen YP, Pope S, Tyler D, Warren GL. Effectiveness of constraint-induced movement therapy on upper-extremity function in children with cerebral palsy: a systematic review and meta-analysis of randomized controlled trials. Clin Rehabil. 2014;28(10):939–53. | Over 2 y of age |
| Chorna O, Heathcock J, Key A, et al. Early childhood constraint therapy for sensory/motor impairment in cerebral palsy: a randomised clinical trial protocol. BMJ Open. 2015;5(12):e010212. | Protocol only |
| Coker-Bolt P, Jarrard C, Woodard F, Merrill P. The effects of oral motor stimulation on feeding behaviors of infants born with univentricle anatomy. Journal of Pediatric Nursing. 2013 Feb 1; 28(1):64–71. | Not motor intervention |
| Dorling J, Hewer O, Hurd M, et al. Two speeds of increasing milk feeds for very preterm or very low-birthweight infants: the SIFT RCT. Health Technol Assess. 2020;24(18):1–94. | Not motor intervention |
| Edwards J, Berube M, Erlandson K, et al. Developmental coordination disorder in school-aged children born very preterm and/or at very low birth weight: a systematic review. J Dev Behav Pediatr. 2011;32(9):678–87. | Over 2 y of age |
| Eliasson AC, Sjostrand L, Ek L, Krumlinde-Sundholm L, Tedroff K. Efficacy of baby-CIMT: study protocol for a randomised controlled trial on infants below age 12 mo, with clinical signs of unilateral CP. BMC Pediatr. 2014;14:141. | Protocol only |
| Eliasson AC, Holmstrom L, Aarne P, et al. Efficacy of the small step program in a randomised controlled trial for infants below age 12 mo with clinical signs of CP; a study protocol. BMC Pediatr. 2016;16(1):175. | Protocol only |
| Ellinger MK, Rempel GR. Parental decision making regarding treatment of hypoplastic left heart syndrome. Advances in Neonatal Care. 2010 Dec 1;10(6):316–22. | Not motor intervention |
| Escobar Jr MA, Flynn-O'Brien KT, Auerbach M, Tiyyagura G, Borgman MA, Duffy SJ, Falcone KS, Burke RV, Cox JM, Maguire SA. The association of nonaccidental trauma with historical factors, examination findings, and diagnostic testing during the initial trauma evaluation. Journal of Trauma and Acute Care Surgery. 2017 Jun 1;82(6):1147–57. | Not motor intervention |
| Goyen TA, Morgan C, Crowle C, Hardman C, Day R, Novak I, Badawi N. Sensitivity and specificity of general movements assessment for detecting cerebral palsy in an Australian context: 2-year outcomes. Journal of pediatrics and child health. 2020 Sep;56(9):1414–8. | Not motor intervention |
| Graham D, Paget SP, Wimalasundera N. Current thinking in the health care management of children with cerebral palsy. Medical Journal of Australia. 2019 Feb;210(3):129–35. | Not systematic review or RCT |

(*continued on next page*)

| Supplemental Table S1 *(continued)* | |
|---|---|
| **Citation** | **Exclusion Rationale** |
| Greaves S, Imms C, Dodd K, Krumlinde-Sundholm L. Assessing bimanual performance in young children with hemiplegic cerebral palsy: a systematic review. Dev Med Child Neurol. 2010;52(5):413–21. | Not motor intervention |
| Holmström L, Eliasson AC, Almeida R, et al. Efficacy of the small step program in a randomized controlled trial for infants under 12 month old at risk of cerebral palsy (CP) and other neurologic disorders. J Clin Med. 2019 Jul 11;8(7):1016. | Included within Systematic Reviews |
| Heineman KR, Hadders-Algra M. Evaluation of neuromotor function in infancy–a systematic review of available methods. Journal of Developmental & Behavioral Pediatrics. 2008 Aug 1; 29(4):315–23. | Not motor intervention |
| Herskind A, Greisen G, Nielsen JB. Early identification and intervention in cerebral palsy. Developmental Medicine & Child Neurology. 2015 Jan;57(1):29–36. | Not motor intervention |
| Hoare BJ, Wallen MA, Thorley MN, et al. Constraint-induced movement therapy in children with unilateral cerebral palsy. Cochrane Database Syst Rev. 2019;4:CD004149. | Over 2 y of age |
| Hoare BJ, Wallen MA, Imms C, Villanueva E, Rawicki HB, Carey L. Botulinum toxin A as an adjunct to treatment in the management of the upper limb in children with spastic cerebral palsy (UPDATE). Cochrane Database Syst Rev. 2010;(1):CD003469. | Not motor intervention |
| Hoare BJ, Imms C, Rawicki HB, et al. Modified constraint-induced movement therapy or bimanual occupational therapy following injection of Botulinum toxin-A to improve bimanual performance in young children with hemiplegic cerebral palsy: a randomised controlled trial methods paper. BMC Neurol. 2010;10:58. | Protocol only |
| Hurley T, Zareen Z, Stewart P, et al. Bisphosphonate use in children with cerebral palsy. Cochrane Database Syst Rev. 2021;7:CD012756. | Not motor intervention |
| Hutchon B, Gibbs D, Harniess P, et al. Early intervention programmes for infants at high risk of atypical neurodevelopmental outcome. Dev Med Child Neurol. 2019 Dec;61(12):1362–7. | Not systematic review or RCT |
| Jackman M, Lannin N, Galea C, Sakzewski L, Miller L, Novak I. What is the threshold dose of upper limb training for children with cerebral palsy to improve function? A systematic review. Aust Occup Ther J. 2020;67(3):269–280. | Over 2 y of age |
| Karatas N, Dalgic AI. Effects of reflexology on child health: A systematic review. Complement Ther Med. 2020;50:102,364. | Not motor intervention |
| Kelly MM, Michalek R. Children born preterm: How are we educating providers? Journal of Nursing Education. 2019 Jun 1;58(6):339–46. | Not motor intervention |
| King AR, Machipisa C, Finlayson F, Fahey MC, Novak I, Malhotra A. Early detection of cerebral palsy in high-risk infants: Translation of evidence into practice in an Australian hospital. Journal of Pediatrics and Child Health. 2021 Feb;57(2):246–50. | Not motor intervention |

*(continued on next page)*

| Supplemental Table S1 *(continued)* | |
|---|---|
| **Citation** | **Exclusion Rationale** |
| Klepper SE, Clayton Krasinski D, Gilb MC, Khalil N. Comparing Unimanual and Bimanual Training in Upper Extremity Function in Children With Unilateral Cerebral Palsy. Pediatr Phys Ther 2017;29(4):288–306. | Over 2 y of age |
| Koly KN, Martin-Herz SP, Islam MS, et al. Parent mediated intervention programmes for children and adolescents with neurodevelopmental disorders in South Asia: A systematic review. PLoS ONE. 2021;16(3):e0247432. | Not motor intervention |
| Kwong AK, Fitzgerald TL, Doyle LW, Cheong JL, Spittle AJ. Predictive validity of spontaneous early infant movement for later cerebral palsy: a systematic review. Developmental Medicine & Child Neurology. 2018 May;60(5):480–9. | Not motor intervention |
| Lakshmanan A, Rogers EE, Lu T, Gy E, Vernon L, Briscoe H, Profit J, Jocson MA, Hintz SR. Disparities and early engagement associated with the 18–36 mo high risk infant follow up visit among very low birthweight infants in California. The Journal of Pediatrics. 2022 May 18. | Not motor intervention |
| Letzkus L, Frazier K, Keim-Malpass J. Assessment of pain and sleep symptoms in children at high risk for cerebral palsy in a pediatric neurodevelopmental clinic: Implications for future quality improvement interventions. Journal of Pediatric Nursing. 2021 Sep 1;60:293–6. | Not motor intervention |
| Lucas BR, Elliott EJ, Coggan S, et al. Interventions to improve gross motor performance in children with neurodevelopmental disorders: a meta-analysis. BMC Pediatr. 2016;16(1):193. | Over 2 y of age |
| Maitre NL, Burton VJ, Duncan AF, et al. Network Implementation of Guideline for Early Detection Decreases Age at Cerebral Palsy Diagnosis. Pediatrics 2020;145(5) | Not motor intervention |
| Mendonça B, Sargent B, Fetters L. Cross-cultural validity of standardized motor development screening and assessment tools: A systematic review. Developmental Medicine & Child Neurology. 2016 Dec;58(12):1213–22. | Not motor intervention |
| Morgan C, Novak I, Dale RC, Guzzetta A, Badawi N. GAME (Goals - Activity - Motor Enrichment): protocol of a single blind randomised controlled trial of motor training, parent education and environmental enrichment for infants at high risk of cerebral palsy. BMC Neurol. 2014;14:203. | Protocol only |
| Morgan C, Novak I, Dale RC, et al. Single blind randomised controlled trial of GAME (Goals - Activity - Motor Enrichment) in infants at high risk of cerebral palsy. Res Dev Disabil. 2016;55:256–67. | Included within systematic review |
| Novak I, Walker K, Hunt RW, et al. Concise Review: Stem Cell Interventions for People With Cerebral Palsy: Systematic Review With Meta-Analysis. Stem cells transl. med. 2016;5(8):1014–25. | Not motor intervention |
| Orton JL, Olsen JE, Ong K, Lester R, Spittle AJ. NICU graduates: The role of the allied health team in follow-up. Pediatric annals. 2018 Apr 1;47(4):e165–71. | Not systematic review or RCT |

*(continued on next page)*

| Supplemental Table S1 *(continued)* | |
|---|---|
| **Citation** | **Exclusion Rationale** |
| Pennington L, Goldbart J, Marshall J. Interaction training for conversational partners of children with cerebral palsy: a systematic review. Int J Lang Commun Disord. 2004;39(2):151–70. | Not motor intervention |
| Pennington L, Goldbart J, Marshall J. Speech and language therapy to improve the communication skills of children with cerebral palsy. Cochrane Database Syst Rev. 2004;(2):CD003466. | Not motor intervention |
| Pepino VC, Mezzacappa MA. Application of tactile/kinesthetic stimulation in preterm infants: a systematic review. Jornal de pediatria. 2015 May;91:213–33. | Not motor intervention |
| Peyton C, Einspieler C. General movements: a behavioral biomarker of later motor and cognitive dysfunction in NICU graduates. Pediatric annals. 2018 Apr 1;47(4):e159–64. | Not motor intervention |
| Plasschaert VF, Vriezekolk JE, Aarts PB, Geurts AC, Van den Ende CH. Interventions to improve upper limb function for children with bilateral cerebral palsy: a systematic review. Developmental Medicine & Child Neurology. 2019 Aug;61(8):899–907. | Over 2 y of age |
| Provasi J, Blanc L, Carchon I. The importance of rhythmic stimulation for preterm infants in the NICU. Children. 2021 Jul 29;8(8):660. | Not motor intervention |
| Raghupathy MK, Rao BK, Nayak SR, Spittle AJ, Parsekar SS. Effect of family-centered care interventions on motor and neurobehavior development of very preterm infants: a protocol for systematic review. Systematic reviews. 2021 Dec;10(1):1–8. | Protocol only |
| Redsell SA, Slater V, Rose J, Olander EK, Matvienko-Sikar K. Barriers and enablers to caregivers' responsive feeding behavior: A systematic review to inform childhood obesity prevention. Obesity Reviews. 2021 Jul;22(7):e13228. | Not motor intervention |
| Richard C, Kjeldsen C, Findlen U, et al. Hearing Loss Diagnosis and Early Hearing-Related Interventions in Infants With or at High Risk for Cerebral Palsy: A Systematic Review. J Child Neurol. 2021;36(10):919–929. | Not motor intervention |
| Roberts G, Grimshaw K, Beyer K, Boyle R, Lack G, Austin M, Garcia-Larsen V, Grabenhenrich L, Halken S, Keil T, Madsen C. Can dietary strategies in early life prevent childhood food allergy? A report from two iFAAM workshops. Clinical & Experimental Allergy. 2019 Dec;49(12):1567–77. | Not motor intervention |
| Rodovanski GP, Reus BA, Damiani AV, et al. Home-based early stimulation program targeting visual and motor functions for preterm infants with delayed tracking: Feasibility of a Randomized Clinical Trial. Res Dev Disabil. 2021 Sep 1;116:104,037. | Not motor intervention |
| Roostaei M, Baharlouei H, Azadi H, et al. Effects of Aquatic Intervention on Gross Motor Skills in Children with Cerebral Palsy: A Systematic Review. Phys Occup Ther Pediatr. 2017;37(5):496–515. | Over 2 y of age |
| Sakzewski L, Ziviani J, Boyd R. Systematic review and meta-analysis of therapeutic management of upper-limb | Over 2 y of age |

*(continued on next page)*

| Supplemental Table S1 (continued) | |
| --- | --- |
| **Citation** | **Exclusion Rationale** |
| dysfunction in children with congenital hemiplegia. Pediatrics. 2009;123(6):e1111–22. | |
| Sakzewski L, Ziviani J, Boyd RN. Efficacy of upper limb therapies for unilateral cerebral palsy: a meta-analysis. Pediatrics. 2014;133(1):e175–204. | Over 2 y of age |
| Sakzewski L, Reedman S, McLeod K, et al. Preschool HABIT-ILE: study protocol for a randomised controlled trial to determine efficacy of intensive rehabilitation compared with usual care to improve motor skills of children, aged 2–5 y, with bilateral cerebral palsy. BMJ Open. 2021;11(3):e041542. | Protocol only |
| Sgandurra G, Beani E, Giampietri M, Rizzi R, Cioni G, CareToy-R Consortium. Early intervention at home in infants with congenital brain lesion with CareToy revised: an RCT protocol. BMC Pediatr. 2018;18(1):295. | Protocol only |
| Seesahai J, Luther M, Church PT, et al. The assessment of general movements in term and late-preterm infants diagnosed with neonatal encephalopathy, as a predictive tool of cerebral palsy by 2 y of age-a scoping review. Syst. rev. 2021;10(1):226. | Not motor intervention |
| Shah TA, Meinzen-Derr J, Gratton T, Steichen J, Donovan EF, Yolton K, Alexander B, Narendran V, Schibler KR. Hospital and neurodevelopmental outcomes of extremely low-birth-weight infants with necrotizing enterocolitis and spontaneous intestinal perforation. Journal of Perinatology. 2012 Jul;32(7):552–8. | Not motor intervention |
| Slattery J, Morgan A, Douglas J. Early sucking and swallowing problems as predictors of neurodevelopmental outcome in children with neonatal brain injury: a systematic review. Developmental Medicine & Child Neurology. 2012 Sep;54(9):796–806. | Not motor intervention |
| Silveira RC, Mendes EW, Fuentefria RN, Valentini NC, Procianoy RS. Early intervention program for very low birth weight preterm infants and their parents: a study protocol. BMC pediatrics. 2018 Dec;18(1):1–1. | Protocol only |
| Spittle AJ, Doyle LW, Boyd RN. A systematic review of the clinimetric properties of neuromotor assessments for preterm infants during the first year of life. Dev Med Child Neurol. 2008;50(4):254–66. | Not motor intervention |
| Sullivan MC, Miller RJ, Fontaine LA, Lester B. Refining Neurobehavioral Assessment of the High-Risk Infant Using the NICU Network Neurobehavioral Scale. Journal of Obstetric, Gynecologic & Neonatal Nursing. 2012 Jan 1;41(1):17–23. | Not motor intervention |
| Tanner A, Dounavi K. The emergence of autism symptoms before 18 mo of age: A systematic literature review. Journal of Autism and Developmental Disorders. 2021 Mar;51(3):973–93. | Not motor intervention |
| Thornton JG, Hornbuckle J, Vail A, Spiegelhalter DJ, Levene M, GRIT study group. Infant wellbeing at 2 y of age in the Growth Restriction Intervention Trial (GRIT): multicentred randomized controlled trial. Lancet. 2004;364(9433):513–20. | Not motor intervention |
| Waddington H, van der Meer L, Sigafoos J. Effectiveness of the Early Start Denver Model: a systematic review. Rev J Autism Dev Dis. 2016 Jun;3(2):93–106. | Not motor intervention |

(continued on next page)

| Supplemental Table S1 (continued) | |
|---|---|
| **Citation** | **Exclusion Rationale** |
| Walshe M, Smith M, Pennington L. Interventions for drooling in children with cerebral palsy. Cochrane Database Syst Rev. 2012;11:CD008624. | Not motor intervention |
| Wasiak J, Hoare B, Wallen M. Botulinum toxin A as an adjunct to treatment in the management of the upper limb in children with spastic cerebral palsy. Cochrane Database Syst Rev. 2004;(4):CD003469. | Not motor intervention |
| Wells H, Marquez J, Wakely L. Garment Therapy does not Improve Function in Children with Cerebral Palsy: A Systematic Review. Phys Occup Ther Pediatr. 2018;38(4):395–416. | Over 2 y of age |
| Whittingham K, Wee D, Boyd R. Systematic review of the efficacy of parenting interventions for children with cerebral palsy. Child Care Health Dev. 2011;37(4):475–83. | Not motor intervention |
| Williams J, Lee KJ, Anderson PJ. Prevalence of motor-skill impairment in preterm children who do not develop cerebral palsy: a systematic review. Dev Med Child Neurol. 2010;52(3):232–7. | Not motor intervention |
| Wilson RB, Enticott PG, Rinehart NJ. Motor development and delay: advances in the assessment of motor skills in autism spectrum disorders. Current opinion in neurology. 2018 Apr;31(2):134. | Not motor intervention |
| Wyckoff MH, Singletary EM, Soar J, Olasveengen TM, et al 2021 international consensus on cardiopulmonary resuscitation and emergency cardiovascular care science with treatment recommendations: summary from the basic life support; advanced life support; neonatal life support; education, implementation, and teams; first aid task forces; and the COVID-19 Working group. Circulation. 2022 Mar 1;145(9):e645–721. | Not motor intervention |
| Yana M, Tutuola F, Westwater-Wood S, Kavlak E. The efficacy of botulinum toxin A lower limb injections in addition to physiotherapy approaches in children with cerebral palsy: A systematic review. NeuroRehabilitation. 2019;44(2):175–189. | Not motor intervention |

# Efficacy of Therapist Supported Interventions from the Neonatal Intensive Care Unit to Home

## A Meta-Review of Systematic Reviews

Dana B. McCarty, PT, DPT[a], Lisa Letzkus, PhD, RN, CPNP-AC[b],
Elaine Attridge, MLS[c], Stacey C. Dusing, PT, PhD[d],*

## KEYWORDS

- High-risk infants • Preterm infants • Cerebral palsy • NICU • Early intervention
- Infant development • Parent mental health

## KEY POINTS

- The transition from neonatal intensive care unit (NICU) to early intervention/outpatient settings results in a disruptive gap in a therapeutic intervention during a period of maximal neuroplasticity and development. Parents of high-risk infants experience significant stress that contributes to poor mental health outcomes.
- Despite the numerous needs of preterm infants and their families, risks of developmental delays, and identified gaps in services, we found that few interventions have been developed and tested that commence in the NICU and transition to the home setting.
- The findings of this meta-review support the development and testing of NICU-to-home interventions that use of key principles of engaging parents with their infants to support motor development and parent-infant interaction to positively impact infant and parent outcomes.

## INTRODUCTION

Infants born preterm or with complicated medical conditions necessitating hospitalization in the neonatal intensive care unit (NICU) are at high risk for long-term developmental disabilities.[1,2] High-risk criteria for developing neurodevelopmental disabilities

[a] Division of Physical Therapy, Department of Health Sciences, The University of North Carolina at Chapel Hill, 3024 Bondurant Hall, CB#7135, Chapel Hill, NC 27599-7135, USA; [b] Division of Neurodevelopmental and Behavioral Pediatrics, Department of Pediatrics, University of Virginia, 101 Hospital Drive, Charlottesville, VA, 22903 USA; [c] Claude Moore Health Sciences Library, University of Virginia, PO Box 800722, Charlottesville, VA 22908, USA; [d] Division of Biokinesiology and Physical Therapy, University of Southern California, 1540 East Alcazar Street, CHP 155, Los Angeles CA 90033, USA
* Corresponding author.
*E-mail address:* Stacey.dusing@pt.usc.edu

Clin Perinatol 50 (2023) 157–178
https://doi.org/10.1016/j.clp.2022.10.004
0095-5108/23/© 2022 Elsevier Inc. All rights reserved.
perinatology.theclinics.com

like cerebral palsy (CP) include low gestational age at birth,[2] intraventricular hemorrhage grade III/IV,[3] periventricular white matter damage,[3] hypoxic-ischemic encephalopathy,[4] or neonatal stroke.[5] During the NICU stay, high risk of infant death and comorbidities contribute to parents' vulnerability to stress and depression[6]—both of which have been linked to worse neurobehavioral outcomes in infants and toddlers,[7,8] altered parent-infant attachment,[9] delayed motor skills,[10] and poor executive functioning in childhood.[11]

### Intervention Before Early Diagnosis Enhances Developmentally Supportive Routines which Improve Infants and Parents' Outcomes

Although the age of early diagnosis is crucial, parents of high-risk infants need support before 3 months of adjusted age. Most care in the NICU is multidisciplinary, with neonatologists, nurses, therapists, and/or other providers working together toward improved family support and neurodevelopmental outcomes for patients. Some therapy interventions provided during the NICU stay and in the first months, post-NICU discharge may be needed to support parent–infant relationships, establish caregiving routines to support development, and enhance neuroplasticity. However, the shift of care from the inpatient, NICU, to the outpatient, Early Intervention (EI), clinic, or school, environment involves changes in service providers and funding sources for therapeutic intervention including physical, occupational, and speech therapy. This requires parents to navigate a fragmented health care system requiring phone, email, and letter by mail communication with new service providers. This transition from the NICU medical model to the EI family-centered education approach is often delayed until a developmental problem is identified. This causes a disruptive gap in therapeutic intervention for high-risk infants during a period when parents are establishing caregiving routings, and of maximal neuroplasticity and developmental change in infants.[12]

Barriers to a Smooth Transition from NICU to Home-based services:

Parents of high-risk infants often find it difficult to balance conflicting priorities: parenting an infant outside of the home, managing or negotiating parental leave time during and after the NICU stay, and/or caring for other children/dependents at home.[13] Parents of healthy newborns routinely interact with their infant multiple times a day through regular feeding, holding, and diapering. In contrast, parents of infants in the NICU see their infants much less frequently, with studies reporting average parent visitation rates between 1 to 4 days per week.[13,14]

Although parents have limited autonomy over their infant's care in the NICU, in preparation for discharge, they must learn and assume care for the complex medical needs of their infant, which may include a specialized feeding plan, medication administration, and/or supplemental oxygen needs in addition to normal infant care needs (ie, holding and diapering). In addition, parents are expected to continue or initiate therapeutic activities as recommended by the physical, occupational, or speech therapist to optimize their infant's development post-discharge while maintaining follow-up appointment schedules for general and specialty care providers.[15] Parents with limited resources (eg, transportation, financial support, employee flexibility) may face significant challenges during this transition, as they experience even greater barriers to accessing health care services.[16] These demands, compounded by the anticipated shift in parenting role and responsibilities further contribute to parents' mental health concerns.[17]

EI services are mandated by the Federal Individuals with Disabilities Education Act and are designed to support the needs of families and infants with or at high risk of disabilities through the provision of "financial assistance to states to develop and implement a statewide, comprehensive, coordinated, multidisciplinary, interagency system that provides EI services for infants and toddlers with disabilities and their families."[18] These services include physical, occupational, speech, developmental, visual, or other specialized therapy evaluation and intervention based on the infant's uniquely identified needs. Despite federal mandates regarding best practice guidelines, individual states determine infant eligibility criteria, infant and family assessment protocols, and model of service provision that results in variability in service delivery between counties and across the country. Initiation of EI services is often delayed after NICU discharge by up to 6 to 12 months.[12,19,20] These delays in service initiation are associated with a variety of factors including miscommunication with the infant's provider, cost or insurance-related issues, and other logistical challenges like missing appointments and illness.[21]

The profound lack of continuity in family support from the NICU to the complex EI system is a barrier to optimizing family psychosocial well-being, which is imperative for infant development[22]; yet, there are few intervention programs that exist to bridge this gap. Therefore, the purpose of this meta-review was to evaluate the evidence from existing systematic reviews (SRs) regarding therapeutic interventions that start in the NICU setting and continue post-discharge with the expressed goals of improving developmental outcomes for infants at high risk for CP and neurodevelopmental conditions. We also evaluated the impact of these interventions on parental mental health outcomes.

## METHODS

The protocol for the review as submitted to PROSPERO and a research librarian (EA) performed a comprehensive literature search of the CINAHL, PubMed, and The Cochrane Database of Systematic Reviews databases using relevant MeSH headings and text words developed in collaboration with investigators (LL and SD) in June 2022. The search retrieval was limited to SRs. All articles published before the search date were eligible for inclusion, and the oldest article returned was published in 1999. Search terms were selected to focus on infants who in the NICU could be considered at high risk for CP; infants born at very early gestational ages (ie, 29 weeks or less),[2] and/or infant with a history of a brain injury (hypoxic ischemic encephalopathy),[4] neonatal stroke,[5] intraventricular hemorrhage grade III/IV and/or periventricular white matter damage.[3] The PICO question for this study was, "In infants at high risk for CP, what are the most effective therapeutic interventions delivered as a collaborative between a Physical Therapist (PT), Occupational Therapist (OT), or Speech Language Pathologist (SLP) and parent, starting in the NICU and continuing post discharge?"

Step one of the review process involved abstract review by 2 independent raters to confirm they met the following inclusion criteria: study was an SR or SR with meta-analyses and a portion of the papers included in the review met the following criteria (1) Because many SRs focused broadly on interventions addressing "neurodevelopmental delay," at least 25% of study samples included were considered to be at high risk for developing CP (as described above) or a subanalysis allowed for comparison of the subsample; (2) the intervention involved at least 1 visit in the NICU and at least 1 visit after NICU discharge, either in the home or outpatient environment; (3) the interventions were provided as a collaboration between therapy (PT, OT, or SLP) and a parent (4) the interventions were focused on improving infant development and/or parent well-being; (5) the review compared the intervention to a comparison or control group receiving usual care; and (5) outcomes were assessed at the end of the intervention period at a minimum. We excluded studies that did not meet the inclusion criteria or did not state explicitly that there was collaboration with parents (therapist delivered exclusively); there was no intervention; the intervention did not take place in the NICU; the intervention did not continue after NICU discharge (in home or outpatient setting). We excluded gray literature, which included studies of unpublished research (ie, dissertations and abstracts from conference proceedings). We also excluded articles that were not published in English.

Step two of the review process involved full-text review of papers by two independent raters with methods consistent with the PRISMA guidelines.[23] Any disagreement about inclusion was discussed and the third reviewer made the final determination (SD, LL, and DM). Data extraction from seven studies was completed using a standardized data extraction form based on recommendations from the Cochrane Collaboration. The AMSTAR checklist[24] for rating the quality of SRs was completed for each included paper, and full agreement between reviewers (SD, LL, DM) was reached after discussion.

## RESULTS
### Study Selection

The initial keyword search produced a total of 510 titles and abstracts. Of these, 461 were excluded because of either discordance with the inclusion criteria or duplication from multiple databases. Full texts of the remaining 49 articles were retrieved. Following full-text screening, 42 articles were further excluded based on our inclusion/exclusion criteria resulting in 7 studies eligible for inclusion (**Fig. 1**). Four studies were SRs with meta-analysis,[25–28] two studies were SRs,[15,29] and one study was a meta-review of SRs.[30]

Because of high variability in the type, duration, and approaches to intervention, variability of outcome measures used, and limited numbers of studies within SRs that met inclusion criteria, we did not perform a meta-analysis. Therefore, the

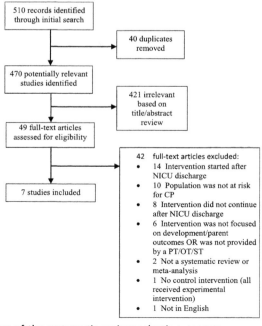

**Fig. 1.** Flow diagram of the systematic review selection process.

extracted data were synthesized narratively according to three main outcomes of interest: infant motor, infant cognitive, and parent outcomes. Effect sizes for interventions meeting inclusion criteria were reported as available.

### Characteristics of the Included Systematic Reviews

Characteristics of included studies are noted in **Table 1**. Two SRs included solely randomized controlled trials,[25,27] whereas the rest included studies irrespective of the design. All studies were conducted in the United Kingdom,[26,30] the United States,[15,29] Australia,[27,28] and Spain.[25] All the included SRs were critically appraised for methodological quality using AMSTAR tool.[24]

### Participants

The majority of the samples included infants born preterm (<37 weeks gestation).[26,28,30,31] Only one SR focused on infants diagnosed or at high risk for CP.[27] Sample sizes ranged from 10 to 915[28] among SRs, and the meta-review analyzed SRs with sample sizes between 1940 and 5556.[30] The SRs did not include other uniform participant characteristics (eg, race, sex, socioeconomic factors).

### Interventions

Eleven interventions across the included SRs had at least one visit in the NICU and one visit at home; met all other inclusion criteria, and are described in **Table 2**.[15,25–27,29,30] The majority of SRs focused on interventions designed to improve infant outcomes, one SR focused on interventions designed to improve parent outcomes,[25] and the meta-review reported on interventions for both infant and parent outcomes.[30] Control groups in SRs were parents or infants who received standard of care or usual care after preterm birth. All studies reported follow up measures between end of the intervention and 12 to 24 months post-intervention, and one study reported parent stress measures up to 7 years post-intervention.[25]

### Effectiveness of Interventions on Infant Outcomes

#### Motor

A variety of measures were used to assess infant motor skills, but the most common standardized assessment was the Psychomotor Developmental Index (PDI) of the Bayley Scales of Infant Development (BSID) II or Motor Scales of the BSID III.[15,26–30] Other assessments included the Test of Infant Motor Performance (TIMP),[15,28] Alberta Infant Motor Skills (AIMS),[15,26,28] Griffiths Developmental Assessments,[15,26,28,30] Neonatal Behavioral Assessment Scale (NBAS),[15,27] Neonatal Neurobehavioral Examination (NNE),[15] Movement Assessment of Infant,[26] Pediatric Evaluation of Disability Inventory (PEDI),[28] and Movement ABC.[26,28]

All SRs reported a small to moderate positive effect (0.19–1.43) in the short-term (<12 months) for motor interventions that commence in the NICU and continue in post-discharge for preterm infants (**Table 3**)[15,26–28,30]; however, of the 5 SRs that reported on motor outcomes at or over 12 months, 4 reported nonsignificant or negative long-term outcomes (eg, >12 months, preschool age). Spittle and colleagues performed a subgroup analysis of infants with brain injury who received developmental early intervention programs and found no significant differences between groups in infancy or preschool age in PDI scores on the BSID-II.[28] Spittle and colleagues also performed a subanalysis examining the efficacy of interventions that commenced in the NICU and continued in the community.[28] Six studies in this subanalysis[32–37] had a slightly greater impact on motor outcomes in infancy (<12 months) than programs

**Table 1**
Systematic review characteristics

| First Author, Year | Study Title | Aim | Study Designs | Included Databases | Number of Studies Cited |
|---|---|---|---|---|---|
| Frolek Clark and Schlabach[29] | Systematic Review of Occupational Therapy Interventions to Improve Cognitive Development in Children Ages Birth–5 y | To determine the evidence for the effectiveness of interventions within the scope of occupational therapy practice to improve cognitive development in children birth to age 5? | RCT, non-RCT experimental, cohort, cross-sectional, SR | Medline, PsyINFO, CINAHL, ERIC, OTseeker, Cochrane Database of Systematic Reviews, Campbell Collaboration | 13 |
| Girabent-Farrés[25] | Effects of Early Intervention on Parenting Stress after Preterm Birth: A Meta-analysis | The goal of this paper is to review the literature on EI programs that impact on the reduction in parenting stress suffered by the parents of a preterm baby. | RCTs | PubMed, Scopus, Web of Science | 10 |
| Hughes[26] | Motor Development Interventions for Preterm Infants: A Systematic Review and Meta-analysis | The aim of the study was to identify interventions that improve the motor development of preterm infants. | RCTs and non-RCT experimental | AMED, CINAHL, Cochrane Central Registry, Embase, ERIC, Maternity, and Infant Care, Medline, PEDro, ProQuest, PsycInfo, PubMed, Science Direct, SCOPUS, Web of Knowledge, Web of Science, EThoS, OpenGrey | 21 |

| Author | Title | Objective | Study designs | Databases | N |
|---|---|---|---|---|---|
| Khurana[15] | Effect of Neonatal Therapy on the Motor, Cognitive, and Behavioral Development of Infants born Preterm: A Systematic Review | To synthesize the existing literature and determine the efficacy of neonatal therapy, starting in the neonatal intensive care unit (NICU), on the motor, cognitive, and behavioral outcomes of infants born preterm | RCTs, non-RCT experimental, cohort | PubMed, Cochrane Database of Systematic Reviews, CINAHL, Web of Science, and PEDro, | 15 |
| Morgan[27] | Enriched Environments and Motor Outcomes in Cerebral Palsy: Systematic Review and Meta-analysis | The objective of this review was to appraise the effectiveness evidence about enriched environments for improving the motor outcomes of infants at high risk of cerebral palsy (CP). | RCTs | Cochrane Database of Systematic Reviews, Cochrane Central Register of Controlled Trials (inclusive of PubMed); the Cumulative Index to Nursing and Allied Health Literature; PsycINFO; Education Resource Information Center; and SocINDEX. | 7 |
| Puthussery[30] | Effectiveness of Early Intervention Programs for Parents of Preterm Infants: A Meta-Review of Systematic Reviews | The aim of this meta-review was to appraise and meta-synthesize the evidence from existing SRs to provide a comprehensive evidence base on the effectiveness of interventions for parents of preterm infants on parental and infant outcomes. | SRs | Cochrane library, Web of science, EMBASE, CINAHL, British Nursing Index, PsycINFO, PubMed/Medline, ScienceDirect, Scopus, IBSS, DOAJ, ERIC, EPPI center, PROSPERO, electronic libraries of the authors' institutions, Google Scholar, WHO Library, and reference list of identified reviews | 11 |

(continued on next page)

**Table 1**
*(continued)*

| First Author, Year | Study Title | Aim | Study Designs | Included Databases | Number of Studies Cited |
|---|---|---|---|---|---|
| Spittle[28] | Early Developmental Intervention Programs Provided Post-Hospital Discharge to Prevent Motor and Cognitive Impairment in Preterm Infants | To compare the effectiveness of early developmental intervention programs provided post-hospital discharge to prevent motor or cognitive impairment in preterm (<37 wk) infants vs standard medical follow-up of preterm infants at infancy (zero to < 3 years), preschool age (3 to < 5 years), school age (5 to < 18 y) and adulthood (≥18 y). | RCTs and non-RCT experimental | Cochrane Central Register of Controlled Trials, MEDLINE Advanced, the Cumulative Index to Nursing and Allied Health Literature, PsycINFO, EMBASE | 25 |

*Abbreviations:* RCT, randomized controlled trial; SR, systematic review.

**Table 2**
Characteristics of interventions that spanned neonatal intensive care unit to home

| Intervention | Reviews | Duration | Delivered by | Description |
|---|---|---|---|---|
| ATVV | Frolek Clark and Schlabach[29] Morgan[27] Spittle[28] | Frequency not specified; Commenced in NICU until 2 mo adjusted age at home | Health care professionals; parents | A multi-sensory stimulation program including auditory, tactile, visual, and vestibular stimuli in response to infant behavioral and physiologic cues. |
| COPE | Puthussery[30] Frolek Clark and Schlabach[29] | One to eight sessions in NICU and 1 session at home. | Nurses | A 4-phase program that consisted of audiotaped and written information and workbooks on infant behavior and parental roles. |
| CC | Puthussery[30] | Five sessions in the NICU, 1 home visit 2–4 wk after discharge | Nurses or clinical psychology graduate students | Designed to teach mothers to (1) recognize signs of their anxiety, (2) use various strategies to alleviate their distress, (3) read their infant's communication cues, and (4) respond sensitively to their infant's cues and distress. |
| DC | Khurana[15] Hughes[26] Frolek Clark and Schlabach[29] | May be considered a unit-wide framework or to be delivered individually by a therapist. To be delivered from time of birth, throughout NICU stay, and at home as appropriate. | Multi-disciplinary | Child- and parent-focused interventions that include regulating the environment and activities the infant is exposed to during general caregiving. DC is based on concepts of synactive theory and family-centered care |
| EI | Puthussery[30] Spittle[28] | First and second components involved three or four 30-min sessions before discharge. At discharge, the intervention group received weekly or biweekly outpatient sessions, each for 40–60 min up to 6 mo of age. | Physical therapists | First component designed to facilitate mother-infant interactions. Second component was presented to parents during visits to the hospital and focused on advising mothers on how to handle their infants according to developmental needs. |

*(continued on next page)*

**Table 2**
*(continued)*

| Intervention | Reviews | Duration | Delivered by | Description |
|---|---|---|---|---|
| MITP | Girabent-Farrés[25] Puthussery[30] Khurana[31] | One session in NICU and four sessions at home. | Nurses | Intervention designed to enhance mother-infant interaction and infant development by teaching mothers to be more sensitive and responsive to infant's physiologic, behavioral and social cues. Delivered by a trained nurse and focused on infant's motor system, state regulation, social interaction, daily care, preparations for home, mutual enjoyment through play and understanding of temperamental patterns |
| M-MITP | Puthussery[30] | Seven visits over 1 wk during NICU stay and four sessions up to 3 mo after discharge at home. | Nurses | Mother-Infant Transaction Program[34] modified[37] to include a physiotherapist and doctor consultation at discharge. Program was implemented by a team of nurses and included education on behavioral cues, parent-infant interaction and appropriate stimulation of the infant |
| PBIP | Girabent-Farrés[25] Puthussery[30] | Intervention commenced from the first weeks after birth in NICU and consisted of weekly 1-h sessions, beginning in hospital, and up to a maximum of 6 sessions at home. | Nurses | Intervention program included strategies to enhance parent-infant interaction, to facilitate attachment, to sensitize parents to their baby's cues and to provide education about developmental care |

| | | | Physical or Occupational Therapists | |
|---|---|---|---|---|
| PDMI | Khurana[15] | Variable | Physical or Occupational Therapists | Teaching a parent or caregiver to provide postural support and opportunities for movement with support during parent–infant interaction to increase infant movement quality and quantity. PDMIs are individualized for each infant with the support of a therapist and delivered through a parent–therapist collaboration. It is theoretically based on action perception and dynamic systems theory |
| SPEEDI | Girabent-Farrés[25] 2021 Puthussery[30] 2018 Khurana[15] 2020 | Intervention has 2 phases: phase 1 in the NICU from 35 wk' gestational age to term; phase 2 in the community from discharge until 3 mo of age. Each family received a minimum of 10 study visits with the therapist, including two parent education sessions | Physical Therapists | Early and intense intervention blended with family support to assist in the transition from hospital to home. |
| TDPCI or PT | Khurana[15] 2020 Hughes[26] 2016 Morgan[27] 2013 | Variable | Physical Therapists | Providing postural support and moving the infant in different positions to provide sensory or motor input. These interventions often involve facilitation of movement by incorporating inputs from tactile, vestibular, and somatosensory receptors within the body. |

*Abbreviations*: ATVV, auditory; tactile, visual; and vestibular intervention; CC, cues and care; COPE, creating opportunities for parent empowerment; DC, developmental care; EI, early intervention program; MITP, mother-infant transaction program; M-MITP, modified mother-infant transaction program; PBIP, parent-baby interaction program; PDMI, parent-delivered motor intervention; PT, physical therapy; SPEEDI, supporting play exploration and early development intervention; TDPCI, therapist-delivered postural control intervention.

**Table 3**
Infant outcomes

| Outcomes | Systematic Review | Participants | Intervention | Effect Size | Additional Information |
|---|---|---|---|---|---|
| **Motor** | | | | | |
| | Hughes[26] | Preterm infants; (majority <34 wk) | Motor development, multidisciplinary, PT, MITP[a] | 3 mo: 1.37 [0.48, 2.27] 6 mo: 0.34 [0.11, 0.57] 12 mo: 0.73 [0.20, 1.26] | Interventions continued beyond neonatal period can positively impact preterm motor development, with the strongest effects before 6 mo. Majority of studies used BSID-II/III |
| | Khurana[15] | Preterm infants (<37 wk) | PDMI | NICU Discharge: 1.04 6 mo: 1.2 12 mo: 1.0 | Most studies too small and heterogeneous to draw conclusions; however, there is preliminary support of daily PDMI to improve short and long-term motor outcomes |
| | | | TDPCI | NICU Discharge: 1.43 | TDPCI provided daily may result in short-term motor gains at NICU discharge with little to no gains post-NICU. Long-term data not available or suggest a lack of efficacy at 6 and > 12 mo |
| | Morgan[27] | Infants with diagnosis of CP or infants with high risk of CP; 2 of 5 interventions in this subgroup analysis spanned from NICU to home. | DC | 6 mo: 0.39 12 mo: 0.70 24 mo: 0.14 | Efficacy on motor and cognitive outcomes is variable, limiting ability to draw definitive conclusions. |
| | | | ATVV[a,36] EI[a,37] | 0.59 [−0.36, 1.54] 0.39 [−0.44, 1.21] | 2 of these studies[36,37] indicated good-quality evidence for a very small but insignificant effect from enrichment interventions in improving motor (BSID-II) for infants with CP. |

| | Participants | Intervention | Effect Size | Additional Information |
|---|---|---|---|---|
| Spittle[28] | Preterm infants born (<37 wk); subgroup of infants with brain injury | Developmental Early Intervention Programs | Infancy: 0.47 [−0.15, 1.10] Preschool: 0.06 [−0.28, 0.40] | 2 studies in this subgroup analysis[36,37] included infants at risk for adverse neurologic outcomes due to PVL or IVH, or both, and showed no significant differences between groups based on BSID-II. |
| Spittle[28] | Preterm infants (<37 wk); subgroup of interventions commenced in the NICU. | Developmental Early Intervention Programs | Infancy: 0.19 [0.05, 0.34] Preschool: 0.06 [−0.28, 0.40] | Infancy: 6 studies in this subanalysis commenced in the NICU[35,36,38-40] and had a slightly greater impact on motor outcomes at infancy than programs that began post hospital discharge. Preschool: One study[38] showed no differences between groups, but another[40] reported significantly higher scores in intervention group at 44 mo (PEDI) |
| Systematic Review | Participants | Intervention | Effect Size | Additional Information |
| Meta-Review Puthussery[30] | | | | |
| Spittle[28] | Preterm infants (<37 wk) | Intervention MITP[a] IHDP[a], M-MITP[a] IBAIP, CBIP, HBIP, SPEEDI[a] | Infancy: 0.10 [0.10, 0.19] Preschool: −0.18 [−0.47, 0.11] | Small significant effect in motor development in infancy. No long-term impact |

Cognition

| | | | | |
|---|---|---|---|---|
| Frolek Clark and Schlabach[29] | Infants and young children from birth to 5 y | Developmental interventions provided by OT in the NICU and home | Not provided | 2 studies[36] considered the effectiveness of interventions spanning NICU to home. Evidence about these programs is inconclusive and have not shown long-term effects. |
| Khurana[15] | Preterm infants (<37 wk) | PDMI | NICU Discharge: 0.8 12 mo: 1.0 | 2 studies reported positive outcomes on BSID-III, but only one of these studies spanned NICU to home. |

(continued on next page)

**Table 3**
*(continued)*

| Outcomes | Systematic Review | Participants | Intervention | Effect Size | Additional Information |
|---|---|---|---|---|---|
| | | | DC | NICU Discharge: 0.35<br>12 mo: 0.70<br>24 mo: 0.50 | Positive effects on mental development were reported at 6[40] and 12 mo, but no effect was found at 6 mo in one study.[37] At 24 mo, effects were inconsistent, with one study reporting improved cognitive scores (BSID-III), but another reporting no cognitive improvements (BSID-II).[40] |
| | Spittle[28] | Preterm infants (<37 wk); subgroup of infants with brain injury | Developmental Early Intervention Programs | Infancy: 0.50 [−0.12, 1.13] | 2 studies in this subgroup analysis[36,37] included infants at risk for adverse neurologic outcomes due to PVL, IVH, or both, and showed no significant differences between groups based on BSID-II |
| | Spittle[28] | Preterm infants (<37 wk); subgroup of interventions commenced in the NICU. | MITP[a] | Infancy: 0.24 [0.08, 0.40]<br>Preschool: 0.51 [0.26, 0.77] | Programs that began while infants were inpatients had a significant impact on cognitive outcome at infancy.<br>Three studies that began in the NICU[35,38] reported a significant effect in favor of the intervention. |
| Outcomes | Systematic Review | Participants | Intervention | Effect Size | Additional Information |
| Meta-Review<br>Puthussery[30] | Systematic Review<br>Spittle[28] | Preterm infants (<37 wk) | MITP[a] IHDP[a] M-MITP[a], IBAIP, CBIP, HBIP, SPEEDI[a] | Infancy: 0.32 [0.16, 0.47]<br>Preschool: 0.43 [0.32, 0.54] | Infancy: Significant improvement in Griffiths Developmental Quotient (P <.001)<br>Preschool: Significant improvement in Intelligence Quotient (P <.001) |

*Abbreviations:* ATVV, auditory; tactile; visual; and vestibular intervention; BSID-II or BSID-III, Bayley Scales of Infant Development; edition 2 or 3; CBIP, clinic-based intervention program; COPE, creating opportunities for parent empowerment; CP, cues program; DC, developmental care; HBIP, home-based intervention program; IHDP, infant health and development program; MITP, mother-infant transaction program; M-MITP, modified mother-infant transaction program; NBAS, neonatal behavioral assessment scale; NIDCAP, newborn individualized developmental & assessment program; PBIP, parent-baby interaction program; PDMI, parent-delivered motor intervention; PEDI, pediatric evaluation of disability index; PT, physical therapy; SPEEDI, supporting play exploration and early development intervention; TDPCI, therapist-delivered postural control intervention; TRT, triadic parent-infant relationship therapy.

[a] Discrete Intervention programs spanning NICU to home.

that began post-discharge, but the impact of these programs at preschool age were inconclusive.

## Cognition

A variety of measures were also used to assess infant cognitive skills, but the most common standardized assessment was the Mental Developmental Index (MDI) of the Bayley Scales of Infant Development (BSID) II or III.[15,26–30] Other assessments included the Early Problem Solving Indicator (EPSI),[15] Griffiths Developmental Assessments,[15,26,28,30] Neonatal Behavioral Assessment Scale (NBAS),[15,27,30] Neonatal Neurobehavioral Examination (NNE),[15] McCarthy Scales of Children's Abilities,[28] and Wechsler Preschool and Primary Scale of Intelligence (WPPSI).[28]

Two SRs reported that Developmental Care (DC) intervention effects on cognition were inconclusive or inconsistent and showed no long-term effects (see **Table 3**).[15,27] Parent-delivered motor interventions (PDMI) and developmental early intervention programs that commenced in the NICU had significant positive effects on cognition in infancy.[15,28] However, Spittle and colleagues also performed a subgroup analysis of infants with brain injury who received developmental early intervention programs and found no significant differences between groups in infancy or preschool age in MDI scores on the BSID-II (see **Table 3**).[28]

### Effectiveness of Interventions on Parent Outcomes

### Self-efficacy and stress

The study by Girabent-Farres et al.[25] was the only SR to examine the efficacy of interventions meeting our inclusion criteria on parent outcomes (**Table 4**). Common measures of parent stress included the Parent Stress Index (PSI), Parent Stress Index-Short Form (PSI-SF), Post-Traumatic Stress Disorder Test (PTSD), and the Perinatal Posttraumatic Stress Disorder Questionnaire (PPQ).[25,30] Parents of preterm infants in this SR had infants with an average gestational age of 29.7 weeks.[25] Of the ten individual interventions this SR examined, three discrete interventions—Triadic Parent-Infant Relationship Therapy (TRT),[38] Mother–Infant Transactional Program (MITP),[35] and Parent Baby Interaction Program (PBIP)[39]—spanned NICU to home in duration. TRT and PBIP showed no improvements on parent stress at 3 months.[25] The MITP produced small to large positive effects on maternal stress at 8 separate time points between 6 months and 9 years, with the greatest effect observed at 18 months (**Table 5**).[25] In the meta-review by Puthussery and colleagues,[30] investigators reported 2 SRs that examined effects of interventions on stress in parents of preterm infants. One SR reporting pooled effects of Creating Opportunities for Parent Empowerment (COPE), Modified-Mother–Infant Transaction Program (M-MITP), PBIP, Neonatal Behavioral Assessment Scale (NBAS), and Infant Behavioral Assessment and Intervention Program (IBAIP) concluded that evidence was lacking to support these interventions for managing parent stress.[30] The other SR reported that COPE, MITP, and Newborn Individualized Developmental & Assessment Program (NIDCAP) reduced stress symptoms immediately post-intervention, but statistical significance was not reported.[30]

### Quality Assessment

The result of the quality appraisal is presented in **Table 5**. The included SRs had a mean AMSTAR score of 8.7 with the majority of studies rated as 'high' (score 8–11) quality,[15,25–28,30] and one SR[29] rated as 'medium' (score 4–7) quality.[24] All the reviews met the AMSTAR criteria 3 (comprehensive literature search conducted).

**Table 4**
Parent outcomes

| Outcomes | Systematic Review | Participants | Intervention | Effect Size | Additional Information |
|---|---|---|---|---|---|
| Stress | Girabent-Farrés[25] | Parents of preterm infants; average gestational age 29.7 wk | TRT[a] MITP[a] PBIP[a] | 3 mo: 0.13 [−0.10, 0.35]<br><br>12 mo: −0.29 [−0.58, −0.11]<br>18 mo: −0.82 [−1.24, −0.40]<br>5 y: −0.41 [−0.66, −0.15] | TRT[41] and PBIP[42] showed no effect on parent stress.<br>Small but significant effect in favor of MITP[47]<br>Large effect size in favor of MITP[47]<br>Moderate effect size in favor of MITP[47] |

| Stress | Meta-Review | Participants | Intervention | Effect Size | Additional Information |
|---|---|---|---|---|---|
| | Puthussery[30] Benzies[48] | Mothers or fathers of preterm infants | M-MITP[a] COPE[a] PBIP[a] IBAIP, NBAS | Pooled effect z = 0.40 (P = .69) | Inconclusive evidence to support these interventions |
| | Brett | Parents of preterm infants | COPE[a] MITP[a] NIDCAP | Not reported | Reduced stress symptoms reported post-intervention. Statistical significance not reported. |

*Abbreviations:* COPE, creating opportunities for parent empowerment; IBAIP, infant behavioral assessment and intervention program; M-MITP, modified mother–infant transaction program; NBAS, neonatal behavioral assessment scale; NIDCAP, newborn individualized developmental & assessment program; PBIP, parent-baby interaction program; TRT, triadic parent-infant relationship therapy; VIBeS plus, Victorian Infant Brain Studies.
[a] Discrete Intervention programs spanning NICU to home.

**Table 5**
AMSTAR[27] quality ratings

| Areas of Quality Assessed | Systematic Reviews | | | | | | |
|---|---|---|---|---|---|---|---|
| | Frolek Clark and Schlabach[29] | Girabent-Farrés[25] | Hughes[26] | Khurana[15] | Morgan[27] | Puthussery[30] | Spittle[28] |
| Was an "a priori" design provided? | 1 | 1 | 1 | 1 | 1 | 1 | 1 |
| Was there duplicate study selection and data extraction? | 1 | 1 | 1 | 1 | 1 | 1 | 1 |
| Was a comprehensive literature search performed? | 1 | 1 | 1 | 1 | 1 | 1 | 1 |
| Was the status of publication (ie, gray literature) used as an inclusion criterion? | 0 | 0 | 0 | 0 | 0 | 0 | 0 |
| Was a list of studies (included) provided? | 0 | 1 | 1 | 1 | 1 | 1 | 1 |
| Was a list of studies (excluded) provided? | 0 | 0 | 0 | 0 | 0 | 0 | 0 |
| Were the characteristics of the included studies provided? | 1 | 0 | 1 | 1 | 1 | 1 | 1 |
| Was the scientific quality of the included studies assessed and documented? | 0 | 1 | 1 | 1 | 1 | 1 | 1 |
| Was the scientific quality of the included studies used appropriately in formulating conclusions? | 1 | 1 | 1 | 1 | 1 | 1 | 1 |
| Were the methods used to combine the findings of studies appropriate? | 1 | 1 | 1 | 1 | 1 | 1 | 1 |
| Was the likelihood of publication bias assessed? | 0 | 1 | 0 | 1 | 0 | 0 | 1 |
| Was the conflict of interest included? | 0 | 1 | 1 | 1 | 1 | 0 | 1 |
| AMSTAR Total | 6 | 9 | 9 | 10 | 9 | 8 | 10 |

AMSTAR TOOL Key: 1 = Yes, 0 = No/Unclear/Not applicable.

## DISCUSSION

Appraised and synthesized of evidence from six SRs and one meta-review were used to address our question "In infants at high risk for CP, what are the most effective therapeutic interventions delivered as a collaborative between a PT, OT, or SLP and parent, starting in the NICU and continuing post discharge?" The efficacy of the interventions was evaluated for eleven discrete interventions that began in the NICU and transitioned into the home or EI setting with differing components delivered in collaboration between therapists and parents.

Although interventions examined for this meta-review were used by a variety of trained health care professionals (eg, nursing, therapists, psychology students), those that most closely align with PT,[40] OT,[41] or SLP[42] current scopes of practice include Therapist-Delivered Postural Control Intervention (TDPCI),[15] Cues and Care (CC),[30] DC,[15,27] Parent-Delivered Motor Intervention (PDMI),[15] and Supporting Play Exploration and Early Development Intervention (SPEEDI).[15,28] Of the interventions focusing on improving movement quality or activities, PDMI,[15] Parent–Baby Interaction Program (PBIP),[25,30] Auditory, Tactile, Visual, Vestibular intervention (ATVV),[33] Early Intervention Program (EI),[28] and SPEEDI,[15,28] showed the greatest positive effects on infant motor and cognitive outcomes, especially during infancy (<12 months of age). Each of these interventions included key principles of involving parents engaging their infants to support preterm infant development. Our results support previous studies recommendations that interventions that promote motor learning, active infant movement, parent engagement, and environmental modifications[28,43]

Other therapy-relevant educational components delivered by trained health care professionals include infant motor skills, state regulation, and social interaction. For example, the original design of the MITP[32] was delivered by a nurse, but the program was updated in 2006[35] to include a PT consult before NICU discharge. MITP is the only intervention reviewed in this meta-review that resulted in positive effects in outcomes for both infants and parents: infant motor,[26,28,30] infant cognition,[28,30] and parent stress[25,44]

Across SRs there was wide variability in timing, dosage, and frequency of interventions provided (see **Table 2**). Varying levels of dosing and intensity may impact infant and parent outcomes of interest. Clear dosing parameters for therapeutic interventions are needed while considering the individual, family, and environmental characteristics.[45]

Despite the numerous needs of preterm infants and their families, risks of developmental delays, and identified gaps in services, we found that few interventions have been developed and tested that commence in the NICU and transition to the home setting with the goals of improving both infant and parent outcomes.[12,21] Although several interventions are currently being evaluated in large-scale clinical trials,[46–48] additional work is needed to evaluate the implementation of interventions that may require support from policy makers.

With increasing efficacy of interventions using similar key principles, the field is primed to begin a consistent effort toward supporting therapy-oriented research; however, there may be several challenges to developing and implementing interventions including determining who will conduct the intervention (which disciplines and inpatient or outpatient providers), cost of intervention, and available payors given the transition from medical to educational systems that occur with NICU to EI transition. In addition, holistic NICU care is guided by neonatologists who are held accountable for the overall growth and development of their patients, due to their expertise and management of physiologic and neurologic health. This endeavor will therefore require collaborative efforts of medical providers and therapists both in research and in clinical practice, to comprehensively address the various complexities and considerations of the population at high-risk for CP and neurodevelopmental conditions.

### Limitations

There are several limitations to this study. Few SRs reported the specific disciplines, credentials, or training requirements of health care providers who performed the interventions. Many SRs reported that the studies evaluated did not provide sufficient detail for replication in research or clinical practice settings, and no studies systematically reported on safety considerations or adverse events (eg, bradycardia, apnea, desaturations, hypothermia, workflow challenges). This lack of information necessary to create safe, sustainable interventions may further hinder the development of effective transitional interventions in research and clinical practice.

## SUMMARY

The findings of this meta-review offer helpful insights toward important aspects of interventions that commence in the NICU and continue at home. When developing NICU-to-home interventions, investigators and clinicians should use key principles of engaging parents with their infants to support motor development *and* parent-infant interaction for a positive impact. Future research should focus on the development and implementation of high-quality RCTs with larger sample sizes evaluating collaborative parent–therapist interventions that integrate these key principles and to determine effectiveness on both infants and their parents. Individual SRs should evaluate interventions on subgroups with a higher risk of preterm birth including Black families and those representing low socioeconomic status.

---

**Best practices**

- When developing NICU to home interventions, investigators and clinicians should employ key principles of engaging parents with their infants to support motor development *and* parent-infant interaction for positive impact.

---

## CLINICS CARE POINTS

---

- We evaluated the efficacy of eleven discrete interventions that began in the NICU and transitioned into the home or EI setting delivered in collaboration between therapists and parents.
- Interventions that focused on improving movement quality or activities demonstrated the greatest positive effects on infant motor and cognitive outcomes when they engaged parents to support their infant's development.
- Results support previous studies' recommendations to employ interventions that promote motor learning, active infant movement, parent engagement, and environmental modifications.

---

## FUNDING

The author's collaboration is funded by a planning grant from the Academy of Pediatric Physical Therapy of the American Physical Therapy Association, United States. Dr D. McCarty's research is funded in part by the Foundation for Physical Therapy

Research, Promotion of Doctoral Studies award. Dr L. Letzkus is an iTHRIV Scholar. The iTHRIV Scholars Program is supported in part by the National Center for Advancing Translational Sciences, United States of the National Institutes of Health, United States under Award Numbers UL1TR003015 and KL2TR003016. Dr S.C. Dusing's research with infants and children with or at high risk of cerebral palsy is funded in part by NICHD R01 HD101900 and R01 HD093624.

## DISCLOSURE

The authors have no interests to disclose.

## REFERENCES

1. Pierrat V, Marchand-Martin L, Arnaud C, et al. Neurodevelopmental outcome at 2 years for preterm children born at 22 to 34 weeks' gestation in France in 2011: EPIPAGE-2 cohort study. BMJ 2017;358:j3448.
2. Kuban KCK, Joseph RM, O'Shea TM, et al. Girls and boys born before 28 Weeks gestation: risks of cognitive, behavioral, and neurologic outcomes at age 10 years. J Pediatr 2016;173:69–75.e1.
3. Siffel C, Kistler KD, Sarda SP. Global incidence of intraventricular hemorrhage among extremely preterm infants: a systematic literature review. J Perinat Med 2021;49(9):1017–26.
4. Danguecan A, El Shahed AI, Somerset E, et al. Towards a biopsychosocial understanding of neurodevelopmental outcomes in children with hypoxic-ischemic encephalopathy: a mixed-methods study. Clin Neuropsychol 2021;35(5):925–47.
5. Elgendy MM, Puthuraya S, LoPiccolo C, et al. Neonatal stroke: clinical characteristics and neurodevelopmental outcomes. Pediatr Neonatol 2022;63(1):41–7.
6. Iob E, Kirschbaum C, Steptoe A. Persistent depressive symptoms, HPA-axis hyperactivity, and inflammation: the role of cognitive-affective and somatic symptoms. Mol Psychiatry 2020;25(5):1130–40.
7. Bozkurt O, Eras Z, Sari FN, et al. Does maternal psychological distress affect neurodevelopmental outcomes of preterm infants at a gestational age of ≤32weeks. Early Hum Dev 2017;104:27–31.
8. Hofheimer JA, Smith LM, McGowan EC, et al. Psychosocial and medical adversity associated with neonatal neurobehavior in infants born before 30 weeks gestation. Pediatr Res 2020;87(4):721–9.
9. Hoffman C, Dunn DM, Njoroge WFM. Impact of postpartum mental illness upon infant development. Curr Psychiatry Rep 2017;19(12):100.
10. Greene MM, Rossman B, Meier P, et al. Elevated maternal anxiety in the NICU predicts worse fine motor outcome in VLBW infants. Early Hum Dev 2018; 116:33–9.
11. de Cock ESA, Henrichs J, Klimstra TA, et al. Longitudinal associations between parental bonding, parenting stress, and executive functioning in toddlerhood. J Child Fam Stud 2017;26(6):1723–33.
12. McManus BM, Richardson Z, Schenkman M, et al. Timing and intensity of early intervention service use and outcomes among a safety-net population of children. JAMA Netw Open 2019;2(1):e187529.
13. Greene MM, Rossman B, Patra K, et al. Maternal psychological distress and visitation to the neonatal intensive care unit. Acta Paediatr 2015;104(7):e306–13.
14. Pineda R, Bender J, Hall B, et al. Parent participation in the neonatal intensive care unit: predictors and relationships to neurobehavior and developmental outcomes. Early Hum Dev 2018;117:32–8.

15. Khurana S, Kane AE, Brown SE, et al. Effect of neonatal therapy on the motor, cognitive, and behavioral development of infants born preterm: a systematic review. Dev Med Child Neurol 2020;62(6):684–92.
16. Robards F, Kang M, Usherwood T, et al. How marginalized young people access, engage with, and navigate health-care systems in the digital age: systematic review. J Adolesc Health 2018;62(4):365–81.
17. Miles MS, Holditch-Davis D, Schwartz TA, et al. Depressive symptoms in mothers of prematurely born infants. J Dev Behav Pediatr 2007;28(1):36–44.
18. Sec. 303.1 Purpose of the early intervention program for infants and toddlers with disabilities - Individuals with Disabilities Education Act. Available at: https://sites.ed.gov/idea/regs/c/a/303.1. Accessed July 8, 2022.
19. Little AA, Kamholz K, Corwin BK, et al. Understanding barriers to early intervention services for preterm infants: lessons from two states. Acad Pediatr 2015; 15(4):430–8.
20. Nwabara O, Rogers C, Inder T, et al. Early therapy services following neonatal intensive care unit discharge. Phys Occup Ther Pediatr 2017;37(4):414–24.
21. Magnusson D, Palta M, McManus B, et al. Capturing unmet therapy need among young children with developmental delay using national survey data. Acad Pediatr 2016;16(2):145–53.
22. Purdy IB, Craig JW, Zeanah P. NICU discharge planning and beyond: recommendations for parent psychosocial support. J Perinatol 2015;35(Suppl 1):S24–8.
23. Rethlefsen ML, Page MJ. PRISMA 2020 and PRISMA-S: common questions on tracking records and the flow diagram. J Med Libr Assoc 2022;110(2):253–7.
24. Bühn S, Ober P, Mathes T, et al. Measuring test-retest reliability (TRR) of AMSTAR provides moderate to perfect agreement - a contribution to the discussion of the importance of TRR in relation to the psychometric properties of assessment tools. BMC Med Res Methodol 2021;21(1):51.
25. Girabent-Farrés M, Jimenez-Gónzalez A, Romero-Galisteo RP, et al. Effects of early intervention on parenting stress after preterm birth: a meta-analysis. Child Care Health Dev 2021;47(3):400–10.
26. Hughes AJ, Redsell SA, Glazebrook C. Motor development interventions for preterm infants: a systematic review and meta-analysis. Pediatrics 2016;138(4). https://doi.org/10.1542/peds.2016-0147.
27. Morgan C, Novak I, Badawi N. Enriched environments and motor outcomes in cerebral palsy: systematic review and meta-analysis. Pediatrics 2013;132(3): e735–46.
28. Spittle A, Orton J, Anderson PJ, et al. Early developmental intervention programmes provided post hospital discharge to prevent motor and cognitive impairment in preterm infants. Cochrane Database Syst Rev 2015;11:CD005495.
29. Frolek Clark GJ, Schlabach TL. Systematic review of occupational therapy interventions to improve cognitive development in children ages birth-5 years. Am J Occup Ther 2013;67(4):425–30.
30. Puthussery S, Chutiyami M, Tseng P-C, et al. Effectiveness of early intervention programs for parents of preterm infants: a meta-review of systematic reviews. BMC Pediatr 2018;18(1):223.
31. Khurana S, Rao BK, Lewis LE, et al. Neonatal PT improves neurobehavior and general movements in moderate to late preterm infants born in India: an RCT. Pediatr Phys Ther 2021;33(4):208–16.
32. Nurcombe B, Howell DC, Rauh VA, et al. An intervention program for mothers of low-birthweight infants: preliminary results. J Am Acad Child Psychiatry 1984; 23(3):319–25.

33. Nelson MN, White-Traut RC, Vasan U, et al. One-year outcome of auditory-tactile-visual-vestibular intervention in the neonatal intensive care unit: effects of severe prematurity and central nervous system injury. J Child Neurol 2001;16(7):493–8.
34. Ohgi S, Fukuda M, Akiyama T, et al. Effect of an early intervention programme on low birthweight infants with cerebral injuries. J Paediatr Child Health 2004;40(12): 689–95.
35. Kaaresen PI, Rønning JA, Ulvund SE, et al. A randomized, controlled trial of the effectiveness of an early-intervention program in reducing parenting stress after preterm birth. Pediatrics 2006;118(1):e9–19. https://doi.org/10.1542/peds.2005-1491.
36. Johnson S, Whitelaw A, Glazebrook C, et al. Randomized trial of a parenting intervention for very preterm infants: outcome at 2 years. J Pediatr 2009;155(4): 488–94.
37. Koldewijn K, Wolf M-J, van Wassenaer A, et al. The Infant Behavioral Assessment and Intervention Program for very low birth weight infants at 6 months corrected age. J Pediatr 2009;154(1):33–8, e2.
38. Castel S, Creveuil C, Beunard A, et al. Effects of an intervention program on maternal and paternal parenting stress after preterm birth: a randomized trial. Early Hum Dev 2016;103:17–25.
39. Glazebrook C, Marlow N, Israel C, et al. Randomised trial of a parenting intervention during neonatal intensive care. Arch Dis Child Fetal Neonatal Ed 2007;92(6): F438–43.
40. Scope of practice | APTA. Available at: https://www.apta.org/your-practice/scope-of-practice. Accessed July 11, 2022.
41. American Occupational Therapy Association. Occupational therapy scope of practice. Am J Occup Ther 2021;75(Supplement_3). https://doi.org/10.5014/ajot.2021.75S3005.
42. Scope of practice in speech-language pathology. Available at: https://www.asha.org/policy/sp2016-00343/. Accessed July 11, 2022.
43. Morgan C, Darrah J, Gordon AM, et al. Effectiveness of motor interventions in infants with cerebral palsy: a systematic review. Dev Med Child Neurol 2016;58(9): 900–9.
44. Landsem IP, Handegård BH, Tunby J, et al. Early intervention program reduces stress in parents of preterms during childhood, a randomized controlled trial. Trials 2014;15:387.
45. Gannotti ME, Christy JB, Heathcock JC, et al. A path model for evaluating dosing parameters for children with cerebral palsy. Phys Ther 2014;94(3):411–21.
46. Dusing SC, Burnsed JC, Brown SE, et al. Efficacy of supporting Play exploration and early development intervention in the first months of life for infants born very preterm: 3-arm randomized clinical trial protocol. Phys Ther 2020;100(8): 1343–52.
47. Baraldi E, Allodi MW, Löwing K, et al. Stockholm preterm interaction-based intervention (SPIBI) - study protocol for an RCT of a 12-month parallel-group post-discharge program for extremely preterm infants and their parents. BMC Pediatr 2020;20(1):49.
48. Deng Q, Li Q, Wang H, et al. Early father-infant skin-to-skin contact and its effect on the neurodevelopmental outcomes of moderately preterm infants in China: study protocol for a randomized controlled trial. Trials 2018;19(1):701.

# Parenting Style Interventions in Parents of Preterm and High-Risk Infants
## Controversies, Cost, and Future Directions

Mary Lauren Neel, MD, MSCI

### KEYWORDS

- Parenting • Preterm • Interventions • Neurodevelopment • Outcomes

### KEY POINTS

- Early parent-child interactions and parenting style can support positive adaptation, resilience, and competence in preterm, and other high-risk, infants.
- Interventions for parents of preterm infants are ongoing and heterogeneous with variability in intervention timing, measured outcomes, program components, and cost.
- Most reported outcomes for parenting style interventions are measured at age less than 2 years; the few studies reporting later child outcomes are overall positive with improved cognition and behavior in prekindergarten/school-aged children.
- Most parenting style interventions to date target parental responsivity/sensitivity; future studies should focus on balanced programs with multiple parenting style axes to avoid an overreliance on a single axis.
- Fewer studies of parenting style interventions report on the outcome of dyadic interaction.

## INTRODUCTION

An ecobiodevelopmental (EBD) framework combines multidisciplinary perspectives, including neuroscience, social science, and genomics, to explain how early experiences and genetics influence lifetime health.[1] When considering childhood adversity, an EBD perspective asserts that stable, safe, and responsive relationships are the most critical buffer to help children restore their stress response system equilibrium, thus avoiding the long-term negative health consequences of toxic stress.[1] The separation of mother and infant after preterm birth is a source of toxic stress.[2] In support of this EBD framework, numerous studies have shown that early parent-child interactions are the most influential environmental factor supporting positive adaptation, resilience, and competence in preterm, and other high-risk, infants.[3–5] Among myriad

The author has nothing to disclose.
Division of Neonatology, Emory University School of Medicine, Children's Healthcare of Atlanta, 1405 Clifton Road Northeast, Atlanta, GA 30322, USA
*E-mail address:* mneel@emory.edu

medical and social factors also associated with outcomes (**Fig. 1**, **Fig. 2**), parenting impacts child development,[3–5] helps mitigate the effects of toxic stress,[1] and is modifiable.[6,7] Even parents with low social resources can be supported by interventions to alter their parenting style behaviors.[8–10] However, current interventions for parents of preterm infants are highly variable in their timing, outcome targets, and resource requirements.[11–13] This variability makes it difficult to draw interstudy conclusions about efficacy and best practices for parenting interventions for parents of preterm infants.

Parenting style is a complex multidimensional construct.[14] Although investigators may use different terminology, 8 major axes, or characteristics, emerge in the literature to comprise the construct of "parenting style" (**Fig. 3**).[14] Although parent-child interactions are undoubtedly bidirectional, studies suggest that the primary direction of influence is from parent to child rather than from child to parent.[3,15] Parenting styles characterized by responsivity, demandingness, and structure have been associated with improved cognitive and behavioral outcomes in former preterm children.[4,16] Furthermore, parenting interventions to improve parenting style, as exemplified by studies of interventions to increase parental responsivity, have effects on child socioemotional[17,18] and cognitive[19] outcomes.

### Other Constructs Studied in Parents of Preterm Infants

Intervention research involving parents of preterm children has targeted many other areas including parental mental health,[5,17] education,[17,20] and self-capacity that may intersect with parenting.[13] Such interventions have focused on provision of psychosocial support

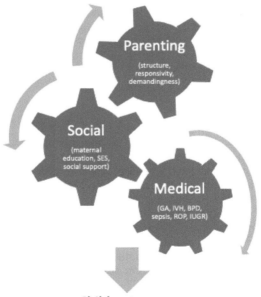

Child outcomes

(cognitive, motor, behavior)

**Fig. 1.** Medical, social, and parenting factors & child outcomes. Medical, social, and parenting factors interact and contribute to neurodevelopmental outcomes in former preterm, and other high-risk, infants. BPD, bronchopulmonary dysplasia; GA, gestational age; IUGR, intrauterine growth restriction; IVH, intraventricular hemorrhage; ROP, retinopathy of prematurity.

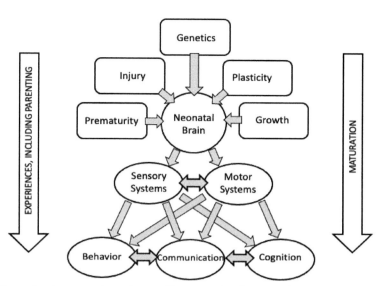

**Fig. 2.** Neurodevelopmental continuum. The neurodevelopmental continuum is not a static process because the neonatal brain is influenced by many dynamic inputs. Sensorimotor development is influenced by medical factors, brain maturation, and infant experience, including environment and parenting factors. Sensorimotor systems develop first, followed by more complex neurobehaviors, including cognition, communication, and behavior. All systems develop in relation to each other and in response to environment, nutrition, maturation, and medical inputs. (*Adapted from* Frosch CA, Fagan MA, Lopez MA, et al. Validation study showed that ratings on the Welch Emotional Connection Screen at infant age 6 months are associated with child behavioural problems at age three years. Acta Paediatr 2019;108(5):889–95 and Neel MLM, Stark AR, Maitre NL. Parenting style impacts cognitive and behavioural outcomes of former preterm infants: A systematic review. Child Care Health Dev 2018;44(4):507–515. Adapted from Maitre 2015[73] Neel 2018.[14])

to promote parental mental health[5,17] and on delivery of parent education, often with the aim of improving child development.[17,20] Parental self-capacity was examined in a previous review of interventions involving parents as active participants,[13] which is critical, but not the focus of this review. Although parental self-capacity, mental health, and education likely influence parenting style and child outcomes, they are not parenting style axes themselves (see **Fig. 3**). Thus, the goal of this review is to highlight the current state of evidence on interventions whose primary purpose is to change parenting style (see **Fig. 3**) in parents of preterm, and other-high risk, infants.

## DISCUSSION

This section highlights some of the more well-studied interventions whose primary purpose is to change an aspect of parenting style in parents of preterm infants. Notably, some of these interventions are limited to the neonatal intensive care unit (NICU) and others to home (post-NICU discharge). However, the vast majority are transitional (starting in the NICU and extending to home).

### Neonatal Intensive Care Unit Interventions

The Parent Baby Interaction Program (PBIP) is the most well-studied parenting intervention in the NICU. The PBIP does include an option for home visits for the first

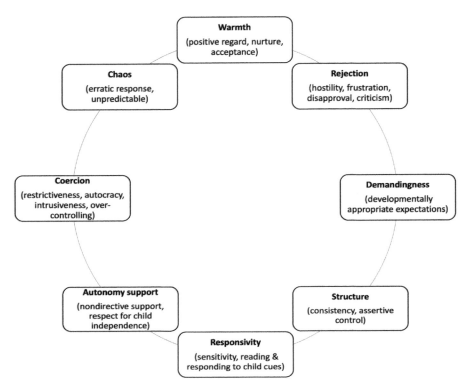

**Fig. 3.** Parenting style axes. The 8 major axes (characteristics) of parenting style and synonyms that emerge across the literature. (*Adapted from* Neel MLM, Stark AR, Maitre NL. Parenting style impacts cognitive and behavioural outcomes of former preterm infants: A systematic review. Child Care Health Dev 2018;44(4):507–15. Adapted from Neel 2018.[14])

6 weeks after discharge, but the program is designed for the NICU and is considered completed at NICU discharge.[21,22] The PBIP aims to increase parental sensitivity to an infant through a nurse-taught, supportive, education curriculum that occurs weekly in the NICU in the first weeks after birth. Session number is variable depending upon the length of time required for content delivery.[21,22] Studies have reported no differences between PBIP and control groups at 3 months corrected gestational age (CGA) in maternal sensitivity (Nursing Child Assessment Teaching Scale [NCATS] sensitivity score 9.6 in intervention group versus 9.5 in control group), parenting stress (Parenting Stress Index [PSI] adjusted mean difference = 3.8; 95% confidence interval [CI], -4.7–12.4), infant neurobehavior (Neurobehavioral Assessment of the Preterm Infant adjusted mean difference = 0.09; 95% CI, -0.06–0.23),[21] or 2-year infant Bayley Scales of Infant Development 2nd edition (Bayley-II) scores (Mental Developmental Index [MDI] group difference −0.9 points; 95% CI, -5 to 3.2; and Psychomotor Developmental Index [PDI] group difference 2.5 points; 95% CI, -3.3–8.4).[22,23]

Other NICU interventions to optimize parenting style have reported some differences in outcomes between intervention and control groups. For example, the "Preterm Infant-Parent Programme for Attachment" includes 3 sessions: reflective interviewing with the mother, mother/trainer observation of infant cues, and video interaction guidance (VIG),[24] a well-defined video feedback strategy focused on parental strengths.[25] After the 3-session intervention in the NICU, parental sensitivity was scored by certified coders using the Child Adult Relationship Evaluation-Index (CARE-Index) at 9 months CGA. This study found no differences between parental sensitivity at 9 months (CARE-Index sensitivity score intervention group mean = 8.33, control group mean = 8.16, $P$ = .969), but did find improved child self-regulation in the intervention group at 12 months (Ages and Stages Questionnaire–Social Emotional Development version [ASQ-SE] intervention group mean = 3.65, control group mean = 6.72, $P$ = .05).[24] Another study using VIG strategy to improve parental sensitivity and decrease parental rejection during parent/child interactions reported increased parental sensitivity and decreased rejection with moderate effect sizes (ES) on video-coded interactions in the first month of life, but this effect faded by 6 months.[26] In summary, although some NICU interventions designed to improve parenting style have been associated with some improved parent or child outcomes, the results are notably mixed. Furthermore, all outcomes are measured at or before 2 years and, at least in some studies improved results are not sustained over time **(Table 1)**.[26]

### Postdischarge (Home) Interventions

The 2 most well-studied home interventions are the Infant Behavioral Assessment and Intervention Program (IBAIP)[30–33] and the Playing and Learning Strategies (PALS) program.[34,35] The IBAIP consists of 6 to 8 intervention sessions, beginning around the time of NICU discharge and continuing until approximately 6 months CGA. The IBAIP targets parental sensitivity as well as structure, by attempting to increase parent sensitivity to infant cues and to teach parents to structure the infant's environment based on infant cues.[30–33] IBAIP randomized controlled trials (RCTs) have demonstrated improvement in parental sensitivity shortly after program completion, at 6 months CGA (intervention vs control group f = 3.8, $P$ = .05 on Maternal Sensitivity and Responsivity Scales).[31] These improvements may or may not be sustained, as another study found no difference in maternal attachment representations at 18 months between IBAIP intervention and control groups.[32] In both groups, ~70% of mothers showed balanced attachment representations and ~30% showed nonbalanced attachment representations on the Working Model of the Child Interview.[32] Nonbalanced attachment representations include disengaged or distorted representations and raise concerns for difficulties with mother/infant attachment and suboptimal infant development.[32]

Similarly, child outcomes after IBAIP are mixed. One study showed that, at 6 months CGA, intervention group Bayley-II cognitive and motor scores were higher than control group scores (intervention vs control adjusted MDI mean = 106 vs 99 ($P$ = .02); adjusted PDI mean = 98 versus 92 [$P$ = .008]).[30] In addition, IBAIP intervention infants showed greater improvement in infant stress and approach behaviors indicating improved regulatory development as measured by the Infant Behavioral Assessment (IBA). IBA approach score increased ($P$ = .001) and IBA stress score decreased ($P$ = .003) in the intervention group compared with controls.[30] In contrast, another study found no differences between infant self-regulation and interactive behaviors at 6 months using the Infant and Caregiver Engagement Phases coding system during parent-infant interaction.[31] The single study that examined longer-term outcomes found significant improvements in motor (ES = 0.355; $P$ = .006), but not cognitive (ES = 0.223; $P$ = .063), outcomes on Movement Assessment Battery for Children, Bayley, and Wechsler Intelligence Scale for Children (WISC) in 5-year-old children whose parents received the IBAIP intervention.[33] Interestingly, children with bronchopulmonary dysplasia (BPD) in the intervention group showed

**Table 1**
Neonatal intensive care unit interventions

| Outcome | Type of Outcome | Age of Outcome Measured | Studies Reporting Improved Outcome in Intervention Group (Intervention Listed) | Studies Reporting Negative/No Outcome Difference Between Intervention (Listed) & Control Groups |
|---|---|---|---|---|
| Cognitive development | Child | <2 y[a] | No studies | Brown et al,[27] 1980 (infant stimulation ± mother training): no difference Bayley cognitive scores at 12 mo[b] (P values not specified) |
| Motor development | Child | <2 y[a] | No studies | Brown et al,[27] 1980 (infant stimulation ± mother training): no difference in Bayley motor scores at 12 mo[b] (P values not specified) |
| Cognitive development | Child | 2 y | No studies | Johnson et al,[22] 2009 (PBIP): no difference in Bayley MDI(-0.4 points; 95% CI, -5.8–5.0) |
| Motor development | Child | 2 y | No studies | Johnson et al,[22] 2009 (PBIP): no difference in Bayley PDI (3.1 points; 95% CI, -3.3–9.6) |
| Behavior or neurobehavior | Child | <2 y[a] | Lawhon et al,[28] 2002 (individualized nursing intervention): APIB median intervention group score = 4.81 at term-corrected age (descriptive study, no historic control for this outcome) Twohig et al,[24] 2021 (PIPPA): improved self-regulation on ASQ-SE at 12 mo CGA (P = .05) | Glazebrook et al,[21] 2007 (PBIP): no difference on NAPI at 35 wk CGA (P = .17) |
| Stress/coping | Parent | <2 y[a] | Browne & Talmi,[29] 2005 (educational demonstration vs educational materials): less stress on PSI 1 mo after NICU discharge (P = .056) | Glazebrook et al,[21] 2007 (PBIP): no difference in PSI at 3 mo CGA (P = .28) |
| Parenting skills | Parent | <2 y[a] | Hoffenkamp et al,[26] 2015 (VIG): more maternal sensitivity and less withdrawal at 6 d and 1 mo CA (P = .001–.01) | Hoffenkamp et al,[26] 2015 (VIG): no difference in maternal sensitivity or withdrawal between control and intervention groups at 6 mo CA (P = .19–.22); no difference between groups for parental intrusiveness at 6 d, 1 mo, or 6 mo CA (P = .38–.96)Twohig et al,[24] 2021 (PIPPA): no difference on CARE-Index maternal sensitivity at 9 mo CGA (P = .8) |

| | | | | |
|---|---|---|---|---|
| Knowledge | Parent | <2 y[a] | Browne & Talmi 2005 (educational demonstration vs educational materials): higher KPIB scores at NICU discharge (P <.001)[29] | No studies |
| Coded interaction | Dyad | <2 y[a] | Browne & Talmi 2005 (educational demonstration vs educational materials): better relationship quality on NCAFS at NICU discharge (P <.05)[29]<br>Lawhon 2002 (individualized nursing intervention): higher NCAFS scores (descriptive study, median intervention parent score = 47 compared with historic control median score = 40 & median intervention infant score = 19.75 compared with historic control median = 17) at term-corrected age[28] | Glazebrook et al,[21] 2007 (PBIP): no difference on NCATS at NICU discharge (P = .43)<br>Brown et al,[27] 1980 (infant stimulation ± mother training): no difference in mother-infant interaction at NICU discharge (P values not specified)<br>Glazebrook et al,[21] 2007 (PBIP): no difference on NCATS at 3 mo CGA (P = .45) |
| HOME scores | Environment | <2 y[a] | No studies | Glazebrook et al,[21] 2007 (PBIP): no difference on HOME scores at 3 mo CGA (P = .46)<br>Brown et al,[27] 1980 (infant stimulation ± mother training): no difference on HOME scores at 9 mo[b] (P values not specified) |

*Abbreviations:* APIB, Assessment of Preterm Infants' Behavior; CA, chronologic age; HOME, Home Observation for Measurement of the Environment; KPIB, knowledge of preterm infant behavior; NAPI, Neurobehavioral Assessment of the Preterm Infant; NCAFS, Nursing Child Feeding Assessment Scale; PIPPA, Preterm Infant-Parent Programme for Attachment.

[a] For the less than 2 y age group, specific ages are listed with the studies.
[b] CA versus CGA not specified.

sustained improvement in both motor and cognitive outcomes (motor ES = 0.896; cognitive ES = 0.681).[33]

The PALS intervention not only primarily targets parental sensitivity but also addresses elements of parental warmth, structure, and lack of rejection.[34,35] This intervention is conducted in the home by a trained facilitator with a curriculum and activities designed to teach parents responsive behaviors in real-life interactions with their high-risk infant through 10 weekly home visits when infant is 6 to 10 months old.[34,35] Short-term results are promising. One study demonstrated that the intervention group maintained responsive parenting skills 3 months after PALS participation, and those who started off weak in parenting domains had increased their skills. In addition, the intervention group parents were more likely to transition from a weaker to a stronger parenting profile.[35] Of those parents in the weakest parenting profile group preintervention, only 17% of intervention parents remained in this profile when compared with 60% of control group parents.[35] Assessments occurred before the first home visit ~6 months CGA, half way through the interventions ~8 months CGA, after the final intervention session ~10 months CGA, and 3 months after the final intervention session ~13 months CGA. Between 6 and 13 months, intervention group parents showed higher contingent responsiveness (d = 0.93) and emotional affective support (d = 0.49), whereas control group parents demonstrated more negative interactive behavior (d = 0.7) on behavioral coding. Furthermore, infants in the intervention group showed lower negative affect (d = 0.7) and greater increases in the use of words (d = 0.75).[34]

Overall, these results from the PALS intervention and others in the home intervention category are encouraging; however, the proximity of the postdischarge home intervention and outcomes less than 2 years highlights the need for further studies of longer-term outcomes after these interventions. The single study of IBAIP that examined outcomes at 5 years demonstrated mixed results, as described earlier.[33] All other studies of home interventions to improve parenting style in parents of former preterm infants included less than 2-year outcomes (**Table 2**).

### Transitional Interventions

The most well-reported transitional parenting intervention for parents of high-risk infants is the Mother Infant Transaction Program (MITP).[43,44] Commensurate with our definition of transitional programs, the MITP begins in the NICU with 7 daily sessions the week of discharge and continues after discharge with 4 home sessions at 3, 14, 30, and 90 days after discharge.[44] The goal of the original MITP is to increase maternal responsivity by sensitizing mothers to their infants' cues and teaching them to respond appropriately.[43,44] Other studies report on modified MITPs; however, the essential program of the original MITP targeting maternal responsivity is unchanged.[45–50] The MITP does appear to increase short-term maternal responsivity in children 3 to 12 months CGA with higher mean values on behaviorally coded mother-child interaction scales, including the Synchrony Scale[50] and the Qualitative Ratings for Parent-Child Interaction at 3 to 15 Months of Age Scale[18] (all $P < .05$). Other maternal outcomes are mixed. One study reports decreased postpartum depression in intervention group mothers at 1 month after NICU discharge (midintervention) measured with the Center for Epidemiologic Studies Depression Scale ($P = .04$),[51] whereas another reports no difference between intervention and control groups on the Edinburgh Postnatal Depression Scale at 3 or 6 months CGA.[50] Other studies describe higher mean scores for intervention parents on measures of maternal role satisfaction (Satisfaction Scale) and self-confidence (Seashore Self-Confidence Rating Paired Comparison Questionnaire [Seashore]) at 6 months

**Table 2**
**After discharge (home) interventions**

| Outcome | Type of Outcome | Age of Outcome Measured | Studies Reporting Improved Outcome in Intervention Group | Studies Reporting Negative/No Outcome Difference Between Intervention and Control Groups |
|---|---|---|---|---|
| Cognitive development | Child | <2 y[a] | Barrera et al,[36] 1986 (parent infant intervention vs developmental care intervention vs control): improved Bayley cognitive scores from 4 to 16 mo CGA (P < .05) <br> McManus et al,[37] 2020 (NBO): improved Bayley communication (b = 1 [0.2, 1.8]), Bayley self-care (b = 2 [0.1, 3.9]), BDI-2 perception/concepts (b = 2 [0.4, 3.6]), BDI-2 attention/memory (b = 3 [0.4, 6]) 6 mo after EI entry (P values ≤ 0.05) <br> Koldewijn et al,[30] 2009 (IBAIP): higher Bayley cognitive scores at 6 mo CGA (P = .02) <br> Landry et al,[34] 2006 (PALS): improved use of words (P = .02) & complex play skills at 6–13 mo CGA (P = .05) | Cho et al,[38] 2013 (JIMHP): no improvement in cognition on KSPD at 12 mo CGA (P value not provided) |
| Cognitive development | Child | PreK/elementary | Van Hus et al,[33] 2016 (IBAIP): children with BPD with sustained cognitive improvement on Bayley & WISC (P = .019) | Van Hus et al,[33] 2016 (IBAIP): no significant longitudinal effects on cognitive outcomes on Bayley & WISC (P = .063) |
| Motor development | Child | <2 y[a] | Koldewijn et al,[30] 2009 (IBAIP): higher Bayley motor scores at 6 mo CGA (P = .008) | Barrera et al,[36] 1986 (parent infant intervention vs developmental care intervention vs control): no significant increase in Bayley PDI scores with intervention from 4-16 mo CGA (P > .05) |

*(continued on next page)*

**Table 2**
*(continued)*

| Outcome | Type of Outcome | Age of Outcome Measured | Studies Reporting Improved Outcome in Intervention Group | Studies Reporting Negative/No Outcome Difference Between Intervention and Control Groups |
|---|---|---|---|---|
| Motor development | Child | PreK/elementary | Van Hus et al,[33] 2016 (IBAIP): improved motor outcomes on Bayley & MABC sustained over 5 y (P = .006) | Cho et al,[38] 2013 (JIMHP): no improvement in child motor outcome on KSPD in intervention vs control group at 12 mo CGA (P value not provided) |
| Behavior or neurobehavior | Child | <2 y[a] | Koldewijn et al,[30] 2009 (IBAIP): higher BRS total scores (P = .004), BRS emotional regulation (P < .001); increased approach behaviors & decreased stress behaviors on IBA (P = .001, P = .003) at 6 mo CGA | Meijssen et al,[31] 2010 (IBAIP): no difference on self-regulation or positive interaction on ICEP at 6 mo CGA (P > .05) |
| Temperament | Child | <2 y[a] | Landry 2006 (PALS): lower negative affect at 6–13 mo CGA (P = .008)[34] Meeks Gardner 2003 (Home visiting intervention): increased cooperation (P < .01) and happiness (P < .05) on Likert scales at 7 mo CA[39] | no studies |
| Problem solving | Child | <2 y[a] | Meeks Gardner 2003 (Home visiting intervention): greater problem solving on "cover test" at 7 mo CA (P < .05)[39] | No studies |
| Mental health | Parent | <2 y[a] | McManus 2020 (NBO): greater decline in maternal depression on CES-D (b = −2.0 [−3.7, −0.3]) at 6 mo post-EI entry (P ≤.05)[37] Cho et al,[38] 2013 (JIMHP): lower ratio of mothers with depression on CES-D at 12 mo CGA (P = .04) | Barlow 2016 (VIG): no difference in parental anxiety (P = .3) or depression (P = .41) on HADS and no difference in PTSD on PC-PTSD (P = .93) after 3 home sessions completed (variable timing)[40] |

| | | | | |
|---|---|---|---|---|
| Parenting skills | Parent | <2 y[a] | Landry et al,[34] 2006 (PALS): higher contingent responsiveness ($P = .001$), higher warm sensitivity ($P = .0001$), & higher verbal scaffolding ($P = .0001$) on standardized coding system at 6–13 mo CGA<br>Guttentag et al,[35] 2006 (PALS): more likely to transition from weaker to stronger profile on standardized video coding (latent class analysis & descriptive analysis, 60% of control group mothers remained in lowest profile group compared with 17% of intervention mothers, $P$ values not provided) at 9–12 mo CGA<br>Meijssen et al,[31] 2010 (IBAIP): increased sensitivity ($P = .05$) & less overcontrolling behaviors ($P = .04$) on MSRS at 6 mo CGA | No studies |
| Attachment | Parent | <2 y[a] | No studies | Meijssen et al,[32] 2011 (IBAIP): no difference in maternal attachment on WMCI at 18 mo CGA ($P = .88$) |
| Social support | Parent | <2 y[a] | No studies | Barnard et al,[41] 1987 (NSTEP-P): no difference in perceived social support on PRQ (high degree of stability in preintervention and postintervention perceived support, $P < .01$ for stability) at 5 mo CGA<br>Cho et al,[38] 2013 (JIMHP): no difference in perceived support from partner, family, or friends at 12 mo CGA ($P$ value not provided) |

(continued on next page)

**Table 2**
*(continued)*

| Outcome | Type of Outcome | Age of Outcome Measured | Studies Reporting Improved Outcome in Intervention Group | Studies Reporting Negative/No Outcome Difference Between Intervention and Control Groups |
|---|---|---|---|---|
| Stress/coping | Parent | <2 y[a] | No studies | Barlow et al,[40] 2016 (VIG): no differences in parental stress on PSI (P = .14) after 3 home sessions completed (variable timing)<br><br>Cho et al,[38] 2013 (JIMHP): no difference in stress on JPSI at 12 mo CGA (P value not provided) |
| Coded interaction | Dyad | <2 y[a] | Barnard 1987 (NSTEP-P): increased mother/infant interaction in almost all categories on NCAFS (P < .01); increased cognitive growth fostering on NCATS (P < .05) at 1 mo–5 mo CGA[41]<br><br>Barlow 2016 (VIG): lower CARE-Index scores for infant difficulty in intervention group (P = .02) after 3 home sessions completed (variable timing).[40]<br><br>Wijnroks[42] 1994 (short-term intervention program): improved mother & infant responsiveness (numbers not available but noted to be "slight improvement" at 6–12 mo[b] (P-values not provided)<br><br>Cho 2013 (JIMHP)– increased maternal interaction on NCAFS at 12 mo CGA (r = 0.57, P < .05)[38]<br><br>Barrera et al,[36] 1986 (parent infant intervention vs developmental care intervention vs control): infants with more verbal independent play (P < .05) & mothers with fewer "no response" to infants (P < .01) at 16 mo CGA | Barnard 1987 (NSTEP-P): no increases on NCATS scores at 3 mo–5 mo CGA (P-value not provided)[41]<br><br>Barlow et al,[40] 2016 (VIG): no significant differences on CARE-Index scores for parental sensitivity, hostility or unresponsiveness (P = .069–.62) or on infant cooperation, compulsiveness, or passivity (P = .01–.4) after 3 home sessions completed (variable timing). However, parental sensitivity and infant cooperation with large effect sizes (d = 0.86, 0.79). |

| HOME scores | Environment | <2 y[a] | Barnard et al,[41] 1987 (NSTEP-P): increased responsivity ($P < .05$) and provision of play materials ($P < .01$) on HOME at 2–4 mo CGA<br>Barrera et al,[36] 1986 (parent infant intervention vs developmental care intervention vs control): higher maternal responsivity & variety of stimulation on HOME ($P < .05$); increased improvement for variety of stimulation & provision of materials on HOME ($P < .05$) at 4–16 mo CGA | No studies |

*Abbreviations:* BDI, Beck Depression Inventory; BRS, Behavioral Rating Scale; CA, chronologic age; CES-D, Center for Epidemiologic Studies Depression Scale; JPSI, Japanese version of the Parenting Stress Index; EI, early intervention; HADS, Hospital Anxiety And Depression Scale; HOME, Home Observation for Measurement of the Environment; JIMHP, Japanese Infant Mental Health Program; KSPD, Kyoto Scale of Psychological Development; MABC, Movement Assessment Battery for Children; MSRS, Maternal Sensitivity and Responsivity Scales; ICEP, Infant and Caregiver Engagement Phases; NBO, Newborn Behavioral Observations System; NSTEP-P, Nursing System Toward Effective Parenting-Premature; PC-PTSD, Primary Care-Post-Traumatic Stress Disorder; PreK, prekindergarten; PRQ, Personal Resources Questionnaire; WMCI, Working Model of the Child Interview.

[a] For the less than 2 y age group, specific ages are listed with the studies.

[b] CA versus CGA not specified.

CGA (~3 months after intervention completion) ($P < .05$).[52] Two studies found that MITP mothers had decreased stress at 3 months (mean difference on PSI = −3.25, $P < .012$)[50] and 2 years (ES = 0.62 on PSI),[46] whereas another study found no differences between MITP and control group mothers' stress at 6 and 12 months on PSI mean total scores ($P$ values = 0.08, 0.46, respectively).[51] A third study reports no difference in maternal anxiety scores on Taylor Manifest Anxiety Scale (Taylor).[52]

Child outcomes after MITP are mixed as well. One study showed improved cerebral white matter microstructure development in MITP intervention group children at term-corrected age.[48] Some studies show improved parent-perceived infant communication skills at 6 to 24 months after MITP on the ASQ (95% CI = 2.8–15.7; $P < .05$)[50] and more advanced communication development on the Communication and Symbolic Behavior Scales Developmental Profile Infant–Toddler Checklist ($P < .05$),[49] whereas other studies report no such improvements using The Pictorial Infant Communication Scales[51] or the Bayley.[46,52] Longer-term child developmental outcomes after MITP have been studied up to 9 years of age.[47,53] Again, these results show variable long-term improvement in child developmental outcomes. One study found no differences between MITP intervention and control group children at 3 years in cognitive or motor outcomes using the Mullen Scale of Early Learning and the ASQ,[54] whereas another found improved scores in the intervention group on the McCarthy Scales of Abilities with a widening intervention gap with age such that by 4 years, intervention preterm group scores were indistinguishable from normal birth weight controls.[52] A third study found insignificant differences in Bayley MDI scores at 3 years, but found that more children in the intervention group (90%) had MDI scores in the normal range when compared with 75% of those in the control group ($P = .03$).[55] Studies of child behavior at 2 and 3 years find no differences between intervention and control groups on the Child Behavior Checklist (CBCL),[46,54] but studies of school-aged children report fewer behavior problems on the CBCL in the intervention group (d = 0.42).[45,53]

School-aged outcomes years after MITP completion are interesting in that one study found no differences in child cognitive outcomes at 7 and 9 years on WISC scores,[47] whereas other studies have found improved cognitive outcomes in intervention groups at 7 and 9 years on the Kaufman Scales.[53,56] These later studies found that low birth weight (LBW) intervention group scores on the Mental Processing Composite of the Kaufman were indistinguishable from normal birth weight controls (means = 107.4 vs 106.1, respectively) and were significantly higher than LBW control scores (mean = 96.6, $P < .001$) at age 7 years,[56] with similar results at 9 years.[53] Two additional studies suggest improved cognitive development in 4- and 5-year-old MITP intervention groups on the McCarthy Scales[52] and the Wechsler Full Scale Intelligence Quotient.[55]

The 3 studies reporting dyadic outcomes of MITP intervention are encouraging.[18,49,50] Results indicate that MITP is associated with improved dyadic interactions, including greater dyadic synchrony on Preterm Mother-Infant Interaction Scale during a bath at term equivalent age ($P < .05$)[49] and higher synchrony ($P < .012$) and mutual attention ($P < .012$) on the Synchrony Scale at 3 to 6 months CGA.[50] A coded dyadic interaction at 12 months CGA found higher maternal responsiveness during interaction with the infant in the intervention group dyads.[18] These consistently improved dyadic interactions after MITP are notable, particularly given the relative lack of coded interactions as outcomes across studies.

Another well-studied transitional parenting intervention is the Creating Opportunities for Parent Empowerment (COPE) Program.[57–59] Although 75% of the COPE program occurs in the NICU, a 1-week postdischarge home visit is a critical component of the intervention.[58] Some versions of COPE include additional postdischarge sessions, for example, at 2, 9, and 18 months CGA.[59] The COPE intervention is multifaceted, but one goal is to sensitize parents to their premature infant's behavior to increase parental responsivity.[57,58] Short-term results of COPE have been promising, with improved 6-month infant cognition on Bayley MDI (ES = 0.72, $P < .05$),[57] stronger parental beliefs about their infant on the Parental Belief Scale (ES 0.47–0.89, $P < .01$),[57,58] and decreased parental stress in the NICU on the Parental Stressor Scale (ES 0.27–0.73, $P < .05$).[57,58] Short-term (0–6 month) maternal anxiety/depression after COPE results are inconsistent. One study found that intervention mothers had less anxiety on the State-Trait Anxiety Inventory (STAI) (ES 0.24, $P = .05$) and depression on the Beck Depression Inventory (ES 0.3, $P = .02$) when compared with control group mothers at 2 months,[58] whereas another study found no group differences between maternal anxiety on STAI or depression on Profile of Mood States Scale at 3 or 6 months.[57] Two-year outcomes after COPE are nuanced with decreased child anxiety measured on the CBCL in children of younger mothers (18–21 years) but not in children of older mothers (children of younger mothers b = −0.26, $P < .05$; children of older mother b = 0.09, $P = $ Not significant [NS]).[59]

A final group of transitional parenting interventions that merit discussion is Neonatal Behavioral Assessment Scale (NBAS)-based interventions.[60–62] These parenting interventions target not only parental responsivity but also elements of parental demandingness by teaching the mother to interact with her infant accounting for the infant's specific development and abilities.[60,61] Some reported outcomes of these interventions up to 12 months are encouraging, with findings of higher infant cognitive scores on Bayley MDI ($P < .05$),[62] improved infant neurobehavior on NBAS ($P < .010$),[60] higher maternal self-efficacy scores on Maternal Self-Efficacy Scale ($P < .05$),[61] and decreased maternal anxiety on STAI ($P = .03$).[60] Other studies have yielded less promising results with no difference between intervention and control groups on less than 12-month Bayley cognitive scores.[60,61] However, to our knowledge, longer-term outcomes of these interventions have not yet been studied.

Across the literature overall, transitional interventions targeting an aspect of parenting style beginning in the NICU and continuing after discharge are the most described. As a result, more outcome data are available for these transitional parenting interventions than for those parenting interventions restricted to either the NICU or the home, individually. A few of these interventions report on school-aged outcomes up to 9 years.[47,53,56] Most studies report improved child cognitive outcomes in the intervention group at preK/school age,[52,53,55,56] and 2 studies report improved child behavioral outcomes at preK/school age.[45,52] These findings suggest that intervention effects may be sustained over time. Almost all the parent outcomes were studied when the child was less than 2 years of age. Although aggregate results suggest that these transitional parenting interventions are associated with improved short-term parental self-confidence[44,60,61] and perception of the infant,[52,57,58] it is not known if these parent outcomes are sustained beyond 2 years. Furthermore, parental mental health outcomes and stress measured when child was less than 2 years of age are notably mixed. Finally, behavioral coding of dyads and environmental Home Observation for Measurement of the Environment scores presented mixed results, with some studies reporting improved maternal responsiveness and positive affect[18,49,50,58] and other studies finding no differences between intervention and control group dyadic interactions (**Table 3**).[40,57,63] However, as mentioned earlier, the dyadic behavioral coding results for the MITP intervention were associated with improved dyadic interactions.[18,49,50]

**Table 3**
Transitional interventions

| Outcome | Outcome Target | Age of Outcome Measured | Studies Reporting Improved Outcome in Intervention Group | Studies Reporting Negative/No Outcome Difference Between Intervention & Control Groups |
|---|---|---|---|---|
| Cognitive development | Child | <2 y | Teti et al,[61] 2009 (EI program with psychoeducational video, infant massage, & serial NBAS): higher Bayley MDI in ELBW subgroup at 3–4 mo CGA (P < .05)<br>Melnyk et al,[57] 2001 (COPE): improved Bayley MDI scores at 3 and 6 mo CGA (ES = 0.6–0.72; P < .05)<br>Zahr,[64] 2000 (home-based intervention): higher Bayley MDI in short intervention at 4 mo CGA (P = .001)<br>Milgrom et al[49] 2013 (Premie Start): more advanced communication on CSBS-DP Infant Toddler Checklist at 6 mo CGA (P < .05)<br>Widmayer and Field,[62] 1981 (Brazelton teaching/NBAS): higher Bayley MDI scores at 12 mo CGA (P < .05)<br>Walker et al,[65] 2004 (psychosocial intervention): higher DQs (P < .05) at 15 mo[b] on Griffiths MDS | Teti et al,[61] 2009 (EI program with psychoeducational video, infant massage, & serial NBAS): no difference in Bayley MDI scores at 3–4 mo CGA (P > .05)<br>Ohgi et al,[60] 2004 (NBAS-based intervention + developmental support): no difference in Bayley MDI scores at 6 mo CGA (P = .07)<br>Rauh et al,[52] 1988 (MITP): no difference on Bayley MDI scores at 6 and 12 mo[b] (P > .05)<br>Ravn et al,[51] 2012 (MITP): no difference on infant communication skills on PICS at 12 mo CGA (P = .86) |
| Cognitive development | Child | 2 y | Walker et al,[65] 2004 (psychosocial intervention): higher performance scores (P < .02) on Griffiths MDS<br>Newnham et al,[50] 2009 (MITP modified): higher communications scores on ASQ (mean difference = 9.27, 95% CI = 2.8–15.7, P > .05)<br>Colditz et al,[66] 2019 (Prem Baby Triple P): improved Bayley cognitive scores (P < .04) | Kaaresen et al,[46] 2008 (MITP modified): no difference on Bayley (P = .14)<br>Rauh et al,[52] 1988 (MITP): no difference on Bayley MDI scores (P > .05)<br>Zahr,[64] 2000 (home-based intervention): control group with higher Bayley MDI (P < .05) |

| Outcome | Target | Age | Findings | No difference |
|---|---|---|---|---|
| Cognitive development | Child | 3 y | Rauh et al,[52] 1988 (MITP): McCarthy scales cognition scores (P < .05)<br>Nordhov et al,[55] 2010 (MITP modified): more normal range Bayley MDI (P = .03) | Kynø et al,[54] 2012 (MITP): no difference on total MSEL (P = .08) & ASQ (P = .34) or any subcategories<br>Nordhov et al,[55] 2010 (MITP modified): no difference on Bayley MDI (P = .06) |
| Cognitive development | Child | PreK/elementary | Rauh et al,[52] 1988 (MITP): improved cognition on McCarthy scales (P < .01)<br>Achenbach et al,[56] 1990 (MITP): improved cognition on Kaufman MPC (P < .001), Sequential (P = .02), and Simultaneous (P = .001) Scales<br>Achenbach et al,[53] 1993 (MITP): improved cognition on Kaufman Total Achievement (P = .022) & Mental Processing Composite (P < .001)<br>Nordhov et al,[55] 2010 (MITP modified): higher FSIQ in intervention group (P = .03) | Hauglann et al,[47] 2014 (MITP modified): no difference in cognitive outcomes on WISC-III (P = .15 at 7 y & P = .45 at 9 y) |
| Motor development | Child | <2 y[a] | Widmayer and Field,[62] 1981 (Brazelton teaching/NBAS): higher tracking, reaching, grasping scores on Denver Developmental Screening at 4 mo CGA (P < .05) | Ohgi et al,[60] 2004 (NBAS-based intervention + developmental support): no difference in Bayley PDI scores at 6 mo CGA (P = .29)<br>Zahr[64] 2000 (home-based intervention): control group with higher Bayley Motor Scale at 8 mo CGA (P < .05)<br>Widmayer and Field,[62] 1981 (Brazelton teaching/NBAS): no difference on Bayley PDI at 12 mo CGA (P > .05) |
| Motor development | Child | 2 y | Colditz et al,[66] 2019 (Prem Baby Triple P): improved Bayley motor scores (P < .001) | Kaaresen et al,[46] 2008 (MITP modified): no difference on Bayley motor scores (P = .66) |
| Motor development | Child | 3 y | No studies | Kynø et al,[54] 2012 (MITP): no difference on total MSEL (P = .08) & ASQ (P = .34) or any subcategories<br>Nordhov et al,[55] 2010 (MITP modified): no difference on Bayley PDI (P = .6) |

(continued on next page)

**Table 3**
*(continued)*

| Outcome | Outcome Target | Age of Outcome Measured | Studies Reporting Improved Outcome in Intervention Group | Studies Reporting Negative/No Outcome Difference Between Intervention & Control Groups |
|---|---|---|---|---|
| Motor development | Child | PreK/elementary | No studies | Nordhov et al,[55] 2010 (MITP modified): no difference in intervention/control groups on McCarthy total scales or grooved pegboard test (P > .05) |
| Behavior or neurobehavior | Child | <2 y[a] | Ohgi et al,[60] 2004 (NBAS-based intervention + developmental support): improved Orientation (P < .01) and State Regulation (P < .01) on NBAS at 1 mo CGA Newnham et al,[50] 2009 (MITP modified): less crying & colic on STSI at 3 mo CGA (P < .012) | Newnham et al,[50] 2009 (MITP modified): no difference on STSI crying or colic at 6 mo CGA (P > .05) |
| Behavior or neurobehavior | Child | 2 y | No studies | Kaaresen et al,[46] 2008 (MITP modified): no difference on CBCL (P = .13–.36) Colditz et al,[66] 2019 (Prem Baby Triple P): no difference on ITSEA (P = .3–.9) or RFOS (P = .7–.9) |
| Behavior or neurobehavior | Child | 3 y | No studies | Kynø et al,[54] 2012 (MITP): no difference on ASQ-SE (P = .83) or CBCL (P = .12–.48) |
| Behavior or neurobehavior | Child | PreK/elementary | Nordhov et al,[45] 2012 (MITP modified): fewer behavior problems on CBCL (d = 0.42; P = .02) & SDQ (d = 0.43; P = .04) Achenbach et al,[53] 1993 (MITP): fewer behavioral problems on CBCL (P = .043) | No studies |

| | | | | |
|---|---|---|---|---|
| Temperament | Child | <2 y[a] | Newnham et al,[50] 2009 (MITP modified): more approach tendencies on STSI at 3 mo CGA (P < .012) | Milgrom et al,[49] 2013 (Premie Start): no difference groups on Short Temperament Scales for Infants at 6 mo CGA (P > .05) Newnham et al,[50] 2009 (MITP modified): no difference on STSI approach tendencies at 6 mo CGA (P > .05) Ravn et al,[51] 2012 (MITP): no improvement in perceived infant temperament on IBQ; only significant P values were increased smiling in control group (P = .006 & P = .022); all other P values > 0.05 at 6 mo and 12 mo CGA |
| Medical (LOS/growth/imaging) | Child | <2 y[a] | Melnyk et al,[58] 2006 (COPE): intervention group with shorter NICU stay (3.8 d) (P = .05) Milgrom et al,[48] 2010 (Premie Start): improved cerebral white matter microstructural development in intervention group on MRI at 40 wk CGA (P = .0006) | Milgrom et al,[49] 2013 (Premie Start): no difference in LOS or respiratory status (P > .05) Teti et al,[61] 2009 (EI program with psychoeducational video, infant massage, & serial NBAS): no intervention/control group differences in anthropometric measurements at 3–4 mo CGA (P > .05) |
| Problem solving | Child | <2 y[a] | No studies | Newnham et al,[50] 2009 (MITP modified): no difference on ASQ Problem Solving between groups at 3–6 mo CGA (P > .05) |
| Child stress/anxiety | Child | 2 y | Oswalt et al,[59] 2013 (COPE): less anxiety on CBCL for children of mothers ≤21 y (b = −0.26, P < .05) | Oswalt et al,[59] 2013 (COPE): no difference in anxiety on CBCL for children of mothers >21 y (b = 0.09, P > .05) |
| Mental health | Parent | <2 y[a] | Ravn et al,[51] 2012 (MITP): less postpartum depression on CES-D 1 mo after NICU discharge (P = .04) Ohgi et al,[60] 2004 (NBAS-based intervention + developmental support): decreased anxiety on STAI at 1 mo CGA (P = .03) | Rauh et al,[52] 1988 (MITP): no difference in maternal anxiety on Taylor Manifest Anxiety Scale at NICU discharge & 4 mo[b] (P > .05) Newnham et al,[50] 2009 (MITP modified): no group difference in maternal depression on EPDS at 3–6 mo CGA (P > .05) |

(continued on next page)

**Table 3**
*(continued)*

| Outcome | Outcome Target | Age of Outcome Measured | Studies Reporting Improved Outcome in Intervention Group | Studies Reporting Negative/No Outcome Difference Between Intervention & Control Groups |
|---|---|---|---|---|
| | | | Melnyk et al,[58] 2006 (COPE): less anxiety on STAI (effect size 0.24, $P = .05$) and depression on BDI at 2 mo CGA (effect size 0.3, $P = .02$)<br><br>Borghini et al,[67] 2014 (transactional preventative intervention): decreased PTSD on PPQ at 12 mo CGA ($P = .001$)<br><br>Oswalt et al,[59] 2013 (COPE): less anxiety on STAI for children of mothers ≤21 y ~18 mo CGA ($B = −0.28$, $P < .05$) | Melnyk et al,[57] 2001 (COPE): no difference on maternal anxiety or depression on STAI or POMS at 3 and 6 mo CGA ($P > .05$)<br><br>Oswalt et al,[59] 2013 (COPE): no difference in anxiety on the STAI for children of mothers >21 y ~18 mo CGA ($B = 0.01$, $P > .05$) |
| Stress/coping | Parent | <2 y[a] | Melnyk et al,[57] 2001 (COPE): decreased maternal stress on PSS before NICU discharge (most often before term age but variable ages of infants) (effect size 0.73, $P < .05$)<br><br>Melnyk et al,[58] 2006 (COPE): decreased maternal stress while in NICU (PSS total score effect size = 0.27, $P = .03$)<br><br>Newnham et al,[50] 2009 (MITP modified): lower maternal stress on PSI at 3 mo CGA ($P < .012$) | Ravn et al,[51] 2012 (MITP): no difference in parental stress on PSI at 6 mo and 12 mo CGA ($P = .08$ & $P = .46$) |
| Stress/coping | Parent | 2 y | Kaaresen et al,[46] 2008 (MITP modified): decreased maternal stress on PSI (ES = 0.62d; $P = .002$) | No studies |
| Parenting skills | Parent | <2 y[a] | No studies | Evans et al,[63] 2017 (Prem Baby Triple P): no differences in maternal responsiveness on MIRI at 6 wk CGA ($P = .935$) or 12 mo CGA ($P = .155$) |

| Outcome | Population | Age | | |
|---|---|---|---|---|
| | | <2 y[a] | | |
| Attachment | Parent | <2 y[a] | No studies | Teti et al,[61] 2009 (EI program with psychoeducational video, infant massage, & serial NBAS): no differences in maternal sensitivity on MBQ at 3–4 mo CGA (P > .05)<br><br>Evans et al,[63] 2017 (Prem Baby Triple P): no difference in attachment on MPAS at 6 wk CGA (P = .61) and lower attachment scores in intervention group at 12 mo CGA (P = .021)<br><br>Brisch et al,[68] 2003 (parent-centered intervention program): no difference on attachment quality on Strange Situation Procedure at 14 mo CGA (P = .084) |
| Social support | Parent | <2 y[a] | Zahr et al,[64] 2000 (home-based intervention): short intervention group with higher social support on ASSIS at 18 mo CGA (P = .004) | No studies |
| Role satisfaction | Parent | <2 y[a] | Rauh et al,[52] 1988 (MITP): higher maternal role satisfaction on Satisfaction Scale at 6 mo[b] (P < .05) | No studies |
| Self-confidence | Parent | <2 y[a] | Ohgi et al,[60] 2004 (NBAS-based intervention + developmental support): increased maternal confidence on LCC at 1 mo CGA (P < .01)<br><br>Zahr et al[64] 2000 (home-based intervention): short intervention group with higher confidence on MCQ at 1 mo CGA (P < .05)<br><br>Teti et al[61] 2009 (EI program with psychoeducational video, infant massage, & serial NBAS): higher maternal self-efficacy on MSES at 3–4 mo CGA (P < .05)<br><br>Rauh et al,[52] 1988 (MITP): higher self-confidence on Seashore Questionnaire at 6 mo[b] (P < .05) | 8 mo CGA Zahr,[64] 2000 (home-based intervention): no difference on competence subscale on PSI (P > .05) |

(continued on next page)

**Table 3**
*(continued)*

| Outcome | Outcome Target | Age of Outcome Measured | Studies Reporting Improved Outcome in Intervention Group | Studies Reporting Negative/No Outcome Difference Between Intervention & Control Groups |
|---|---|---|---|---|
| Perception of infant | Parent | <2 y[a] | Melnyk et al,[57] 2001 (COPE): stronger beliefs PBS before NICU discharge (most often before term age but variable ages of infants) (ES = 0.89, P < .01)<br>Melnyk et al,[58] 2006 (COPE): stronger beliefs on PBS during NICU stay (ES = 0.47, P < .001)<br>Rauh et al,[52] 1988 (MITP): lower negative perception of infant temperament on CITQ at 6 mo[b] (P < .01) | No studies |
| Breastfeeding | Parent | <2 y[a] | Ravn et al,[51] 2012 (MITP): increased breastfeeding on WHO breastfeeding categories at 9 mo CGA (P = .02) | No studies |
| Coded interaction | Dyad | <2 y[a] | Melnyk et al,[58] 2006 (COPE): more positive parent-infant interactions (mother ES = 0.26, P = .04; father/coparent ES = 0.55, P = .003) in NICU<br>Milgrom et al,[49] 2013 (Premie Start): more sensitivity synchrony & decreased infant stress during bath (P < .05) on PREMIIS at term equivalent age<br>Kang et al,[9] 1995 (SM ± NSTEP-P vs active control): improved mother/infant interaction scores on NCAFS (P = .01–.04) & NCATS (P = .01–.05) at 1.5 mo CGA<br>Newnham et al,[50] 2009 (MITP modified): more maternal responsiveness (P < .05), attentiveness (P < .012) & alertness (P < .012); dyads with more synchrony (P < .012) & mutual attention (P < .012) on Synchrony Scale at 3–6 mo CGA | Melnyk et al,[57] 2001 (COPE): no difference on NCAFS at 3 and 6 mo CGA (P > .05)<br>Evans et al,[63] 2017 (Prem Baby Triple P): no difference in quality of mother-infant relationship using EA at 6 wk CGA (P = .418–.979) or 12 mo CGA (P = .194–.955)<br>Borghini et al,[67] 2014 (transactional preventative intervention): no difference between intervention/control group on CARE-Index for maternal controlling/unresponsiveness or infant compliance/passivity at 4–5 mo CGA (P > .05)<br>Zahr[64] 2000 (home-based intervention): no differences between intervention and control groups on NCAFS & NCATS scores at 1, 8, or 18 mo CGA (P > .05) |

| Outcome measure | Unit of analysis | Age | | |
|---|---|---|---|---|
| Coded interaction | Dyad | <2 y[a] | Widmayer and Field,[62] 1981 (Brazelton teaching/NBAS): improved mother-infant interaction scores on standardized rating scale at 4 mo CGA (P < .05)<br>Borghini et al,[67] 2014 (transactional preventative intervention): increase in maternal sensitivity (P < .05) & infant cooperation (P < .001) on CARE-Index at 4–5 mo CGA<br>Ravn et al,[18] 2011 (MITP): higher sensitivity/responsiveness on coded interaction at 12 mo CGA (P = .05) | Zahr,[64] 2000 (home-based intervention): no differences between intervention and control groups on NCATS scores (P > .05) |
| Coded interaction | Dyad | 2 y | No studies | |
| HOME scores | Environment | <2 y[a] | Walker et al,[65] 2004 (psychosocial intervention): higher HOME scores (P < .05), avoidance of restriction (P < .01), punishment and maternal involvement (subscale P < .01) on HOME at 12 mo[b] | Melnyk et al,[57] 2001 (COPE): no difference on HOME scores at 3 and 6 mo CGA (P > .05)<br>Zahr,[64] 2000 (home-based intervention): no differences between intervention and control groups on HOME scores at 4 and 18 mo CGA (P > .05) |
| HOME scores | Environment | 2 y | No studies | Zahr,[64] 2000 (home-based intervention): no differences between intervention and control groups on HOME scores (P > .05) |

*Abbreviations:* ASSIS, Arizona Social Support Interview Schedule; BDI, Beck Depression Inventory; CA, Chronologic age; CES-D, Center for Epidemiologic Studies Depression Scale; CITQ, Carey Infant Temperament Questionnaire; CSBS-DP Infant Toddler Checklist; Communication and Symbolic Behavior Scales Developmental Profile Infant–Toddler Checklist; DQ, developmental quotient; EA, emotional availability scales; EI, early intervention; ELBW, extremely low birth weight; EPDS, Edinburgh Postnatal Depression Scale; FSIQ, Wechsler Full Scale Intelligence Quotient; HOME, Home Observation for Measurement of the Environment; IBQ, Infant Behavior Questionnaire; ITSEA, Infant And Toddler Social Emotional Adjustment Scale; LCC, lack of confidence in caregiving; LOS, length of stay; MBQ, Maternal Behavioral Q-Set; MCQ, Maternal Confidence Questionnaire; MDS, mental developmental scales; MIRI, Maternal Infant Responsiveness; MOC, Mental Processing Composite; MPAS, Maternal Postnatal Attachment Scale; MPC, Mental Processing Composite; MSEL, Mullen Scale of Early Learning; MSES, Maternal Self-Efficacy Scale; NSTEP-P, Nursing System Toward Effective Parenting-Premature; PICS, Pictorial Infant Communication Scales; PBS, Parental Belief Scale; POMS, Profile of Mood States Scale; PPQ, Perinatal Posttraumatic Stress Disorder Questionnaire; Prem Baby Triple P, Baby Triple P for Preterm Infants; PREMIIS, Preterm Mother-Infant Interaction Scale; PSS, Parental Stressor Scale; RFOS, Revised Family Observation Schedule; SDQ, Strengths & Difficulties Questionnaire; Seashore Questionnaire, Seashore Self-Confidence Rating Paired Comparison Questionnaire; SM, state modulation; STSI, The Short Temperament Scale for Infants; WHO, World Health Organization.

[a] For the less than 2 y age group, specific ages are listed with the studies.

[b] CA versus CGA not specified.

**Supplementary Table 1**
Parenting style intervention timing, type and parenting style axis targeted.

| Author | Year | Timing | Intervention Name | Parenting Axis |
|---|---|---|---|---|
| Barlow et al[40] | 2006 | Home | VIG | Sensitivity |
| Barnard et al[41] | 1987 | Home | NSTEP-P | Sensitivity, structure |
| Barrera et al[36] | 1986 | Home | Parent infant intervention vs developmental care intervention vs control groups | Sensitivity |
| Cho et al[38] | 2013 | Home | JIMHP | Sensitivity |
| Guttentag et al[35] | 2006 | Home | PALS | Sensitivity, warmth, rejection, structure |
| Koldewijn et al[30] | 2009 | Home | IBAIP | Sensitivity |
| Landry et al[34] | 2006 | Home | PALS | Sensitivity, warmth, rejection, structure |
| Landry et al[88] | 2008 | Home | PALS | Sensitivity, warmth, rejection, structure |
| McManus et al[37] | 2020 | Home | NBO | Sensitivity |
| Meeks-Gardner et ak[39] | 2003 | Home | Home visiting intervention based on a program from the Mental Health Department of the WHO | Sensitivity, structure |
| Meijssen et al[31] | 2010 | Home | IBAIP | Sensitivity, structure |
| Meijssen et al[32] | 2011 | Home | IBAIP | Sensitivity, structure |
| Van Hus et al[33] | 2016 | Home | IBAIP | Sensitivity, structure |
| Wijnroks[89] | 1994 | Home | Short-term intervention program | Sensitivity |
| Brown et al[27] | 1980 | NICU | 3 intervention groups: infant stimulation, mother training, both, and control group | Sensitivity |
| Browne & Talmi[29] | 2005 | NICU | Group 1 demonstration of infant reflexes, attention, motor skills, sleep/wake state vs Group 2 educational materials | Sensitivity |

| Study | Year | Setting | Intervention | Outcome |
|---|---|---|---|---|
| Glazebrook et al[21] | 2007 | NICU (optional extension for 6 wk) | PBIP | Sensitivity |
| Hoffenkamp et al[26] | 2015 | NICU | VIG | Sensitivity, rejection |
| Johnson et al[22] | 2009 | NICU (optional extension for 6 wk) | PBIP | Sensitivity |
| Lawhon[28] | 2002 | NICU | Individualized nursing intervention | Sensitivity |
| Twohig et al[24] | 2021 | NICU | Preterm Infant-Parent Programme for Attachment: reflective interview, observation of infant cues and VIG | Sensitivity |
| Achenbach et al[56] | 1990 | Transitional | MITP | Sensitivity |
| Achenbach et al[53] | 1993 | Transitional | MITP | Sensitivity |
| Borghini et al[67] | 2014 | Transitional | transactional preventive intervention | Sensitivity, demandingness |
| Brisch et al[68] | 2003 | Transitional | Parent centered intervention program with 4 parts: parent group, psychotherapy, home visit, parent sensitivity training | Sensitivity |
| Colditz et al[66] | 2019 | transitional | Prem Baby Triple P | Sensitivity, structure, demandingness, warmth, autonomy support |
| Evans et al[63] | 2017 | Transitional | Prem Baby Triple P | Sensitivity, structure, demandingness, warmth, autonomy support |
| Hauglann et al[47] | 2014 | Transitional | MITP modified | Sensitivity |
| Kaaresen et al[46] | 2008 | Transitional | MITP modified | Sensitivity |
| Kang et al[9] | 1995 | Transitional | SM ± NSTEP-P vs active control | Sensitivity, structure |
| Kyno[54] | 2012 | Transitional | MITP | Sensitivity |
| Melnyk et al[57] | 2001 | Transitional | COPE | Sensitivity |
| Melnyk et al[58] | 2006 | Transitional | COPE | Sensitivity |
| Milgrom et al[48] | 2010 | Transitional | Premie Start (MITP modified) | Sensitivity |
| Milgrom et al[49] | 2013 | Transitional | Premie Start (MITP modified) | Sensitivity |

(continued on next page)

**Supplementary Table 1 (continued)**

| Author | Year | Timing | Intervention Name | Parenting Axis |
|---|---|---|---|---|
| Newnham et al[50] | 2009 | Transitional | MITP modified | Sensitivity |
| Nordhov et al[55] | 2010 | Transitional | MITP modified | Sensitivity |
| Nordhov et al[45] | 2012 | Transitional | MITP modified | Sensitivity |
| Nurcombe et al[43] | 1984 | Transitional | MITP | Sensitivity, structure |
| Ohgi et al[60] | 2004 | Transitional | NBAS-based intervention plus developmental support | Sensitivity, demandingness, structure |
| Oswalt et al[59] | 2013 | Transitional | COPE | Sensitivity |
| Rauh et al[52] | 1988 | Transitional | MITP | Sensitivity |
| Rauh et al[44] | 1990 | Transitional | MITP | Sensitivity |
| Ravn et al[18] | 2011 | Transitional | MITP | Sensitivity |
| Ravn et al[51] | 2012 | Transitional | MITP | Sensitivity |
| Teti et al[61] | 2009 | Transitional | EI program with psychoeducational video, infant massage and serial NBAS | Sensitivity, demandingness |
| Walker et al[65] | 2004 | Transitional | Psychosocial intervention | Sensitivity |
| Widmayer et al[62] | 1981 | Transitional | Brazelton teaching/NBAS | Sensitivity |
| Zahr[64] | 2000 | Transitional | Home-based intervention | Sensitivity |

COPE, Creating Opportunities for Parent Empowerment; EI, early intervention; IBAIP, Infant Behavioral Assessment and Intervention Program; JIMHP, Japanese Infant Mental Health Program; MITP, Mother Infant Transaction Program; NBAS, Neonatal Behavioral Assessment Scale; NBO, Newborn Behavioral Observations System; NSTEP-P, Nursing System Toward Effective Parenting- Premature; PALS, Playing And Learning Strategies; PBIP, Parent Baby Interaction Program; Prem Baby Triple P, Baby Triple P for Preterm Infants; SM, state modulation; VIG, video interaction guidance; WHO, World Health Organization.

## Intervention Targets

Across NICU, home, and transitional interventions, most parenting style interventions target parental responsivity (synonymous with sensitivity) (see **Fig. 3**; **Supplementary Table 1**). A previous review of interventions in preterm infants found that the most successful interventions supported parental responsivity.[11] In addition, programs after discharge that support responsive parenting and sensitive parent-infant interactions may be highly effective in supporting child developmental gains.[3,19] Although parental responsivity forms a basis for high-quality parent-infant interactions[3] and is important for later child outcomes,[69] parental responsivity is not the only parenting characteristic that is important to optimize child development.[4,16,70] Specifically, parental demandingness (often defined as developmentally appropriate expectations) and parental structure have both been linked with improved developmental outcomes in former preterm children.[4,16]

## Reported Outcomes

Most studies on parenting style interventions report short-term outcomes at less than 2 years of life; however, a few studies did include longer-term outcomes to school age (see **Tables 1–3**). Child outcomes (cognitive, behavior, stress) were reported most frequently, followed by parent outcomes (mental health, stress, role satisfaction). Relatively fewer studies report on dyadic interactions or home environment as outcomes. The Nursing Child Feeding Assessment Scale (NCAFS) and NCATS[41] were the most frequently reported measures of dyadic interaction (see **Tables 1–3**). The NCAFS and NCATS are self-reported questionnaires with yes/no responses regarding typical interactions between caregiver and infant during a feeding or simple teaching activity, respectively.[41] Dyadic interactions are critical, because parent-infant interactions are foundational for child development.[71] A recent tool, the Welch Emotional Connection Screen, has been validated in late preterm infants as a measure of mother-infant relational health.[72] This screen can be used during a 5-minute parent-child interaction and does not rely on parental report or extensive coding systems.[72,73] Other novel measures of parent-infant dyadic interactions include electroencephalography measures of frontal connectivity[74] and frontal alpha asymmetry,[75] among others.

## CONTROVERSIES

### Timing of Interventions and Outcome Measures

As discussed, parenting style interventions for parents of preterm infants occur in the NICU, at home, and spanning both locations. A Cochrane review of early developmental interventions found that programs that begin in the NICU were associated with the most long-term improvement in cognition at school age compared with programs that began after discharge.[20] Although this Cochrane review does not specifically address parenting style interventions as we do here, early interventions have been associated with improved parent-child interactions moving forward, before suboptimal dynamics can be cemented.[19,76]

Early intervention impacts downstream development,[65] and the earlier the intervention, the greater the return on investment.[77] One study found that intervention shortly after birth was associated with improved problem-solving skills at 7 months.[65] These shorter-term outcomes were then associated with improved child developmental quotients at 15 and 24 months.[65] Thus, even if intervention is associated with short-term outcome improvement, these short-term outcomes may lay the foundation for improved longer-term outcomes. Other studies have suggested that interventions need to continue after discharge because the longer-term benefits of NICU interventions are less clear.[3,5] A review of interventions for parents of preterm infants found that most effective interventions included multiple contacts over 1 year and actively involved parents in the intervention.[11]

## Cost

Although long-term sustained contact with parents of formerly preterm infants may be most ideal, the issue of feasibility emerges. Long-term, high-contact programs are expensive and time consuming and may not be feasible for researchers, hospitals, and families. Most of the parenting style interventions included in this review required a full-time specially trained staff member (often a registered nurse with previous NICU experience).[21,22,44,78] Furthermore, sessions targeting parenting style require time and repetition, sometimes 1 to 2 h/wk until 6 months CGA or beyond.[34,60,64] Home visits are time and resource intensive, particularly in centers with large catchment areas. The requirements of these intervention programs may also limit their generalizability, because parents who have limited parental leave, other children, and/or lack of family support may have difficulty participating in these programs. These time and resource constraints for both intervention providers and families may limit the number of parents and children who could benefit from these programs. Although daunting, there is evidence that low-cost programs can still impact child outcomes. For example, a home visiting intervention in Jamaica with 8 weekly 1-hour visits and costing $70 total per child (including trainer, travel, and toys) was associated with improved infant problem-solving skills and behaviors at 7 months.[39] The investigators conclude that even "limited inputs can have benefits."[39] For all interventions, the cost, benefit, generalizability, and return on investment must be at the forefront of the program design discussion.[77,79]

## Parenting Style Targets

Most interventions to date have targeted parental responsivity (see **Supplementary Table 1**). However, the 8 parenting style characteristics are often not clearly separated.[14] For example, many studies describe parental responsivity with inclusion of an element of parental structure as well. As parents notice their child's cues and respond by structuring the child's environment, elements of both parental responsivity and parental structure to support the child are seen.[14,60] Other parenting style constructs are defined by their combination of several of the 8 parenting style characteristics. For example, Baumrind's[80,81] typology of Authoritarian, Authoritative, and Permissive parenting styles are defined based on the degree of parental responsivity and parental demandingness.[82] Permissive parenting is characterized by high responsivity and low demandingness.[16,80–82] Permissive parenting style has been associated with worse behavioral, sensory, cognitive, and motor outcomes in former preterm children,[4,16] thus highlighting the dangers of an over-reliance on a single parenting axis, not balanced by another axis. Parenting style is a complex and multidimensional construct. We do not yet know the most ideal, yet feasible, combination of parenting style characteristic targets to optimize outcomes in former preterm infants, together with their families.

## FUTURE DIRECTIONS

Since the 1990s, researchers have noted a lack of mechanistic understanding regarding why certain parenting interventions work.[11] Although recent work on resilience and positive adaptation have expanded our conceptual framework,[4,83] we need to better characterize the mechanistic underpinnings and early infant response to parenting style interventions to better assess the efficacy of our interventions in real time. To this end, novel measures of parent/infant dyadic interactions, as described earlier, may prove useful.

Studies of neuroscience and economics would suggest that the earlier the intervention, the greater the impact.[77,84,85] To take advantage of brain neuroplasticity, the intervention must begin as early as possible.[86] Such data may shift the cost-benefit equation of early parenting interventions. Most studies to date have not adequately studied the longer-term impact of the earliest parenting interventions.[3]

We must focus on studies that target parenting characteristics beyond responsivity alone. Such characteristics, in combination, may be uniquely important for formerly preterm children.[4] Furthermore, we need to focus on groups of preterm infants who might benefit most from interventions, to narrow the disparity gap.[33,59,61] Such groups might include those with particular medical comorbidities, such as BPD or intraventricular hemorrhage, nonwhite infants, or those with lower maternal education levels. Finally, all interventions targeting parenting should be based on a strong theoretic framework, tested in pilot studies, and followed by RCTs.[69]

## SUMMARY

"Intervene early, intervene often, and intervene effectively," JF Mustard.[87] To intervene effectively we must examine the mechanistic underpinnings of parenting style interventions, novel measures of dyadic interactions, combinations of parenting style characteristic targets, how different subsets of preterm infants benefit differentially, and longer-term outcomes of parenting style interventions. These data, in combination, will advance our goal as practitioners to support evidence-based parenting styles, so that parents can best augment the development of their formerly preterm children.

## BEST PRACTICES

*What is the current practice for parenting style interventions for parents of preterm, and other high-risk, infants?*

Parenting style interventions can alter parenting style, and parenting style impacts child neurodevelopmental outcomes. Although critical to optimize child neurodevelopment, parenting style interventions for parents of high-risk infants to date are heterogeneous, with variable timing and with most outcomes reported at less than 2 years of age.

Major recommendations
Future research on parenting style interventions for parents of high-risk infants should include:
- examination of the mechanistic underpinnings of parenting style interventions
- novel measures of dyadic interactions
- combinations of parenting style characteristic targets
- longer-term outcomes of parenting style interventions
- careful consideration of the cost, benefit, generalizability, and return on investment in intervention design
- intervention design based on theoretic framework and tested in pilot studies followed by randomized controlled trials

## REFERENCES

1. Child CoPAo, Family Health CoEC, Adoption, Dependent Care, et al. Early childhood adversity, toxic stress, and the role of the pediatrician: translating developmental science into lifelong health. Pediatrics 2012;129(1):e224–31.

2. Bergman NJ. Birth practices: maternal-neonate separation as a source of toxic stress. Birth defects Res 2019;111(15):1087–109.
3. Guralnick MJ. Preventive interventions for preterm children: effectiveness and developmental mechanisms. J Developmental Behav Pediatr 2012;33(4):352.
4. Neel ML, de Silva A, Taylor HG, et al. Exceeding expectations after perinatal risks for poor development: associations in term-and preterm-born preschoolers. J Perinatol 2022,;42(4),):491–8.
5. Spittle A, Treyvaud K. The role of early developmental intervention to influence neurobehavioral outcomes of children born preterm. Elsevier 2016;542–8.
6. Berlin LJ, Brooks-Gunn J, McCarton C, et al. The effectiveness of early intervention: examining risk factors and pathways to enhanced development. Prev Med 1998;27(2):238–45.
7. Feldman R, Eidelman AI, Sirota L, et al. Comparison of skin-to-skin (kangaroo) and traditional care: parenting outcomes and preterm infant development. Pediatrics 2002;110(1):16–26.
8. White-Traut RC, Nelson MN. Maternally administered tactile, auditory, visual, and vestibular stimulation: relationship to later interactions between mothers and premature infants. Res Nurs Health 1988;11(1):31–9.
9. Kang R, Barnard K, Hammond M, et al. Preterm infant follow-up project: a multisite field experiment of hospital and home intervention programs for mothers and preterm infants. Public Health Nurs 1995;12(3):171–80.
10. Pridham KA, Lutz KF, Anderson LS, et al. Furthering the understanding of parent–child relationships: a nursing scholarship review series. Part 3: interaction and the parent–child relationship—Assessment and intervention studies. J Specialists Pediatr Nurs 2010;15(1):33–61.
11. Patteson DM, Barnard KE. Parenting of low birth weight infants: a review of issues and interventions. Infant Ment Health J 1990;11(1):37–56.
12. Evans T, Whittingham K, Sanders M, et al. Are parenting interventions effective in improving the relationship between mothers and their preterm infants? Infant Behav Dev 2014;37(2):131–54.
13. Vanderveen J, Bassler D, Robertson C, et al. Early interventions involving parents to improve neurodevelopmental outcomes of premature infants: a meta-analysis. J perinatology 2009;29(5):343–51.
14. Neel MLM, Stark AR, Maitre NL. Parenting style impacts cognitive and behavioural outcomes of former preterm infants: a systematic review. Child Care Health Dev 2018;44(4):507–15.
15. Treyvaud K, Doyle LW, Lee KJ, et al. Parenting behavior at 2 years predicts school-age performance at 7 years in very preterm children. J Child Psychol Psychiatr 2016;57(7):814–21.
16. Neel ML, Slaughter JC, Stark AR, et al. Parenting style associations with sensory threshold and behavior, a prospective cohort study in term/preterm infants. Acta Paediatr 2019;108(9):1616–23.
17. Benzies KM, Magill-Evans JE, Hayden KA, et al. Key components of early intervention programs for preterm infants and their parents: a systematic review and meta-analysis. BMC pregnancy and childbirth 2013;13(1):1–15.
18. Ravn IH, Smith L, Lindemann R, et al. Effect of early intervention on social interaction between mothers and preterm infants at 12 months of age: a randomized controlled trial. Infant Behav Development 2011;34(2):215–25.
19. van Wassenaer-Leemhuis AG, Jeukens-Visser M, van Hus JW, et al. Rethinking preventive post-discharge intervention programmes for very preterm infants and their parents. Developmental Med Child Neurol 2016;58:67–73.

20. Spittle A, Orton J, Anderson PJ, et al. Early developmental intervention programmes provided post hospital discharge to prevent motor and cognitive impairment in preterm infants. Cochrane Database Syst Rev 2015;11:1–84.
21. Glazebrook C., Marlow N., Israel C., et al., Randomised trial of a parenting intervention during neonatal intensive care, Arch Dis Child Fetal Neonatal Ed, 92 (6), 2007, F438-F443.
22. Johnson S, Whitelaw A, Glazebrook C, et al. Randomized trial of a parenting intervention for very preterm infants: outcome at 2 years. J Pediatr 2009;155(4): 488–94. e1.
23. Platt MPW. A good idea that doesnt work the Parent Baby Interaction Programme. Arch Dis Childhood-Fetal Neonatal Edition 2007;92(6):F427–8.
24. Twohig A, Murphy JF, McCarthy A, et al. The preterm infant–parent programme for attachment—PIPPA Study: a randomised controlled trial. Pediatr Res 2021; 90(3):617–24.
25. Kennedy H, Landor M, Todd L. Video interaction guidance. London, UK: Jessica Kingsley; 2011.
26. Hoffenkamp HN, Tooten A, Hall RA, et al. Effectiveness of hospital-based video interaction guidance on parental interactive behavior, bonding, and stress after preterm birth: a randomized controlled trial. J Consulting Clin Psychol 2015; 83(2):416.
27. Brown J, LaRossa M, Aylward G, et al. Nursery-based intervention with prematurely born babies and their mothers: are there effects? J Pediatr 1980;97(3): 487–91.
28. Lawhon G. Facilitation of parenting the premature infant within the newborn intensive care unit. J perinatal neonatal Nurs 2002;16(1):71–82.
29. Browne JV, Talmi A. Family-based intervention to enhance infant–parent relationships in the neonatal intensive care unit. J Pediatr Psychol 2005;30(8):667–77.
30. Koldewijn K, Wolf M-J, van Wassenaer A, et al. The Infant Behavioral Assessment and Intervention Program for very low birth weight infants at 6 months corrected age. J Pediatr 2009;154(1):33–8. e2.
31. Meijssen D, Wolf MJ, Koldewijn K, et al. The effect of the Infant Behavioral Assessment and Intervention Program on mother–infant interaction after very preterm birth. J Child Psychol Psychiatry 2010;51(11):1287–95.
32. Meijssen D, Wolf M-J, van Bakel H, et al. Maternal attachment representations after very preterm birth and the effect of early intervention. Infant Behav Development 2011;34(1):72–80.
33. Van Hus J, Jeukens-Visser M, Koldewijn K, et al. Early intervention leads to long-term developmental improvements in very preterm infants, especially infants with bronchopulmonary dysplasia. Acta Paediatr 2016;105(7):773–81.
34. Landry SH, Smith KE, Swank PR. Responsive parenting: establishing early foundations for social, communication, and independent problem-solving skills. Developmental Psychol 2006;42(4):627.
35. Guttentag CL, Pedrosa-Josic C, Landry SH, et al. Individual variability in parenting profiles and predictors of change: effects of an intervention with disadvantaged mothers. J Appl Dev Psychol 2006;27(4):349–69.
36. Barrera M, Rosenbaum P, Cunningham C. Early home intervention with low-birth-weight infants and their parents. Child development 1986;20–33.
37. McManus BM, Blanchard Y, Murphy NJ, et al. The effects of the Newborn Behavioral Observations (NBO) system in early intervention: a multisite randomized controlled trial. Infant Ment Health J 2020;41(6):757–69.

38. Cho Y, Hirose T, Tomita N, et al. Infant mental health intervention for preterm infants in Japan: promotions of maternal mental health, mother–infant interactions, and social support by providing continuous home visits until the corrected infant age of 12 months. Infant Ment Health J 2013;34(1):47–59.
39. Gardner JM, Walker SP, Powell CA, et al. A randomized controlled trial of a home-visiting intervention on cognition and behavior in term low birth weight infants. J Pediatr 2003;143(5):634–9.
40. Barlow J, Sembi S, Underdown A. Pilot RCT of the use of video interactive guidance with preterm babies. J Reprod infant Psychol 2016;34(5):511–24.
41. Barnard KE, Hammond MA, Sumner GA, et al. Helping parents with preterm infants: field test of a protocol. Early Child Development Care 1987;27(2):255–90.
42. Wijnroks L. Early maternal stimulation and the development of cognitive competence and attention of preterm infants. Early Development Parenting: An Int J Res Pract 1998;7(1):19–30.
43. Nurcombe B, Howell DC, Rauh VA, et al. An intervention program for mothers of low-birthweight infants: preliminary results. J Am Acad Child Psychiatry 1984; 23(3):319–25.
44. Rauh VA, Nurcombe B, Achenbach T, et al. The Mother-Infant Transaction Program. The content and implications of an intervention for the mothers of low-birthweight infants. Clin perinatology 1990;17(1):31–45.
45. Nordhov SM, Rønning JA, Ulvund SE, et al. Early intervention improves behavioral outcomes for preterm infants: randomized controlled trial. Pediatrics 2012; 129(1):e9–16.
46. Kaaresen PI, Rønning JA, Tunby J, et al. A randomized controlled trial of an early intervention program in low birth weight children: outcome at 2 years. Early Hum Dev 2008;84(3):201–9.
47. Hauglann L, Handegaard BH, Ulvund SE, et al. Cognitive outcome of early intervention in preterms at 7 and 9 years of age: a randomised controlled trial. Arch Dis Childhood-Fetal Neonatal Edition 2015;100(1):F11–6.
48. Milgrom J, Newnham C, Anderson PJ, et al. Early sensitivity training for parents of preterm infants: impact on the developing brain. Pediatr Res 2010;67(3):330–5.
49. Milgrom J, Newnham C, Martin PR, et al. Early communication in preterm infants following intervention in the NICU. Early Hum Dev 2013;89(9):755–62.
50. Newnham CA, Milgrom J, Skouteris H. Effectiveness of a modified mother–infant transaction program on outcomes for preterm infants from 3 to 24 months of age. Infant Behav Dev 2009;32(1):17–26.
51. Ravn IH, Smith L, Smeby NA, et al. Effects of early mother–infant intervention on outcomes in mothers and moderately and late preterm infants at age 1 year: a randomized controlled trial. Infant Behav Development 2012;35(1):36–47.
52. Rauh VA, Achenbach TM, Nurcombe B, et al. Minimizing adverse effects of low birthweight: four-year results of an early intervention program. Child Development 1988;59:544–53.
53. Achenbach TM, Howell CT, Aoki MF, et al. Nine-year outcome of the Vermont intervention program for low birth weight infants. Pediatrics 1993;91(1):45–55.
54. Kynø NM, Ravn IH, Lindemann R, et al. Effect of an early intervention programme on development of moderate and late preterm infants at 36 months: a randomized controlled study. Infant Behav Development 2012;35(4):916–26.
55. Nordhov SM, Rønning JA, Dahl LB, et al. Early intervention improves cognitive outcomes for preterm infants: randomized controlled trial. Pediatrics 2010; 126(5):e1088–94.

56. Achenbach TM, Phares V, Howell CT, et al. Seven-year outcome of the Vermont intervention program for low-birthweight infants. Child Development 1990;61(6): 1672–81.
57. Melnyk BM, Alpert-Gillis L, Feinstein NF, et al. Improving cognitive development of low-birth-weight premature infants with the COPE program: a pilot study of the benefit of early NICU intervention with mothers. Res Nurs Health 2001;24(5): 373–89.
58. Melnyk BM, Feinstein NF, Alpert-Gillis L, et al. Reducing premature infants' length of stay and improving parents' mental health outcomes with the Creating Opportunities for Parent Empowerment (COPE) neonatal intensive care unit program: a randomized, controlled trial. Pediatrics 2006;118(5):e1414–27.
59. Oswalt KL, McClain DB, Melnyk B. Reducing anxiety among children born preterm and their young mothers. MCN Am J Matern Child Nurs 2013;38(3):144–9.
60. Ohgi S, Fukuda M, Akiyama T, et al. Effect of an early intervention programme on low birthweight infants with cerebral injuries. J paediatrics child Health 2004; 40(12):689–95.
61. Teti DM, Black MM, Viscardi R, et al. Intervention with African American premature infants: four-month results of an early intervention program. J Early Intervention 2009;31(2):146–66.
62. Widmayer SM, Field TM. Effects of Brazelton demonstrations for mothers on the development of preterm infants. Pediatrics 1981;67(5):711–4.
63. Evans T, Boyd RN, Colditz P, et al. Mother-very preterm infant relationship quality: RCT of baby triple P. J Child Fam Stud 2017;26(1):284–95.
64. Zahr LK. Home-based intervention after discharge for Latino families of low-birthweight infants. Infant Ment Health J 2000;21(6):448–63.
65. Walker SP, Chang SM, Powell CA, et al. Psychosocial intervention improves the development of term low-birth-weight infants. J Nutr 2004;134(6):1417–23.
66. Colditz PB, Boyd RN, Winter L, et al. A randomized trial of baby triple P for preterm infants: child outcomes at 2 years of corrected age. J Pediatr 2019;210: 48–54. e2.
67. Borghini A, Habersaat S, Forcada-Guex M, et al. Effects of an early intervention on maternal post-traumatic stress symptoms and the quality of mother–infant interaction: the case of preterm birth. Infant Behav Development 2014;37(4): 624–31.
68. Brisch KH, Bechinger D, Betzler S, et al. Early preventive attachment-oriented psychotherapeutic intervention program with parents of a very low birthweight premature infant: results of attachment and neurological development. Attachment Hum Dev 2003;5(2):120–35.
69. Olds DL, Sadler L, Kitzman H. Programs for parents of infants and toddlers: recent evidence from randomized trials. J Child Psychol Psychiatry 2007; 48(3-4):355–91.
70. Hall R, Hoffenkamp H, Tooten A, et al. Longitudinal associations between maternal disrupted representations, maternal interactive behavior and infant attachment: a comparison between full-term and preterm dyads. Child Psychiatry Hum Development 2015;46(2):320–31.
71. Hane A, N. LaCoursiere J, Mitsuyama M, et al. The Welch Emotional Connection Screen (WECS): Validation of a brief mother-infant relational health screen, Acta Paediatr, 2019;108(4):615–625.
72. Hane AA, LaCoursiere JN, Mitsuyama M, et al. The Welch Emotional Connection Screen: validation of a brief mother–infant relational health screen. Acta Paediatr 2019;108(4):615–25.

73. Frosch CA, Fagan MA, Lopez MA, et al. Validation study showed that ratings on the Welch Emotional Connection Screen at infant age six months are associated with child behavioural problems at age three years. Acta Paediatr 2019;108(5): 889–95.

74. Perone S, Gartstein MA. Relations between dynamics of parent-infant interactions and baseline EEG functional connectivity. Infant Behav Development 2019;57: 101344.

75. Perone S, Gartstein MA, Anderson AJ. Dynamics of frontal alpha asymmetry in mother-infant dyads: Insights from the Still Face Paradigm. Infant Behav Development 2020;61:101500.

76. Hall RA, Hoffenkamp HN, Tooten A, et al. The quality of parent–infant interaction in the first 2 years after full-term and preterm birth. Parenting 2015;15(4):247–68.

77. Heckman JJ. Skill formation and the economics of investing in disadvantaged children. Science 2006;312(5782):1900–2.

78. Welch MG, Hofer MA, Brunelli SA, et al. Family nurture intervention (FNI): methods and treatment protocol of a randomized controlled trial in the NICU. BMC Pediatr 2012;12(1):14.

79. Welch MG, Myers MM. Advances in family-based interventions in the neonatal ICU. Curr Opin Pediatr 2016;28(2):163–9.

80. Baumrind D. Child care practices anteceding three patterns of preschool behavior, Genet Psychol Monogr, 1967;75(1):43–88.

81. Baumrind D. Patterns of parental authority and adolescent autonomy. New Directions Child Adolescent Development 2005;2005(108):61–9.

82. Maccoby EE, Martin JA. In: Mussen PH, Hetherington EM, editors. Handbook of Child Psychology, 4. New York: Socialization, Personality, and Social Development; 1983. p. 1–101.

83. de Silva A, Neel ML, Maitre N, et al. Resilience and vulnerability in very preterm 4-year-olds. Clin Neuropsychol 2021;35(5):904–24.

84. DeMaster D, Bick J, Johnson U, et al. Nurturing the preterm infant brain: leveraging neuroplasticity to improve neurobehavioral outcomes. Pediatr Res. 2019;85(2):166-175.

85. Daelmans B, Darmstadt GL, Lombardi J, et al. Early childhood development: the foundation of sustainable development. Lancet 2017;389(10064):9–11.

86. Maitre NL. Neurorehabilitation after neonatal intensive care: evidence and challenges. Arch Dis Child - Fetal Neonatal Edition 2015;100(6):F534–40. https://doi.org/10.1136/archdischild-2013-305920.

87. Mustard JF. Experience-based brain development: Scientific underpinnings of the importance of early child development in a global world. Paediatrics Child Health 2006;11(9):571–2.

88. Landry SH, Taylor HB, Guttentag C, et al. Responsive parenting: Closing the learning gap for children with early developmental problems. Int Rev Res Ment Retard 2008;36:27–60.

89. Wijnroks A. Dimensions of mother-infant interaction and the development of social and cognitive competence in preterm infants. Groningen, Netherlands: University of Groningen; 1994.

## BIBLIOGRAPHIC SOURCE(S):

Evans T, Whittingham K, Sanders M, Colditz P, Boyd RN. Are parenting interventions effective in improving the relationship between mothers and their preterm infants? Infant behavior and development 2014;37(2):131–54.

Heckman JJ. Skill formation and the economics of investing in disadvantaged children. Science 2006;312(5782):1900–2.

Kang R, Barnard K, Hammond M. Preterm infant follow-up project: A multi-site field experiment of hospital and home intervention programs for mothers and preterm infants. *Public Health Nurs.* 1995;12(3):171–80.

Gardner JM, Walker SP, Powell CA, Grantham-McGregor S. A randomized controlled trial of a home-visiting intervention on cognition and behavior in term low birth weight infants. The Journal of pediatrics 2003;143(5):634–9.

Guralnick MJ. Preventive interventions for preterm children: effectiveness and developmental mechanisms. *Journal of Developmental and Behavioral Pediatrics.* 2012;33(4):352–64.

Neel ML, de Silva A, Taylor HG, Benninger K, Busch T, Hone E, Moore-Clingenpeel M, Pietruszewski L, Maitre NL. Exceeding expectations after perinatal risks for poor development: associations in term-and preterm-born preschoolers. *Journal of Perinatology.* 2021;42:1–8.

Neel MLM, Stark AR, Maitre NL. Parenting style impacts cognitive and behavioural outcomes of former preterm infants: A systematic review. Child: care, health and development 2018;44(4):507–15.

Olds DL, Sadler L, Kitzman H. Programs for parents of infants and toddlers: recent evidence from randomized trials. Journal of Child Psychology and Psychiatry 2007;48(3-4):355–91. https://doi.org/10.1111/j.1469-7610.2006.01702.

Patteson DM, Barnard KE. Parenting of low birth weight infants: A review of issues and interventions. *Infant Mental Health Journal.* 1990;11(1):37–56.

Pridham KA, Lutz KF, Anderson LS, Riesch SK, Becker PT. Furthering the understanding of parent–child relationships: A nursing scholarship review series. Part 3: Interaction and the parent–child relationship—Assessment and intervention studies. Journal for Specialists in Pediatric Nursing 2010;15(1):33–61.

Spittle A, Treyvaud K. The role of early developmental intervention to influence neurobehavioral outcomes of children born preterm. Elsevier; 2016. p. 542–8.

Vanderveen J, Bassler D, Robertson C, Kirpalani H. Early interventions involving parents to improve neurodevelopmental outcomes of premature infants: a meta-analysis. Journal of perinatology 2009;29(5):343–51.

Welch MG, Myers MM. Advances in family-based interventions in the neonatal ICU. Current opinion in pediatrics 2016;28(2):163–9.

White-Traut RC, Nelson MN. Maternally administered tactile, auditory, visual, and vestibular stimulation: Relationship to later interactions between mothers and premature infants. Research in nursing & health 1988;11(1):31–9.

# Beyond Survival

## Challenges and Opportunities to Improve Neurodevelopmental Outcomes of Preterm Birth in Low- and Middle-Income Countries

Samudragupta Bora, PhD

### KEYWORDS

- Global health • Health equity • High-risk infant • Low-and middle-income countries
- Neonatal follow-up • Neurodevelopment • Resource-limited settings

### KEY POINTS

- Low- and middle-income countries have some of the highest rates of preterm birth, account for the largest proportion of preterm births globally, and have significantly lower survival rates than high-income countries.
- Limited evidence exists regarding neurodevelopmental consequences of preterm birth in low- and middle-income countries, with predominantly methodologically weak research designs leading to uncertainty of evidence, along with almost no data from many of these resource-constrained settings.
- Understanding of short- and long-term neurodevelopmental outcomes of preterm birth are biased by findings from high-income countries with access to high quality of care, strong health care infrastructure, and a lower burden of preterm birth.
- To reduce existing inequities, development of sustainable and scalable models of neonatal follow-up, codesigned with local stakeholders and families of infants born preterm, needs to be prioritized while ensuring the same standards of care as in high-income countries and outcomes meaningful to them.
- Advocacy efforts should broaden from reduction of mortality of preterm birth in low- and middle-income countries to improving neurodevelopmental outcomes of these high-risk infants and their families.

## INTRODUCTION

Preterm birth, defined as a live birth before 37 completed weeks of gestation, is a leading global child health concern. Based on recent estimates, approximately 15 million infants are born preterm every year worldwide, although considerable disparities exist

University Hospitals Rainbow Babies & Children's Hospital, Case Western Reserve University School of Medicine, Cleveland, Ohio, USA; Mater Research Institute, Faculty of Medicine, The University of Queensland, Brisbane, Queensland, Australia
*E-mail address:* Samudragupta.Bora@UHhospitals.org

Clin Perinatol 50 (2023) 215–223
https://doi.org/10.1016/j.clp.2022.11.003
0095-5108/23/© 2022 Elsevier Inc. All rights reserved.
perinatology.theclinics.com

in prevalence and neonatal mortality between countries.[1,2] Survivors of preterm birth are at risk for a range of neurodevelopmental challenges across cognitive, language, socioemotional, behavioral, and motor domains that may adversely impact their quality of life, academic achievement, occupational success, and other life-course outcomes.[3–5] Most of the evidence to date concerning neurodevelopmental consequences of preterm birth originates from a few selected high-income countries with advanced health care systems, including Australia, Canada, New Zealand, United Kingdom, United States, and countries in Western Europe. There is limited evidence from South Asia and sub-Saharan Africa, although they have some of the highest rates of preterm birth and account for 60% to 80% of preterm births globally.[1,2] Consequently, there is limited understanding of neurodevelopmental outcomes of survivors of preterm birth within resource-constrained settings.

This article highlights the current evidence on preterm birth in low- and middle-income countries, focusing particularly on neurodevelopmental outcomes, and discusses challenges and opportunities to the delivery of and access to neonatal follow-up in those settings. The goal is to accelerate progress by identifying priority areas to address unmet needs necessary for improving neurodevelopmental outcomes of preterm birth in these vulnerable communities.

## LOW- AND MIDDLE-INCOME COUNTRIES

The World Bank categorizes countries based on Gross National Income per capita into four income classes every fiscal year. These classes and their 2023 thresholds are low- (≤US$1,085), lower-middle- (US$1,086–$4,255), upper-middle- (US$4,256–$13,205), and high- (US$≥$13,205) income economies.[6] Two-thirds of the countries are categorized as low- and middle-income economies; however, there is variability within classes, and an income-based classification alone may not fully capture sociopolitical complexities including health policy, state of the infrastructure, technological advancements, and economic growth, all of which are relevant for the delivery of and access to high-quality health care. Although there is caution around the misuse/overuse of this income-based classification in global health,[7] it is a useful framework and permits comparability with the existing literature.

## PRETERM BIRTH IN LOW- AND MIDDLE-INCOME COUNTRIES

Challenges to ascertaining the global prevalence and incidence of preterm birth result from the paucity of reliable data in many countries, particularly from South Asia and sub-Saharan Africa. Based on recent estimates, 10.6% of all live births worldwide in 2014 were preterm, with regional rates ranging from 8.7% in Europe to 13.4% in North Africa.[1] Furthermore, 81.1% of these preterm births are from countries in South Asia and sub-Saharan Africa, disproportionately overrepresented within the low- and middle-income categories. Of the top 10 countries with the highest number of preterm births,[1] one is low-, six are lower-middle-, and two are upper-middle-income economies. Similar statistics were reported based on national estimates for 2010 across 184 countries,[2] the first country-level preterm birth estimates. Of the top 10 countries with the highest rates of preterm birth (>15%) in 2010,[2] (as opposed to the highest numbers), two are low-, six are lower-middle-, and two are upper-middle-income economies. Nonetheless, rates of preterm birth vary widely within geographic regions and income classes.

In the absence of reliable data, estimates of preterm birth rates rely on studies with imprecise gestational age. To overcome this challenge, gestational age dating based on the gold standard early ultrasound was undertaken in a recent population-based study across five countries in South Asia and sub-Saharan Africa.[8] In 9,974 live births, preterm birth rates were 3.2%, 4.9%, 7.4%, 11.7%, and 15.7% in Ghana, Tanzania, Zambia, Bangladesh, and Pakistan, respectively. Furthermore, 13.8% of these infants died during the neonatal period, with a death rate of 62.2% (n = 61/98) for very preterm (<32 weeks gestation), 20.8% (n = 30/144) for moderate preterm (32–33 weeks), and 5.9% (n = 43/732) for late preterm (34–36 weeks).

Regardless of discrepancies in reported preterm birth rates, the highest prevalence and survival of preterm birth are evident among moderate to late preterm infants, across high- and low-resource settings. Globally, approximately 85% of preterm births are moderate to late preterm, 10% are very preterm, and only 5% are extremely preterm (<28 weeks gestation).[1,2]

Neonatal mortality at lower gestational ages has declined over the last three decades in high-income countries and those with advanced health care systems, with greater than 85% survival to discharge for those born extremely preterm at 26 to 28 weeks gestation.[9] Nonetheless, neonatal mortality for those born extremely and very preterm remains elevated in low- and middle-income countries. Survival to discharge was 39% in a recent meta-analysis of 66 studies with a pooled sample of 8,412 infants born extremely preterm in low- and middle-income countries, with a consistent increase in survival across income classes (13% low-, 28% lower-middle-, 48% upper-middle-income economies).[10] However, some single-center studies reported survival rates of up to 60% in upper-middle-income countries and 67% in one lower-middle-income country.

Despite the lower risk of mortality among moderate to late preterm infants, there is strong emerging evidence of neonatal morbidities and long-term neurodevelopmental challenges among this preterm birth subgroup relative to those born at term.[11–13] Even a slight increase in their relative risk can lead to a significant public health burden, because they account for the largest proportion of preterm births globally. Furthermore, infants born preterm and small for gestational age, highly prevalent in low- and middle-income countries, are at even higher risk of adverse neurodevelopment.[14,15] Based on recent estimates, 22% of moderate to late preterm infants in low- and middle-income countries in 2010 were small for gestational age.[16]

## NEURODEVELOPMENTAL OUTCOMES OF PRETERM BIRTH IN LOW- AND MIDDLE-INCOME COUNTRIES

Current evidence is limited to few resource-constrained settings, with almost no data available for more than half of the low- and middle-income countries. Studies in high-resource countries may suggest that preterm birth is a major risk factor for poor childhood neurodevelopment in low- and middle-income countries; however, risk magnitude is imperfectly understood, because of the scarcity of research and methodologic weaknesses of available studies. Furthermore, the extent to which well-established associations between gestational age and neurodevelopmental outcomes in high-income countries can be generalized to low- and middle-income countries remains unknown: the interplay of multiple prenatal and postnatal risk factors for poor neurodevelopment, over and above preterm birth, is unclear in those low- and middle-income countries. Despite methodologic limitations, the current state of research from relevant systematic reviews and meta-analyses is summarized next, highlighting the knowledge gaps.

### Cognition

In the meta-analysis by Sania and colleagues,[17] children younger than 7 years of age who were born late preterm demonstrated lower cognitive scores than their term-born peers (standardized mean difference [SMD], −0.21; 95% confidence interval [CI], −0.39 to −0.04; $P$ = .04), after adjusting for sex, age, maternal education, and household wealth across pooled data from eight studies. Similar associations were not evident for those born early preterm at less than 34 weeks gestation (SMD, −0.16; 95% CI, −0.34 to 0.31; $P$ = .15); however, there were moderate to high levels of heterogeneity in effect sizes across these studies. Furthermore, stratification of the preterm group into small (n = 5 studies) and appropriate (n = 8 studies) for gestational age demonstrated significantly lower cognitive scores for both subgroups compared with their term-born appropriate for gestational age peers. Reported associations for gestational age groups may be imprecise because most studies determined gestation based on recall of the last day of the menstrual period rather than ultrasound.

There is also wide variability in reported rates of cognitive impairment among the preterm population in low- and middle-income countries. For example, Milner and colleagues[18] reported a pooled median prevalence of 16.3% (interquartile range [IQR], 6.3%–29.6%) across 18 studies (n = 3,422) of children born preterm and/or low birthweight aged primarily between 12 and 48 months (1 study at 13 years). In contrast, Pascal and colleagues[19] reported a prevalence of 47% (95% CI, 41.7%–52.4%) based on pooled data from two studies (n = 332) of 8- to 24-month-old very preterm and/or very low birthweight children in upper-middle income countries. This discrepancy may partly be accounted for by differences in the gestational age of the samples.

### Motor Function

In the meta-analysis by Sania and colleagues,[17] there were no differences in motor scores of children born late preterm (SMD, −0.14; 95% CI, −0.33 to 0.04; $P$ = .17; n = 8 studies), early preterm (SMD, −0.26; 95% CI, −0.53 to 0.006; $P$ = .10; n = 7 studies), and their term-born peers, after accounting for sex, age, maternal education, and household wealth. Further stratification of the preterm group demonstrated lower motor scores for the preterm-born appropriate for gestational age (SMD, −0.23; 95% CI, −0.42 to −0.03; $P$ = .05; n = 9 studies) but not for small for gestational age (SMD, −0.15; 95% CI, −0.40 to 0.09; $P$ = .29; n = 5 studies) group, compared with their term-born appropriate for gestational age peers. Regarding rates of motor impairment, Pascal and colleagues[19] reported a prevalence of 33.4% (95% CI, 26.9%–40.6%) based on pooled data from two studies (n = 332) of 8- to 24-month-old very preterm and/or very low birthweight children in upper-middle income countries.

Furthermore, as reported by Pascal and colleagues,[19] the pooled prevalence of cerebral palsy was 4.9% (95% CI, 2.5%–9.1%) for upper-middle-income (n = 980; 3 studies) and 9.5% (95% CI, 3.9%–21.1%) for lower-middle-income (n = 115; 2 studies) countries. Similarly, Milner and colleagues[18] reported a pooled median prevalence of 11.2.% (IQR, 5.9%–16.%) across 21 studies of 12- to 48-month-old children born preterm and/or low birthweight. In contrast, the prevalence of cerebral palsy was reported as 3% (95% CI, 1%–9%) at 18 to 24 months corrected age in a recent meta-analysis[10] of two studies (n = 105) of children born extremely preterm in low- and middle-income countries. This low rate despite the inclusion of the highest risk gestational group is inconsistent with existing literature. Moreover, the certainty of the evidence was graded as low.

### Language

In the meta-analysis by Sania and colleagues,[17] there were no differences in language scores of children born late preterm (SMD, −0.05; 95% CI, −0.23 to 0.13; $P$ = .64;

n = 5 studies), or those born early preterm (SMD, −0.20; 95% CI, −0.55 to 0.15; $P$ = .35; n = 4 studies) and their term-born peers, after adjusting for sex, age, maternal education, and household wealth. Furthermore, unlike cognitive and motor outcomes, there were no differences in language scores of preterm and term-born appropriate for gestational age comparison (SMD, −0.02; 95% CI, −0.23 to 0.19; $P$ = .87; n = 4 studies). Regarding rates of language impairment, Milner and colleagues[18] reported prevalence ranging from 2.6% to 20% across five studies (n = 679) of children born preterm and/or low birthweight aged 12 to 36 months.

### Neurodevelopmental Impairment

Prevalence of neurodevelopmental impairment at 18 to 24 months corrected age was reported as 29% (95% CI, 23%–37%) in a recent meta-analysis of four studies (n = 243) of children born extremely preterm in low- and middle-income countries[10]; however, the certainty of the evidence was graded as very low. A lower median prevalence of 21.4% (IQR, 11.6%–30.8%) was reported by Milner and colleagues[18] across 16 studies (n = 2,906) of 12- to 48-month-old children born preterm and/or with low birthweight. This discrepancy can partly be explained by the inclusion of samples born at higher gestational ages in the meta-analysis by Milner and colleagues.[18]

In summary, findings from these studies highlight inconclusive evidence concerning neurodevelopmental outcomes in survivors of preterm birth in low- and middle-income countries. They also emphasize the challenges of assessing the true impact of preterm birth on neurodevelopmental outcomes within these resource-constrained settings. Concerningly, as consistently identified across these studies, most research designs are methodologically weak, leading to the uncertainty of evidence. In addition, there are challenges associated with heterogeneous exposure and outcome classifications, diverse assessment instruments with varying psychometric properties, small sample sizes, and broad age ranges. There are limited data beyond early childhood and for outcomes in behavior, socioemotional adjustment, executive function, and academic achievement, all recognized as major concerns in studies from high-income countries.

## NEONATAL FOLLOW-UP IN LOW- AND MIDDLE-INCOME COUNTRIES

The development and strengthening of neonatal follow-up programs to deliver high-quality neurodevelopmental care are of prime importance in low- and middle-income countries. It can provide a robust platform for generating reliable data for research and benchmarking, to guide improvements in clinical care.[20] Additionally, neonatal follow-up can facilitate early detection of neurodevelopmental impairments, which with timely intervention has the potential to optimize outcomes and quality of life.

Many lower- and upper-middle-income countries have some form of neonatal follow-up program, although they may be less structured and focus primarily on neurosensory than the more widely prevalent neurodevelopmental impairments in this high-risk population.

This section outlines some of the challenges to neonatal follow-up in low- and middle-income countries, based on existing literature and the author's field experience in Ghana since 2018 and a workshop conducted in a remote public hospital setting in India in 2019. The section concludes by identifying opportunities to improve neonatal follow-up in resource-limited settings.

### Challenge 1: Lack of Consensus on Who, When, What, and How to Assess

There are limited guidelines and best practice recommendations for neonatal follow-up of infants born preterm. Of the few that exist, most are from high-income countries developed to meet the needs and priorities of their population and health care systems, with a few lower-middle- and upper-middle-income countries adapting or developing similar guidelines. Nonetheless, there are discrepancies regarding eligibility for follow-up, neurodevelopmental domains of interest, and assessment approaches (surveillance vs screening vs evaluation). This is further complicated in low- and middle-income countries for the following reasons: lack of adequate relevant data; considerable variability in neonatal survival, clinical, and social risk profiles; poor health care infrastructure; and inadequate investment in health care, thereby limiting the adoption or adaptation of guidelines and recommendations from other settings. Finally, as previously acknowledged by other researchers,[21] studies in low- and middle-income countries have used narrow frameworks for understanding neurodevelopment in this high-risk population, with limited focus on outcomes, such as behavioral and socioemotional adjustment, executive function, adaptive behavior, and learning skills, recognized as highly relevant in these children.

### Challenge 2: Lack of Standardized Assessments and Reference Criteria

There is a scarcity of standardized and validated neurodevelopmental instruments to meet the unique sociocultural, economic, and specialist training requirements of low- and middle-income countries. Furthermore, the lack of relevant normative data and reference standards for instruments free of cross-cultural bias has been consistently identified as one of the most predominant barriers to neonatal follow-up. Lastly, the prohibitive cost of standardized instruments and their associated training of multidisciplinary professionals has been identified as a major barrier.

### Challenge 3: Lack of Suitable Infrastructure

The acute shortage of health care professionals, particularly multidisciplinary specialists in low- and middle-income countries, coupled with poor health care infrastructure make it logistically, economically, and ethically difficult to invest limited available resources in neonatal follow-up (typically characterized by high prevalence and low severity impairments) over life-threatening or other severe chronic conditions.

### Challenge 4: Lack of Awareness Regarding the Value of Early Detection and Intervention

There is limited awareness and knowledge among health care professionals and families in low- and middle-income countries regarding the value of early detection of neurodevelopmental impairments. This is further exacerbated by risks of the stigma associated with neurodevelopmental impairments that are widely prevalent in some of these settings. Additionally, it remains difficult to prioritize early detection in the absence of opportunities for accessing early intervention and support services, typical in most low- and middle-income countries.

### Challenge 5: Lack of Focus on Developing Novel Models of Care Delivery

There is increasing recognition worldwide, including in high-income countries, that the current models of neonatal follow-up for infants born preterm are obsolete and do not meet the changing demands of the communities and health care systems. Further challenges with financial sustainability and scalability have always been a concern. There has been recent interest in developing novel care delivery models in high-income countries. Nonetheless, there are limited documented efforts to establish models of neonatal follow-up for the preterm population that are appropriate to low- and middle-income countries, accounting for their resource limitations, fragile health care systems, and economic, political, and sociocultural contexts.

### Challenge 6: Lack of Engagement with Stakeholders to Identify Meaningful Outcomes

Many countries, primarily Australia, Canada, New Zealand, United Kingdom, and countries in Western Europe have increasingly engaged with parents of children born preterm and other relevant stakeholders to identify outcomes that are meaningful to them and their communities. Such efforts are crucial to facilitating the uptake of neonatal follow-up and opportunities to enhance strategic investment. Nonetheless, such efforts have not yet been widely adopted in low- and middle-income countries. Given the unique needs of families in low- and middle-income countries, it is even more important that we have a strong understanding of outcomes, systems, and processes that are feasible, relevant, and acceptable for their specific contexts.

### Challenge 7: Lack of Implementation Science Focus

Although there has been an increasing focus on implementation science for efficient and effective translation of evidence into practice, including cost-benefit and cost-effectiveness evaluations, they are still in their infancy in low- and middle-income countries. It can be argued that there is little scope for implementation research within the context of neonatal follow-up in low- and middle-income countries given the current state of evidence relevant to those settings; however, there is no doubt that it needs to be prioritized to accelerate progress.

### Opportunities

Given the absence of relevant reliable data, it is challenging to identify eligibility for neonatal follow-up in low- and middle-income countries. Until high-quality local data become available for risk stratification in those settings, one approach is to screen annually all infants born preterm for neurosensory, cognitive, language, and motor development at least for the first 3 years of their life. Given the interplay of a multitude of risk factors in those settings, restricting neonatal follow-up to a few preterm birth subgroups may not be optimal based on current evidence. Another potential approach is to establish a general neonatal follow-up guideline, specific to meet the needs of low- and middle-income countries, which is adapted easily to different contexts based on a consensus of local experts.

Inadequate access to standardized instruments for neurodevelopmental assessment is a well-recognized barrier. The development and/or utilization of instruments that are free of cross-cultural biases and consideration for a universally applicable preterm birth-specific neonatal follow-up toolbox are recommended. Furthermore, coordination of efforts is indicated to establish normative data for commonly used standardized instruments in high-income settings that have robust psychometric properties and can be used in low- and middle-income countries.

It is important to consider capacity building and long-term mentorship of multidisciplinary health care professionals to deliver the highest standards of neonatal follow-up care even in resource-limited settings. To address challenges associated with the shortage of health care professionals, engaging community health workers for high-risk neurodevelopmental screening and creating appropriate referral pathways would also be beneficial.

Stronger partnership with diverse, relevant local stakeholders including families of infants born preterm is of utmost priority. This will facilitate the identification of meaningful neurodevelopmental outcomes specific to their settings and help codesign sustainable, scalable, high-quality models of neonatal follow-up addressing their unique needs.

## SUMMARY

Ultimately a multipronged approach across clinical care, research, education, and advocacy is needed to improve neurodevelopmental outcomes of survivors of preterm birth in resource-limited settings. Although the World Bank's income-based classification of countries provides a framework to recognize some of the common challenges faced by low- and middle-income countries, a more targeted global framework specific to neonatal and developmental medicine may accelerate progress. Advocacy is critical to recognize optimal neurodevelopment as a priority health outcome along with the reduction of mortality in low- and middle-income countries.

## BEST PRACTICES

What is the current practice for neonatal follow-up of infants born preterm in low- and middle-income countries?
There are neonatal follow-up programs in many low- and middle-income countries, though they may be less structured and concentrate more on neurosensory than neurodevelopmental impairments. What changes in current practice are likely to improve outcomes?

- It is critical to collect methodologically sound, high-quality data from low- and middle-income countries to inform clinical practice because the magnitude of the risk associations between gestational age and neurodevelopmental outcomes varies depending on country income classifications and resource constraints.
- Determine neurodevelopmental outcomes that are important to a variety of local stakeholders, including families of infants born preterm.
- Prioritize the development of novel neonatal follow-up models to address the specific challenges of low- and middle-income countries while maintaining the same standards of care as high-income countries.

## DISCLOSURE

There is no relevant financial relationship to disclose.

## CONFLICT OF INTEREST

There is no potential, perceived, or real conflict of interest to disclose.

## REFERENCES

1. Chawanpaiboon S, Vogel JP, Moller AB, et al. Global, regional, and national estimates of levels of preterm birth in 2014: a systematic review and modelling analysis. Lancet Glob Health 2019;7(1):e37–46.
2. Blencowe H, Lee AC, Cousens S, et al. Preterm birth-associated neurodevelopmental impairment estimates at regional and global levels for 2010. Pediatr Res 2013;74(Suppl 1):17–34.
3. Allotey J, Zamora J, Cheong-See F, et al. Cognitive, motor, behavioural and academic performances of children born preterm: a meta-analysis and systematic review involving 64 061 children. BJOG 2018;125(1):16–25.
4. Fitzallen GC, Sagar YK, Taylor HG, et al. Anxiety and depressive disorders in children born preterm: a meta-analysis. J Dev Behav Pediatr 2021;42(2):154–62.

5. de Gamarra-Oca LF, Ojeda N, Gómez-Gastiasoro A, et al. Long-term neurodevelopmental outcomes after moderate and late preterm birth: a systematic review. J Pediatr 2021;237:168–76.

6. World Bank country and lending groups – World Bank data help desk [Internet]. Available at: https://datahelpdesk.worldbank.org/knowledgebase/articles/906519-world-bank-country-and-lending-groups. Accessed June 30, 2022.

7. Lencucha R, Neupane S. The use, misuse and overuse of the 'low-income and middle-income countries' category. BMJ Glob Health 2022;7(6):e009067.

8. The Alliance for Maternal and Newborn Health Improvement (AMANHI) GA Study Group. Population-based rates, risk factors and consequences of preterm births in South-Asia and sub-Saharan Africa: a multi-country prospective cohort study. J Glob Health 2022;12:04011.

9. Helenius K, Sjörs G, Shah PS, et al. Survival in very preterm infants: an international comparison of 10 national neonatal networks. Pediatrics 2017;140(6): e2017126.

10. Ramaswamy VV, Abiramalatha T, Bandyopadhyay T, et al. ELBW and ELGAN outcomes in developing nations: systematic review and meta-analysis. PLoS One 2021;16(8):e0255352.

11. Cheong JL, Doyle LW, Burnett AC, et al. Association between moderate and late preterm birth and neurodevelopment and social-emotional development at age 2 years. JAMA Pediatr 2017;171(4):e164805.

12. Huff K, Rose RS, Engle WA. Late preterm infants: morbidities, mortality, and management recommendations. Pediatr Clin North Am 2019;66(2):387–402.

13. Woythaler M. Neurodevelopmental outcomes of the late preterm infant. Semin Fetal Neonatal Med 2019;24(1):54–9.

14. Sacchi C, Marino C, Nosarti C, et al. Association of intrauterine growth restriction and small for gestational age status with childhood cognitive outcomes: a systematic review and meta-analysis. JAMA Pediatr 2020;174(8):772–81.

15. Arcangeli T, Thilaganathan B, Hooper R, et al. Neurodevelopmental delay in small babies at term: a systematic review. Ultrasound Obstet Gynecol 2012;40(3): 267–75.

16. Lee AC, Katz J, Blencowe H, et al. National and regional estimates of term and preterm babies born small for gestational age in 138 low-income and middle-income countries in 2010. Lancet Glob Health 2013;1(1):e26–36.

17. Sania A, Sudfeld CR, Danaei G, et al. Early life risk factors of motor, cognitive and language development: a pooled analysis of studies from low/middle-income countries. BMJ Open 2019;9(10):e026449.

18. Milner KM, Neal EF, Roberts G, et al. Long-term neurodevelopmental outcome in high-risk newborns in resource-limited settings: a systematic review of the literature. Paediatr Int Child Health 2015;35(3):227–42.

19. Pascal A, Govaert P, Oostra A, et al. Neurodevelopmental outcome in very preterm and very-low-birthweight infants born over the past decade: a meta-analytic review. Dev Med Child Neurol 2018;60(4):342–55.

20. Doyle LW, Anderson PJ, Battin M, et al. Long term follow up of high risk children: who, why and how. BMC Pediatr 2014;14:279.

21. Milner KM, Lawn JE. Counting every small and sick newborn: better data, better care. Arch Dis Child 2020;105:105–6.

# High-Risk Infant Follow-Up After NICU Discharge

## Current Care Models and Future Considerations

Jonathan S. Litt, MD, MPH, ScD[a,b,c,]*, Deborah E. Campbell, MD[d,e]

### KEYWORDS

- Infants • High-risk infant follow-up • Care models
- Children with medical complexity • Developmental delay

### KEY POINTS

- Preterm and other infants needing intensive care after birth are at increased risk for health and developmental problems in infancy, childhood, and later life.
- Specialized follow-up programs provide periodic health and developmental surveillance and link infants with needed therapeutic services and supports.
- There is no standard of follow-up care for high-risk infants.
- The future of follow-up will focus on infant and family needs, address gaps in the equitable distribution of postdischarge services, and provide training and support for all members of the care team including clinicians, early intervention providers, and educators.

## INTRODUCTION

Infants born preterm (<37 weeks' gestational age) commonly experience chronic respiratory disease, poor feedi1ng and growth, neurosensory impairments, and delays in cognitive and motor development through infancy and early childhood.[1–7] Perinatal morbidities such as necrotizing enterocolitis and intracranial hemorrhage may amplify these risks.[8] Therefore, it is not surprising that high-risk infants experience high rates of special health care needs, using health services, prescription medication, and medical technology at rates far greater than their term-born peers.[9] Even preterm infants without significant morbidities require specialized follow-up by multiple providers— primary care pediatricians, high-risk infant follow-up (HRIF) programs, early intervention (EI) providers, and audiologists, to name but a few.[10,11]

[a] Department of Neonatology, Beth Israel Deaconess Medical Center, 330 Brookline Avenue, Boston, MA 02215, USA; [b] Department of Pediatrics, Harvard Medical School; [c] Department of Social and Behavioral Sciences, Harvard TH Chan School of Public Health; [d] Division of Neonatology, Children's Hospital at Montefiore, Weiler Einstein Campus, 1601 Tenbroeck Avenue, Bronx, NY 10461, USA; [e] Department of Pediatrics, Albert Einstein College of Medicine
* Corresponding author.
*E-mail address:* jlittt@bidmc.harvard.edu

Clin Perinatol 50 (2023) 225–238
https://doi.org/10.1016/j.clp.2022.11.004
0095-5108/23/© 2022 Elsevier Inc. All rights reserved.

**perinatology.theclinics.com**

HRIF programs provide periodic surveillance of medical and developmental sequelae of preterm birth and link infants and families to needed supportive and therapeutic services. Despite their ubiquity, there is significant variability in the patient populations served, team structure, and frequency and duration of follow-up provided.[12] Follow-up may be performed in an academic medical center, private hospital, or community-based clinic. Although typically considered within the scope of Neonatal practice, and a core competency for trainees in neonatal-perinatal medicine, follow-up may be provided by general pediatricians with special interest in HRIF, developmental pediatricians, neurologists, complex care programs, or any number of pediatric subspecialists. With the advent of widely available Internet and telemedicine technologies, some programs offer online health and developmental screening and may include virtual visits or a hybrid in-person/virtual approach.[13,14]

A workshop held jointly by the National Institute of Child Health and Development and the National Institute of Neurologic Diseases and Stroke in 2002 provided an evidence-based review of the benefits of HRIF, a description of optimal methods and ages to assess outcomes, and identifying barriers to tracking patients over time.[15] Yet, the workshop report did not offer specific guidance for performing clinical follow-up.

An expert panel was convened in 2006 to develop a set of quality indicators for HRIF.[16] The resulting report included 70 quality indicators in a range of domains: general care, physical, neurosensory, behavioral and developmental, and psychosocial assessments, and a range of interventions. This comprehensive compendium of metrics, while helpful in informing the content of follow-up visits, does not comment on optimal delivery models.

The American Academy of Pediatrics (AAP) Committee on Fetus and Newborn issued a policy statement on hospital discharge of the high-risk neonate in 2008.[17] In this statement, the AAP emphasized the importance of periodic evaluation for evolving health and developmental challenges and timely implementation of EI services. The recommendations also include guidance regarding assessing caregiver needs, access to services, and the home setting, acknowledging the influence of the postdischarge environment on later outcomes. Yet, the policy statement does not specify the provider responsible for follow-up care nor the location or structure of visits.

There is currently no evidence base that supports one model of follow-up care over another. In this review, we aim to describe common HRIF models, identify opportunities and challenges to providing clinical follow-up care in the twenty-first century, and offer recommendations for improving postdischarge care for high-risk infants.

## Current Models of Follow-Up Care

### Primary care pediatric practice

Community-based primary care pediatric providers offer first-line care after NICU discharge, serving as the child's medical home in supporting growth and nutrition, sleep and temperament, developmental milestones, and routine health care maintenance.[18] They typically serve as the first point of contact for caregivers, often leading to lasting and trusting relationships. Although primary care practitioners are well-equipped to provide care to infants and toddlers, some may look to neonatologists or other subspecialists for guidance in the care of more medically complex patients.[19]

The family-centered medical home has been the recommended model of pediatric primary care for at least five decades.[20,21] With an emphasis on care coordination and enhanced communication among care team members, receiving care within a family-centered medical home has been associated with reduced odds of having unmet care needs[22] and improved functional outcomes.[23]Al Although children born preterm often have complex medical and developmental needs, they are less likely to have a medical home compared with term-born peers.[24] Although the traditional medical home model has been shown to mediate racial and ethnic disparities in unmet needs among children with medical complexity, notable inequities remain.[25]

### Subspecialty and multidisciplinary clinics

Subspecialty and multidisciplinary models of follow-up are heterogeneous. The subspecialty HRIF clinic may be directed by a neonatologist, developmental pediatrician, neurologist, or general pediatrician with special interest in HRIF or complex care. Programs may support comanagement of high-risk infant care by community physicians, facilitate continuity of care, provide anticipatory guidance, make referrals for subspecialty care and EI, and perform outcomes research and trainee education. The scope of care varies from a singular focus on neurodevelopment to provide surveillance of infant health and development to comprehensive primary care integrating routine health care maintenance, sick child visits, and enhanced health and developmental care needs for infants with medical complexity or technology dependence.[12,26] Comprehensive HRIF programs use a medical home model of integrated, coordinated, medical, and developmental follow-up care that reduces care fragmentation and enhances family satisfaction. The support structure of the subspecialty HRIF clinic may include a patient care coordinator, nurses, nurse practitioners, and/or social workers.

The cardiac neurodevelopmental follow-up program is another type of subspecialty HRIF clinic that focuses on health and developmental screening and management for infants with complex congenital heart disease requiring intervention during the first year of life or extracorporeal membrane oxygenation.[27] The cardiologist works collaboratively with a neonatologist or developmental pediatrician to provide developmental surveillance in addition to managing the child's growth, feeding difficulties, and cardiac medications. As with traditional HRIF programs, there is significant variability in the scope and timing of routine screening and objective testing in these programs.[28]

Multidisciplinary HRIF clinics integrate allied health professionals, physical, and occupational therapists, speech–language pathologists, dietitians, social workers, psychologists, infant development and family support specialists, care coordinators, and if needed specific subspecialty physicians to provide holistic, "one-stop" access to comprehensive care for the high-risk infant and family.[29–32]

### Novel approaches

The Transition Home Program designed by Dr Betty Vohr and colleagues is an innovative set of interventions to improve care in the first year following NICU discharge. The program enhanced routine clinic-based follow-up with intensive predischarge education and coordination and postdischarge care including a follow-up call within a day, a home visit in the first week, and access to round-the-clock on call by study physicians up to 90 days postdischarge. Program participation was associated with lower odds of hospital readmission within 90 days of discharge.[33] Expanding to include late preterm and term infants discharged from the NICU was associated with lower postdischarge health service utilization and cost.[34]

For individuals with multimorbid chronic conditions, the conceptualization of the medical home may need to be broadened to a "medical neighborhood" that integrates the primary care setting with community-based services and medical subspecialists.[35–37] Care must be integrated across these settings emphasizing bidirectional communication, child- and family-centered goal-setting, minimizing family burden, and optimizing team functioning.[35,38] Alternative payment models that focus on integrating care across settings and populations have been shown to improve quality, reduce costs, and address social determinants that drive inequities in health.[39] A ~~demonstration project using this value-based, population health management approach for HRIF is underway at Boston Children's Hospital, funded by Massachusetts Medicaid~~.

## Considerations

### Eligibility

As there are no standard eligibility criteria for HRIF, infants referred encompass a spectrum of infants requiring intensive or specialized neonatal care including infants born at varying gestational ages, birth weights, and illness severity. There are many approaches to defining risk that serve both research and clinical purposes. Risk stratification for HRIF of infants born preterm may be categorized as high (<29 weeks' gestation), moderate (29–32 weeks) and lower risk (>32 weeks). Although the greatest focus of health and developmental surveillance is on infants born less than 32 weeks' gestation or very low birth weight, population-based studies have identified higher rates of mortality and morbidity, including neurodevelopmental impairments and poorer school age outcomes among infants born moderate and late preterm and early term (37–38 weeks' gestation).[40–43] In reality, gestational age is only one indicator of risk for adverse health and developmental outcomes, and often an unreliable predictor at that.[44] Term-born infants considered at high risk include babies affected by neonatal encephalopathy/hypoxic ischemic encephalopathy, neonatal stroke, critical congenital heart disease, congenital diaphragmatic hernia, and infants with genetic disorders, or major malformations. A third category of infants who benefit from enhanced follow-up are babies with high social risk, particularly infants exposed to substances in utero.

### Visit timing

There is no fully established evidence base to guide the optimal visit frequency, time between visits, and length of follow-up. The frequency of visits may be dictated by degree of medical complexity and developmental and/or social risk. Significant variability in the timing of the initial HRIF appointment exists, moderated by HRIF program scope, purpose, and finances. Some follow-up programs see the infant for the initial visit 1 to 6 weeks after NICU discharge focusing on the transition home, infant growth and feeding, and technology dependence. Most HRIF programs assess eligible infants 2 to 6, 8 to -12, 18 to 24, and 30 to 36 months corrected age. Many programs offer annual assessments through the age of 5 years.[12,15]

Programs engaged in research may offer annual follow-up into later childhood or adolescence. An HRIF visit between 2 and 6 months corrected age provides an opportunity for assessment of growth adequacy, nutrition, feeding skills, infant temperament and infant integration into the family unit, need for rehospitalization and emergency department use, receipt of recommended specialty care and community-based services, screening parental mental health and need for additional resources, and evaluation for early identification of high risk for cerebral palsy (CP).[45] In fact, the 2017 international guidelines for early detection of CP recommends assessments validated for this early time period,[46] the systematic implementation of which have been shown to decrease the age of diagnosis.[47]

A novel Canadian HRIF program focuses on specific developmental touchpoints for the child and family.[48] Touchpoints are described as moments of child development that may cause family disruption. Three guiding principles include (1) surveillance for the traditional outcomes is necessary to identify outcomes associated with disability, (2) filling gaps in the care system without duplicating services, and (3) identifying the preterm behavioral phenotype which manifests inconsistently, support this framework. Collaboration with communities, schools, and families is essential to avoid duplication and maintain consistency in messaging and care. Easily accessible, interactive communication networks for parents and the clinical team along with informational and educational resources and tools for parents are an integral component. This cost-effective approach links families with health care and community entities.

## Visit logistics

Visits may be in-person, conducted by telehealth, include online parent-reported outcomes or be a hybrid that encompasses all or some of these modalities. The COVID pandemic led to a rapid implementation and growth of telehealth visits by telephone or video link.[49] There are advantages and disadvantages to each visit type. In-person visits afford the clinical team the chance to physically assess the child and identify subtle differences or atypias not as easily discerned during a telehealth visit or from parent report. During a telehealth visit, some parts of the physical examination and standardized testing beyond visual observation are not possible. The use of standardized test materials and forms can be difficult as is the ability to assess the child–clinician interaction. Investigators have offered strategies to facilitate assessment, including testing that focuses on child functioning rather than solely on performance.[13]

The logistics and costs of travel, childcare, and time off from work are barriers to recommended follow-up, particularly for children with medical complexity, numerous specialty care appointments, and whose families also need to navigate EI and other community-based services. Telehealth visits provide an opportunity to increase access to HRIF for vulnerable infants and their families, facilitating assessment of the infant in their natural environment and providing a window into the child's home environment and the parent/caregiver–infant interaction and family dynamics. Darrah and colleagues offer a comprehensive review of the literature on the use of telehealth in NICU follow-up and discussion of the drawbacks and advantages elsewhere in this issue.

## Financing

Financing is a limitation in the availability, accessibility, and scope of HRIF care within a hospital or community. Heterogeneity in funding sources and variable reimbursement create challenges in developing and sustaining programs. HRIF is often funded through a complex array of reimbursements from private and public payers, State Children's Health Insurance Program combined with hospital, foundation, and/or grant funding. Through State Title V Maternal and Child Health Services Block Grant program funding several states, such as California and Utah, have implemented statewide models of NICU follow-up care.[50] Title V funding also supports the "Babies Can't Wait," Georgia EI program[51] and the Tennessee Early Intervention System[52] that emphasizes early identification of at risk infants, particularly infants born preterm, who required neonatal intensive care. Tennessee also stipulates referral for high-risk infant follow-up for eligible infants treated in state designated level III and IV (regional) neonatal units.[53]

Parents identify financial concerns about the costs of health care, durable medical equipment, lost wages, and out-of-pocket expenses, such as transportation and childcare, as causes of significant worry after their child's NICU discharge.[54] Supplemental security insurance can help support some of these out-of-pocket expenses, though access is variable. Underinsurance is an additional factor, particularly for lower income families with private insurance, who experience high deductibles, and limited prescription and subspecialty provider coverage. The Affordable Care Act and its subsidiary programs (Accountable Care Organizations (ACOs) and Health Homes) have not focused on the population of high risk and preterm children with special health care needs. Individual states like Georgia[55] and California[56] have passed legislation making Medicaid services available to children with functional impairments regardless of family finances.

### Equity

Achieving equity in access and utilization of HRIF requires exploration of factors that impede family participation. Social and demographic inequities—and their political and economic drivers—are associated with poor HRIF participation. Inequities in referral at NICU discharge contribute to inconsistent participation in HRIF even in states and communities with access to HRIF programs.[57] Maternal race/ethnicity and infant gestational age or birth weight are associated with missed referral. Differences in personnel, resources, and approaches among HRIF clinics as well as variations in NICU discharge planning, the approach to developmental care team involvement and knowledge of HRIF eligibility criteria and referral processes influence referral rates.[12,26,58]

Being born to a Black mother or a family with limited English proficiency and residing in a very low child opportunity index neighborhood are factors in low HRIF participation.[59] Public insurance coverage, rural residence, or a distance from the clinic have also been shown to be associated with poorer HRIF participation.[60] Extremely low birth weight, EI enrollment, and timely attendance at the first HRIF visit increase subsequent follow-up participation. Sustained participation is also improved when families connect earlier in their child's post-NICU follow-up care.[61] Parents identify better communication and care coordination as key to improved satisfaction with postdischarge follow-up care.[62] Limited support and resources, lower socioeconomic status, travel logistics, and costs contribute to challenges adhering to recommended follow-up.[63–65] A recently published quality improvement initiative demonstrated the effectiveness of a "bundle" that included NICU provider education, discharge planning, and parent education in increasing attendance at HRIF clinic visits.[66] (For further discussion, see "Health Care Disparities in High-Risk Neonates" by Johnson, and colleagues, elsewhere in this issue.)

### Recommendations

In light of the myriad program types and configurations, and the challenges to providing high-quality, high-value, equitable follow-up care, the authors offer the following general recommendations. Far from being prescriptive, the authors have identified concepts and considerations that apply to follow-up programs regardless of setting or location.

### Clinical care

1. *Follow-up care should center families and be responsive to their needs and values.* HRIF programs use standardized neurodevelopmental assessments that require specialized training to administer and interpret and unreliably predict later outcomes. Preterm infants are at risk for behavior and learning problems that emerge in early school-age and cannot be assessed with tests commonly used in the first years of life. The results of standardized tests, while helpful for diagnostic and research purposes, may not measure the outcomes most important to families. Parents have reported their preferred outcomes including such topics as family integration and functional outcomes that impact a child's and family's daily life.[67]

Given these notable limitations to current practice, the HRIF community must provide information, guidance, and services that reflect families' ongoing needs after NICU discharge. This can only be accomplished by first engaging parents as partners in the establishing of the mission and design of follow-up programs.

2. *Goals should be clear, transparently communicated, and aligned with family values.* Every clinical encounter should have an explicitly expressed purpose. Follow-up for its own sake—without clearly stated objectives and actionable goals—can lead to confusion, conflicting expectations, and low-value care. Families may not know the reason for referral for HRIF or understand the different roles of follow-up, primary care, and EI services. Follow-up programs may perform enhanced developmental screening, facilitate and coordinate care, or even provide direct therapeutic services. Regardless of the program model, the directives must be clearly articulated to the family and entire care team from the time of referral. Goals of care should be discussed with the family at every opportunity and plans developed with time-bound activities and contingencies.

3. *Hybrid approaches offer flexibility, increase opportunity for participation, and may reduce waste.* Many programs adopted telehealth platforms for providing continued support to their high-risk NICU graduates at the start of the COVID-19 pandemic.[13] This strategy uncovered several opportunities and challenges.[14] Although clinics were eventually able to safely offer in-person visits, many programs have opted to transition to hybrid in-person/telehealth models. Despite the notable hurdles, a hybrid approach offers flexibility for families and staff in a pandemic with an uncertain trajectory. Groups at both Emory[68] and the Children's Hospital of Philadelphia[13] have successfully implemented virtual approaches to augment their developmental follow-up programs. Care must be taken to ensure that all families have needed access to telehealth services and assure virtual visits are of the same quality and value as their in-person counterparts.

4. *No matter the route of data collection, programs should strive to assess similar outcomes using similar tools to facilitate benchmarking and inter-hospital comparisons.* No two HRIF programs are alike.[12] Variability in the complement of providers, array of assessments, and timing of visits make comparing outcomes among programs—and populations—impossible. Care should be patient-centered and driven by the needs and goals of infants and their families. However, some attempt at harmonizing approaches can allow for collaborative learning and coordinated efforts to improve the care we provide, both in the NICU and after discharge.[69]

### Education

To assure appropriate surveillance of high-risk infants, it is necessary to identify: (1) health and developmental outcomes important to infants' well-being and optimal functioning, (2) parent education, resource, and support needs, and (3) gaps in the systems of care. This requires discipline-specific education and interprofessional development for professionals and community workers who engage with children and families in addition to parent education and empowerment.

1. *Pediatric Primary Care Clinicians.* Pediatric primary care professionals (PCP) include pediatricians, family physicians, nurse practitioners, and physician assistants who require education regarding follow-up care needs of high risk and medically complex infants and children. This is particularly important given the variability in families' access to HRIF care either as an independent program or through comanagement with the child's PCP. Kuo and colleagues[37] proposed a care system redesign for preterm children after discharge from the NICU. This will require

residency and postgraduate training and continuing medical educational offerings for practicing clinicians about care of the child with medical complexity provided within a framework that is condition-specific and whole-child centric. There should be attention to how conditions interact with environmental and personal modifiers and the medical neighborhood.

2. *Trainees in Neonatology, Developmental and Behavioral Pediatrics, and Child Neurology.* American Board of Pediatrics and American College of Graduate Medical Education specifications for training in follow-up care for high-risk NICU graduates offers limited expectations without well-delineated goals and objectives for training and education in HRIF care.[70] Cicalese and colleagues, on behalf of the AAP Section on Neonatal Perinatal Medicine Organization of Neonatal Training Program Directors, comment on the clinical educational and experiential "essentials" of neonatal perinatal fellowship, noting the increased survival among infants born at the cusp of viability or with complex congenital malformations and the necessity to transition from neonatal focused to long-term pediatric complex medical care. In addition, advanced communication skills are imperative as parents increasingly access health information and medical advice from Websites, apps, and social media.[71]

3. *Early Intervention Providers.* To more optimally support families whose infants are referred for EI and facilitate more effective evaluations, an understanding of the developmental trajectories and therapeutic needs of preterm infants and babies with medical complexity is required for EI evaluators and providers. Neonatologists and pediatricians with special interest in HRIF are encouraged to partner with their state/county EI programs to build awareness about the health and developmental needs of high-risk infants and challenges particularly in the first year to meet state eligibility requirements for services when thresholds are variable and automatic eligibility varies from state to state.

4. *Educators and School Systems.* As with EI, there are no standard guidelines or recommendations regarding the need for teachers knowing the birth history of their students and the unique educational and behavioral challenges that many of these children experience that can impact their school performance, functioning, and success.[72] The United Kingdom and Canada have developed guidance and resources for schools and educators, parents, and health professionals.[73-75]

### Equity and follow-through

There are considerable barriers to HRIF access and participation that need to be addressed to ensure all preterm infants have the opportunity to thrive as they transition from the NICU to home. These include inequities by material deprivation, race/ethnicity,[61] language proficiency, and neighborhood opportunity.[76] Horbar and colleagues[77] have offered a comprehensive framework for providing equitable "follow-through" care for all NICU graduates and a compendium of potentially better practices. Here, we highlight and expand on four high-impact elements of equity-focused follow-through.

1. *Standard screening for social determinants of health can help identify and resolve material needs.* There are multiple tools with which to screen families for material needs like housing, food, and utilities. These range from a two-question screener for food insecurity to lengthier clinician-directed interviews. Regardless of the measure, programs should take a systematic approach to screening all families, reinforcing that answering sensitive questions about income and public assistance is entirely voluntary, and having a plan for addressing needs uncovered by the screening.

2. *Acknowledging biases and deploying interventions to mitigate their effects can reduce racial and ethnic inequities in care.* All humans carry with them biases about

the people and world around them. Regardless if we are aware of these biases (explicit) or not (implicit), our preconceptions drive how we act toward and behave around others. In health care, bias about individuals from minoritized communities has been associated with patient–provider interactions, treatment decisions, and patient psychosocial outcomes.[78] Although pervasive, many providers are unaware of their biases and how they affect patient care.[79] There are novel interventions to help health care providers become aware of their biases and reduce the negative impact of racial biases on care.[80,81]

3. *Health literacy environment assessments can help identify improvement opportunities.* Organizational health literacy, defined as "the degree to which an organization implements policies, practices, and systems" to enable people to use information and services in caring for their health,[82] is part of the US Department of Health and Human Services Healthy People 2030 priorities. Individual-level interventions can be highly effective, such as ensuring written materials are presented in clear, plain language and available in a family's preferred language. Yet, HRIF programs, often housed within large medical centers, must also have institutional policies and supports to make clinical spaces usable for all—including clearly posted and legible signage, widely available wayfinding aids, and universal access to medical interpretation for families with limited English proficiency. Assessment tools like the Walking Interview Tool[83] and the Health Literacy Environment of Hospitals and Health Centers[84] can help identify gaps and guide interventions to improve the health literacy environment of follow-up programs.

4. *Drivers of barriers to follow-up by neighborhood opportunity, local resources, and state-level policies should be explored and eliminated.* Local, state, and federal health, education, and social policy helps shape the availability of medical and developmental support services for high-risk infants. Although addressing such far-reaching policies is beyond the scope of this review, we cannot ignore the effect that these structural drivers have on the inequitable distribution of health and health care. Working locally and through national organizations such as the AAP, follow-up providers can advocate for programs and policies that broaden health, educational, and economic opportunities for all infants and their families.

## SUMMARY

HRIF is a cornerstone of health and developmental support after NICU discharge and vital to fulfilling our obligation to providing follow-through for our patients and their families. There are many models of follow-up care, and at present, there is no evidence base to favor one approach over another. Rigorous studies are needed to help inform strategies for potentially better practices for HRIF. There are, however, several precepts that apply regardless of the content of follow-up visits or model of care delivery. Elevating the needs of infants and the values of families, all with a commitment to closing equity gaps, is paramount to providing a high-quality, high-value follow-up care.

## BEST PRACTICES

What is the current practice for high-risk infant follow-up (HRIF)?

Current practices in HRIF are highly variable with respect to the patient populations served, the content and cadence of visits, and duration of follow-up care. There are currently no practice guidelines or potentially better practices to inform program development. And There are significant inequities in access to and participation in HRIF programs.

What changes in current practice are likely to improve outcomes?

Shift focus from standardized testing to functional outcomes assessments and child- and family-centered goal-setting. Solicit the input of families and multiple stakeholders across disciplines.

Consider the impact of parental mental health, stress, and trauma on child outcomes and family functioning. Address social and structural determinants of health to close gaps in access and participation.

(Kuppala V.S., Tabangin M., Haberman B., et al., Current state of high-risk infant follow-up care in the United States: results of a national survey of academic follow-up programs, J Perinatol, 32, 2012, 293–298.; Litt J.S. and Hintz S.R., Quality improvement for NICU graduates: feasible, relevant, impactful, Semin Fetal Neonatal Med, 26, 2021, 101205.; Garg A., Sandel M., Dworkin P.H., et al., From medical home to health neighborhood: transforming the medical home into a community-based health neighborhood, J Pediatr, 160, 2012, 535–536 e531.; Lakshmanan A., et al. Kubicek K., Williams R., et al., Viewpoints from families for improving transition from NICU-to-home for infants with medical complexity at a safety net hospital: a qualitative study, BMC Pediatr, 19, 2019, 223.; Horbar J.D., Edwards E.M. and Ogbolu Y., Our responsibility to follow through for NICU infants and their families, Pediatrics, 146, 2020, doi:10.1542/peds.2020-0360.)

## CONFLICTS OF INTEREST

Dr Litt and Dr Campbell have no financial conflicts of interest to disclose.

## REFERENCES

1. Botting N, Powls A, Cooke RW, et al. Cognitive and educational outcome of very-low-birthweight children in early adolescence. Dev Med Child Neurol 1998;40:652–60.
2. Doyle LW, Casalaz D, Victorian Infant Collaborative Study G. Outcome at 14 years of extremely low birthweight infants: a regional study. Arch Dis Child Fetal Neonatal Ed 2001;85:F159–64.
3. Grunau RE, Whitfield MF, Fay TB. Psychosocial and academic characteristics of extremely low birth weight (< or =800 g) adolescents who are free of major impairment compared with term-born control subjects. Pediatrics 2004;114:e725–32.
4. Isaacs EB, Edmonds CJ, Chong WK, et al. Brain morphometry and IQ measurements in preterm children. Brain 2004;127:2595–607.
5. Johnson A, Bowler U, Yudkin P, et al. Health and school performance of teenagers born before 29 weeks gestation. Arch Dis Child Fetal Neonatal Ed 2003;88:F190–8.
6. Saigal S, Hoult LA, Streiner DL, et al. School difficulties at adolescence in a regional cohort of children who were extremely low birth weight. Pediatrics 2000;105:325–31.
7. Taylor HG, Klein N, Minich NM, et al. Middle-school-age outcomes in children with very low birthweight. Child Dev 2000;71:1495–511.
8. McCormick MC, Litt JS, Smith VC, et al. Prematurity: an overview and public health implications. Annu Rev Public Health 2011;32:367–79.
9. Hack M, Taylor HG, Drotar D, et al. Chronic conditions, functional limitations, and special health care needs of school-aged children born with extremely low-birth-weight in the 1990s. JAMA 2005;294:318–25.
10. Follow-up care of high-risk infants. Pediatrics 2004;114:1377–97.

11. American Academy of Pediatrics Committee on F, Newborn. Hospital discharge of the high-risk neonate. Pediatrics 2008;122:1119–26.
12. Kuppala VS, Tabangin M, Haberman B, et al. Current state of high-risk infant follow-up care in the United States: results of a national survey of academic follow-up programs. J Perinatol 2012;32:293–8.
13. DeMauro SB, Duncan AF, Hurt H. Telemedicine use in neonatal follow-up programs - what can we do and what we can't - lessons learned from COVID-19. Semin Perinatol 2021;45:151430.
14. Litt JS, Mercier CE, Edwards EM, et al. Follow-through care for high-risk infants during the COVID-19 pandemic: lessons learned from the Vermont Oxford Network. J Perinatol 2021;41:2625–30.
15. Follow-up care of high-risk infants. Pediatrics 2004;114:1377–97.
16. Wang CJ, McGlynn EA, Brook RH, et al. Quality-of-care indicators for the neurodevelopmental follow-up of very low birth weight children: results of an expert panel process. Pediatrics 2006;117:2080–92.
17. Fetus Co, Newborn. Hospital discharge of the high-risk neonate. Pediatrics 2008;122:1119–26.
18. McCourt MF, Griffin CM. Comprehensive primary care follow-up for premature infants. J Pediatr Health Care 2000;14:270–9.
19. Voller SMB. Follow-up care for high-risk preterm infants. Pediatr Ann 2018;47:e142–6.
20. Medical home initiatives for children with special needs project advisory committee. American Academy of, P. The medical home. Pediatrics 2002;110:184–6.
21. Council on Children with, D. & Medical Home Implementation Project Advisory, C. Patient- and family-centered care coordination: a framework for integrating care for children and youth across multiple systems. Pediatrics 2014;133:e1451–60.
22. Boudreau AA, et al. Care coordination and unmet specialty care among children with special health care needs. Pediatrics 2014;133:1046–53.
23. Litt JS, McCormick MC. Care coordination, the family-centered medical home, and functional disability among children with special health care needs. Acad Pediatr 2015;15:185–90.
24. Litt JS, McCormick MC. Preterm infants are less likely to have a family-centered medical home than term-born peers. J Perinatol 2018;38:1391–7.
25. Bennett AC, Rankin KM, Rosenberg D. Does a medical home mediate racial disparities in unmet healthcare needs among children with special healthcare needs? Matern Child Health J 2012;16(Suppl 2):330–8.
26. Bockli K, Andrews B, Pellerite M, et al. Trends and challenges in United States neonatal intensive care units follow-up clinics. J Perinatol 2014;34:71–4.
27. Marino BS, Lipkin PH, Newburger JW, et al. Neurodevelopmental outcomes in children with congenital heart disease: evaluation and management: a scientific statement from the American Heart Association. Circulation 2012;126:1143–72.
28. Miller TA, Sadhwani A, Sanz J, et al. Variations in practice in cardiac neurodevelopmental follow-up programs. Cardiol Young 2020;30:1603–8. https://doi.org/10.1017/S1047951120003522.
29. Orton JL, Olsen JE, Ong K, et al. J. NICU graduates: the role of the allied health team in follow-up. Pediatr Ann 2018;47:e165–71.
30. Feehan K, et al. Development of a multidisciplinary medical home program for NICU graduates. Matern Child Health J 2020;24:11–21.
31. Broyles RS, et al. Comprehensive follow-up care and life-threatening illnesses among high-risk infants: a randomized controlled trial. JAMA 2000;284:2070–6.

32. Lipner HS, Huron RF. Developmental and interprofessional care of the preterm infant: neonatal intensive care unit through high-risk infant follow-up. Pediatr Clin North Am 2018;65:135–41.

33. Vohr B, et al. Impact of a transition home program on rehospitalization rates of preterm infants. J Pediatr 2017;181:86–92 e81.

34. Liu Y, et al. Transition home plus program reduces Medicaid spending and health care use for high-risk infants admitted to the neonatal intensive care unit for 5 or more days. J Pediatr 2018;200:91–97 e93.

35. Garg A, Sandel M, Dworkin PH, et al. From medical home to health neighborhood: transforming the medical home into a community-based health neighborhood. J Pediatr 2012;160:535–536 e531.

36. Greenberg JO, Barnett ML, Spinks MA, et al. The "medical neighborhood": integrating primary and specialty care for ambulatory patients. JAMA Intern Med 2014;174:454–7.

37. Kuo DZ, Houtrow AJ, Council. On children with, D. Recognition and management of medical complexity. Pediatrics 2016;138. https://doi.org/10.1542/peds.2016-3021.

38. Antonelli RC, Turchi RM. Care management for children with medical complexity: integration is essential. Pediatrics 2017;140. https://doi.org/10.1542/peds.2017-2860.

39. Langer CS, Antonelli RC, Chamberlain L, et al. Evolving federal and state health care policy: toward a more integrated and comprehensive care-delivery system for children with medical complexity. Pediatrics 2018;141:S259–65.

40. de Jong M, Verhoeven M, van Baar AL. School outcome, cognitive functioning, and behaviour problems in moderate and late preterm children and adults: a review. Semin Fetal Neonatal Med 2012;17:163–9.

41. McLaurin KK, Hall CB, Jackson EA, et al. Persistence of morbidity and cost differences between late-preterm and term infants during the first year of life. Pediatrics 2009;123:653–9.

42. Downs-Canner S, Shaw PH. A comparison of clinical trial enrollment between adolescent and young adult (AYA) oncology patients treated at affiliated adult and pediatric oncology centers. J Pediatr Hematol Oncol 2009;31:927–9.

43. Dempsey AG, Goode RH, Colon MT, et al. Variations in criteria for eligibility determination for early intervention services with a focus on eligibility for children with neonatal complications. J Dev Behav Pediatr 2020;41:646–55.

44. McCormick MC, Litt JS. The outcomes of very preterm infants: is it time to ask different questions? Pediatrics 2017;139.

45. Novak I, Morgan C, Adde L, et al. Early, accurate diagnosis and early intervention in cerebral palsy: advances in diagnosis and treatment. JAMA Pediatr 2017;171: 897–907.

46. Novak I, Morgan C, Adde L, et al. Early, accurate diagnosis and early intervention in cerebral palsy: advances in diagnosis and treatment. JAMA Pediatr 2017;171: 897–907.

47. Maitre NL, et al. Network implementation of guideline for early detection decreases age at cerebral palsy diagnosis. Pediatrics 2020;145.

48. Church PT, et al. The E-Nurture project: a hybrid virtual neonatal follow up model for 2021. Children (Basel) 2021;8. https://doi.org/10.3390/children8020139.

49. Albayrak B, Dathe AK, Cordier L, et al. Clinical experience on video consultation in preterm follow-up care in times of the COVID-19 pandemic. Pediatr Res 2021; 89:1610–1.

50. Association of Maternal & Child Health Programs. Partnering to Promote Follow-Up Care for Premature Infants. 2013. Available at: www.amchp.org. Accessed September 10, 2022.

51. Georgia Medicaid. Tax Equity and Fiscal Responsibility Act/TEFRA (P.L. 97-248), the Katie Beckett Medicaid Program (KB).2018). Available at: https://medicaid. georgia.gov/programs/all-programs/tefrakatie-beckett. Accessed on September 16, 2022.

52. Tennessee Department of Education. Physician's and Tennessee's Early Intervention System. 2004. Available at: efaidnbmnnnibpcajpcglclefindmkaj/https://files. eric.ed.gov/fulltext/ED500377.pdf. Accessed on September 15, 2022.

53. Tennessee Department of Health. Guidelines for Regionalization, Hospital Care Levels, Staffing and Facilities. 2014. Available at: efaidnbmnnnibpcajpcglcle-findmkaj/https://www.tn.gov/content/dam/tn/health/documents/Regionalization_ Guidelines_Approved_2014.pdf. Accessed on September 15, 2022.

54. Lakshmanan A, et al. The financial burden experienced by families of preterm infants after NICU discharge. J Perinatol 2022;42:223–30.

55. Medicaid G. TEFRA/Katie beckett. 2022. Available at: https://medicaid.georgia. gov/programs/all-programs/tefrakatie-beckett.

56. Services, C. D. o. H. C. CCS program overview. 2022. Available at: https://www. dhcs.ca.gov/services/ccs/Pages/ProgramOverview.aspx.

57. Hintz SR, et al. Referral of very low birth weight infants to high-risk follow-up at neonatal intensive care unit discharge varies widely across California. J Pediatr 2015;166:289–95.

58. Synnes AR, Lefebvre F, Cake HA. Current status of neonatal follow-up in Canada. Paediatr Child Health 2006;11:271–4.

59. Fraiman YS, Stewart JE, Litt JS. Race, language, and neighborhood predict high-risk preterm Infant Follow up Program participation. J Perinatol 2022;42:217–22.

60. Fuller MG, Lu T, Gray EE, et al. Rural residence and factors associated with attendance at the second high-risk infant follow-up clinic visit for very low birth weight infants in California. Am J Perinatol 2021. https://doi.org/10.1055/s-0041-1729889.

61. Lakshmanan A, Rogers EE, Lu T, et al. Disparities and early engagement associated with the 18- to 36-month high-risk infant follow-up visit among very low birth-weight infants in California. J Pediatr 2022. https://doi.org/10.1016/j.jpeds.2022. 05.026.

62. Seppanen AV, et al. Parents' ratings of post-discharge healthcare for their children born very preterm and their suggestions for improvement: a European cohort study. Pediatr Res 2021;89:1004–12.

63. Lakshmanan A, Kubicek K, Williams R, et al. Viewpoints from families for improving transition from NICU-to-home for infants with medical complexity at a safety net hospital: a qualitative study. BMC Pediatr 2019;19:223.

64. Ballantyne M, Benzies K, Rosenbaum P, et al. Mothers' and health care providers' perspectives of the barriers and facilitators to attendance at Canadian neonatal follow-up programs. Child Care Health Dev 2015;41:722–33.

65. Harmon SL, Conaway M, Sinkin RA, et al. Factors associated with neonatal intensive care follow-up appointment compliance. Clin Pediatr (Phila) 2013;52:389–96.

66. Brachio SS, et al. Improving neonatal follow-up: a quality improvement study analyzing in-hospital interventions and long-term show rates. Pediatr Qual Saf 2020;5:e363.

67. Janvier A, Farlow B, Baardsnes J, et al. Measuring and communicating meaningful outcomes in neonatology: a family perspective. Semin Perinatol 2016;40:571–7.

68. Maitre NL, et al. Standardized neurodevelopmental surveillance of high-risk infants using telehealth: implementation study during COVID-19. Pediatr Qual Saf 2021;6:e439.

69. Litt JS, Hintz SR. Quality improvement for NICU graduates: feasible, relevant, impactful. Semin Fetal Neonatal Med 2021;26:101205.

70. Medicine, T. A. B. o. P. C. O. N.-P. 2020 ACGME program requirements for GME in neonatal perinatal medicine. 2020. Available at: https://www.acgme.org/globalassets/PFAssets/ProgramRequirements/329_NeonatalPerinatalMedicine_2020.pdf?ver=2020-06-29-162707-410&ver=2020-06-29-162707-410.

71. Cicalese E, et al. Essentials of Neonatal-Perinatal Medicine fellowship: part 2 - clinical education and experience. J Perinatol 2022;42:410–5.

72. Church PT, Cavanagh A, Lee SK, et al. Academic challenges for the preterm infant: parent and educators' perspectives. Early Hum Dev 2019;128:1–5.

73. Excellence, N. I. f. H. a. C. Developmental follow-up of children and young people born preterm. 2018. Available at: www.nice.org.uk/guidance/qs169.

74. Professionals, P. B. I. f. E. PRISM premature infants' skills in mathematics. Available at: www.nottingham.ac.uk/helm/dev/prism.

75. Health, P. C. f. M. a. C. Neonatal follow-up implementation strategy. Available at: www.pcmch.on.ca/wp-content/uploads/2022/02/NNFUImplementationWorkGroupFinalReport_2017NOV09.pdf.

76. Fraiman YS, Litt JS, Davis JM, et al. Racial and ethnic disparities in adult COVID-19 and the future impact on child health. Pediatr Res 2021;89:1052–4.

77. Horbar JD, Edwards EM, Ogbolu Y. Our responsibility to follow through for NICU infants and their families. Pediatrics 2020;146. https://doi.org/10.1542/peds.2020-0360.

78. Hall WJ, et al. Implicit racial/ethnic bias among health care professionals and its influence on health care outcomes: a systematic review. Am J Public Health 2015;105:e60–76.

79. Maina IW, Belton TD, Ginzberg S, et al. A decade of studying implicit racial/ethnic bias in healthcare providers using the implicit association test. Soc Sci Med 2018;199:219–29.

80. Ruben M, Saks NS. Addressing implicit bias in first-year medical students: a longitudinal, multidisciplinary training program. Med Sci Educ 2020;30:1419–26.

81. Tajeu GS, et al. Development of a multicomponent intervention to decrease racial bias among healthcare staff. J Gen Intern Med 2022;37:1970–9.

82. Brega AG, Hamer MK, Albright K, et al. Organizational health literacy: quality improvement measures with expert consensus. Health Lit Res Pract 2019;3:e127–46.

83. Lloyd J, Dougherty L, Dennis S, et al. Culturally diverse patient experiences and walking interviews: a Co-design approach to improving organizational health literacy. Health Lit Res Pract 2019;3:e238–42.

84. Bremer D, Klockmann I, Jass L, et al. Which criteria characterize a health literate health care organization? - a scoping review on organizational health literacy. BMC Health Serv Res 2021;21:664.

# Intensive Multidisciplinary Feeding Intervention for High-Risk Infants

William G. Sharp, PhD[a,b]

## KEYWORDS

- Avoidant/restrictive food intake disorder • Pediatric feeding disorder • Nutrition
- Tube weaning

## KEY POINTS

- Infants born premature or other medical complex infants are at high risk for developing long-term feeding problems that extends beyond infancy.
- Multiple factors contribute to this increased risk, including dysfunction of multiple systems, delayed exposure to food, and conditioned food aversion.
- Intensive multidisciplinary feeding intervention (IMFI) represents the standard of care for children with chronic and severe feeding issues, with a team that should involve, at a minimum, psychology, medicine, nutrition, and feeding skill expertise.
- IMFI seems to hold benefit for preterm and medically complex infants; however, there remains a need to develop and investigate new therapeutic pathways to reduce the number of patients who likely require this level of care.

## INTRODUCTION

Infants born premature and other infants with medical complexities (eg, congenital or acquired respiratory, cardiac, and gastrointestinal [GI] problems) frequently experience chronic feeding concerns.[1,2] For these medically complex children, tube feeding represents a common and potentially lifesaving medical solution for delivering nutrition when oral feeding is unsafe (eg, aspiration), not feasible (eg, poor coordination of a suck-swallow-breath pattern), and/or limited due to food refusal. Prolonged tube feeding, however, also circumvents key sensory, developmental, physiologic, and social processes associated with eating and may result in delayed feeding milestones and/or elevated risk for developing a feeding disorder.[3,4] Feeding disorders in children are often complicated by predisposing medical conditions, oral-motor delays or deficits, dietary deficiencies, and/or psychosocial dysfunction that perpetuate

[a] Department of Pediatrics, Emory University School of Medicine, Atlanta, GA, USA; [b] Center for Advanced Pediatrics, Children's Healthcare of Atlanta, 1400 Tullie Road NE, Atlanta, GA 30329, USA
*E-mail address:* William.sharp@choa.org

Clin Perinatol 50 (2023) 239–251
https://doi.org/10.1016/j.clp.2022.10.005
0095-5108/23/© 2022 Elsevier Inc. All rights reserved.

restricted food intake.[5] Children with this level of feeding concern benefit most from a multidisciplinary approach to assessment and intervention.[4,6] The standard treatment of complex feeding problems involves the multidisciplinary team coordinating treatment at a day hospital or inpatient setting.[6] In this article, we review the factors contributing the emergence and maintenance of feeding problems in high-risk infants, describe the intensive multidisciplinary feeding intervention (IMFI) model of care, and assess outcomes associated with both preterm and full-term infants.

### Risk Factors for Feeding Concerns in Pediatric Populations

With advances in maternal and newborn care, increased survival of children born premature or other infants with serious medical complexities present the challenge of mitigating downstream medical, developmental, and behavioral complications.[7] Problematic feeding is a well-recognized and common morbidity associated with prematurity as well as other medical conditions that interfere with the mechanics of normal feeding.[5] A nationwide prevalence survey suggested annual prevalence of feeding disorders between 1 in 3 and 1 in 5 among children aged younger than 5 years with a chronic disease (eg, congenital or acquired respiratory, cardiac, and GI problems).[8] A meta-analysis estimated 42% of preterm infants experience significant feeding problems in the first 4 years of life.[1] In a more focused analysis of ~2500 extremely preterm infants (ie, <28 weeks gestational age at birth), the prevalence increased to 46% for this more vulnerable subgroup.

Among preterm infants, difficulty with oral feeding often begins at birth due to the underdevelopment of neurologic, cardiorespiratory, GI, and/or oral-motor systems.[3] Dysfunction of these systems presents challenges with feeding due to safety (eg, aspiration), oral-motor coordination, and/or feeding fatigue.[9] Other medically complex children may experience increased risk of GI conditions (eg, motility disease; gastroesophageal reflux disease, GERD) or neurologic conditions (eg, cerebral palsy) that may place limits on feeding volume or make it difficult to achieve nutritional needs through oral intake due to underdeveloped feeding skill (respectfully). In addition, medical conditions—such as infants born with congenital heart disease—may require prolonged hospitalization with surgical and other critical care interventions that delay or subvert oral feeding.[5,10] Until a developmental shift occurs to support efficient and safe oral intake, tube feeding is frequently required in medically fragile pediatric populations.

Transitioning off tube feeding and achieving adequate oral intake is a critical milestone for medically complex infants to promote growth and provide nutrition to support cognitive, motor, and sensory development.[11] Discharge from the hospital often depends on an infant's ability to safely and reliably feed, and problematic feeding is a common reason for extended length of stay.[1,9] In cases where an infant is unable to achieve full oral feeding, the use of a surgically placed gastrostomy tube (G-tube) represents an alternative vehicle for delivering nutrition at home.[9] Risk factors for oral feeding problems and eventual G-tube placement include younger gestational age and lower birth weight.[11] Children with younger gestational age often require G-tube placement due to complications associated with prematurity, such as respiratory disease[10]; low birth weight infants present with lower energy reserves despite having higher energy requirements compared with full-term infants.[11]

Length of tube feeding also portends elevated risk for long-term feeding problems. This includes cases involving both the inability to advance oral feeding due to medical complications as well as patients unwilling to consume food.[4,11] Although many children requiring G-tube feeding eventually achieve full oral feeding during infancy, a subset will develop feeding tube dependence. For example, in a retrospective cohort of 194 preterm infants with feeding difficulties referred to a neonatal feeding disorders program, 40% (n = 77) were discharged on G-tube feedings.[12] Of this cohort, 78% continued to rely on tube feeding fully (40%) or partially (38%) 1 year later. When feeding problems persist, resolution and/or effective management of underlying medical concerns may not improve oral intake due to active and persistent food refusal.[4] Although early feeding problems generally involve symptoms that include drooling, uncoordinated suck-swallow-breathe, gagging, choking, or coughing during feeding,[1,11] the topography of active food refusal in later infancy/childhood involves behaviors—such as pushing away food, crying, and turning the head away from food—aimed at avoiding and/or restricting contact with food.[6] This type of food refusal is posited to be driven (in large part) by conditioned food aversion—that is, pairing unpleasant consequences with eating. This includes medical conditions (eg, GERD) associated with pain, as well as the very lifesaving medical procedures aimed at reducing mortality (eg, mechanical ventilation and/or recurring endotracheal suctioning) that contribute to noxious orofacial sensory stimulation.[13]

Regardless of what factors contribute to the emergence of food refusal, behaviorally based feeding concerns involve a learning process on both sides of the parent–child dyad (**Fig. 1**). On the child side, there is a well-established body of literature suggesting many longstanding feeding problems function as a means for the child to escape aversive feeding experiences.[14] Caregiver responses to problem behaviors often include both negative reinforcement (eg, removing food and/or ending the meal due to problem behavior) and positive reinforcement (eg, attention in the form on prompting or coaxing) that inadvertently shape and strengthen problem behaviors overtime.[15] Through this process, the child learns that food—an aversive stimulus based on a history of pain, discomfort, or fatigue—is removed in response to problem behavior, which in turn increases the likelihood these behaviors will occur during future meals.

On the parent side, a similar learning process occurs. When food is removed, the caregiver learns that food removal results in rapid cessation of an aversive event

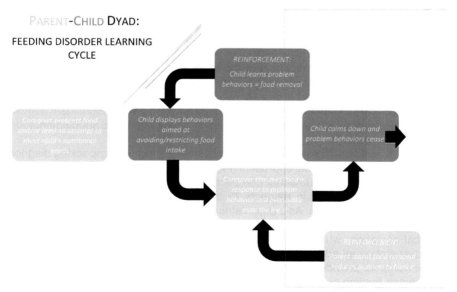

**Fig. 1.** The learning cycle across the parent–child dyad for behaviorally based feeding concerns.

(eg, their child crying or displaying other disruptive mealtime behaviors). Food removal and/or ending the meal is subsequently negatively reinforced, making this form of behavior management more likely to occur when faced with problem behavior during future meals. Without intervention, this cycle is maintained or increases in frequency and severity overtime, resulting in limited contact with food for the child and high levels of stress with conducting meals on the part of the caregiver.[4,16]

### Diagnostic Nomenclature

Historically, lack of a formal definition encompassing the complexity and heterogeneity of disrupted food intake in high-risk infants has affected clinical and research activities and delayed early recognition and formal diagnosis in pediatric settings. Case in point, the average age for accessing specialized care for a feeding problem is 2 years or greater; however, parents frequently report a much earlier age of onset.[17] For example, Sharp and colleagues[6] reported outcomes for a cohort of 81 patients requiring treatment of feeding tube dependence. The median age at admission was 40 months (range: 10–230) despite 68% of parents reporting that the feeding problem was present at birth. Lack of clarity is due—in part—on divergent theoretic underpinnings and terms used to describe the cause, assessment, diagnosis, and treatment by the various disciplines called on to care for children with feeding challenges. Current and past diagnostic classifications include terms such as failure to thrive (medical/nutrition), infantile anorexia (psychiatry), dysphagia (speech language pathology, SLP), and food refusal (behavior).[17]

Recent developments in diagnostic systems move beyond the limitations of single-discipline nomenclature and adopt a broader multidisciplinary framework to support clinical and research activities. Pediatric feeding disorder (PFD) is a new consensus definition describing a complex and heterogeneous disturbance in oral intake associated with dysfunction in medical and nutritional status, feeding skill and safety, and/or psychosocial functioning.[5] In doing so, PFD identifies 4 primary domains (medical, nutritional, feeding skill, and psychosocial) as potentially contributing to the emergence and maintenance of feeding problems in pediatric populations. Preterm and other medically complex infants with medical and/or developmental conditions preventing safe, painless, and/or efficient consumption meet diagnostic criteria for PFD. When disruptive mealtime behaviors (eg, crying, tantrums) emerge and maintain food refusal despite the resolution of the medical concern, the broader psychiatric diagnosis of avoidant/restrictive food intake disorder (ARFID) captures cases where failure to meet nutrition and/or energy needs is the result of avoidance or restriction of food. Clinical manifestations of ARFID include faltering growth, significant nutritional deficiencies, and/or the need for enteral feeding or oral nutritional supplementation to meet energy needs.[18]

The introduction of these new classification systems requires unpacking diagnostic overlap and intended clinical end-users (**Fig. 2**). Both ARFID and PFD involve psychosocial dysfunction and nutritional complications as core diagnostic features. The 2 systems, however, differ in respects to their relationship with underlying medical and feeding skill concerns. As a psychiatric/behavioral diagnosis, ARFID explicitly excludes cases where the feeding/eating disturbance is better attributed a concurrent medical condition, whereas PFD incorporates medical and developmental feeding skill dysfunction as additional etiologic features. In doing so, PFD provides a diagnostic home for providers managing the medical, nutritional, and skill-based aspects of pediatric feeding concerns. ARFID, by contrast, is intended for mental health providers (eg, psychologists) more likely called on to manage behaviorally based mealtime difficulties.

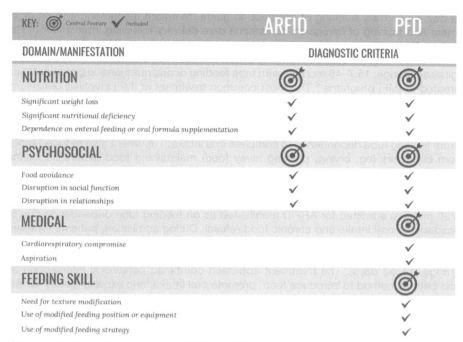

Fig. 2. Core diagnostic features of ARFID and PFD.

## Multidisciplinary Feeding Assessment and Intervention

When an infant or child is not eating beyond the neonatal period, best clinical practice involves adopting a multidisciplinary framework to assess etiologic and maintaining factors across medical, nutritional, feeding skill, and behavioral domains.[4] This process begins with a detailed GI workup to identify and treat any underlying medical conditions that may be contributing to unsafe or painful eating. In complex cases, it should also involve instrumental assessment of swallowing (eg, fiberoptic evaluation of swallowing) to evaluate the anatomy and function of aerodigestive structures,[15] a process frequently overseen by SLP. A skill-based provider, such as an SLP, will also assess how the child moves its mouth and tongue and observe how the child picks up food, chews, swallows, and drinks.[19] A registered dietitian focuses on providing nutrition education and guidance for advancing oral intake and managing formula volume via tube if oral intake improves.[6] Finally, a psychologist with expertise in feeding disorders can oversee exposure-based treatment aimed at overcoming avoidance and promote learning to consume food when it no longer has adverse consequences.[20]

The standard of care for young children with complex feeding concerns (eg, ARFID) frequently involves IMFI delivered at day hospital program or inpatient settings. These programs aim to expand oral intake, improve nutritional status, and/or reduce dependence on oral or enteral nutrition supplementation.[4] IMFI provides a common clinical umbrella for the multidisciplinary team—which most often includes psychologists, physicians, dietitians, SLPs, and social work—to coordinate treatment and monitor potential complications with the introduction of food (eg, aspiration, marked weight loss, allergic reactions). This treatment model also permits multiple therapeutic meals a day, close/daily tracking of progress to guide treatment refinement, and engagement and training of caregivers to assume care delivery following intervention.[6] The extant literature suggests positive outcomes associated with IMFI. This includes a meta-analysis of 11 studies reporting outcomes for 593 patients (314 boys and 279 girls; age range, 15.7–48 months) with tube feeding or oral nutritional supplementation treated at IMFI programs.[4] The most common treatment at IMFI involved behavioral intervention (eg, exposure, reinforcement) to structure the introduction of new foods followed by rapid weaning from tube feedings to promote hunger. Findings indicated that 71% of patients (95% confidence interval: 54%–83%) successfully transitioned from feeding tube dependence to complete oral intake. Treatment also reduced problem behaviors (eg, crying, pushing away food) maintaining food avoidance during meals.

In a more recent retrospective study, Sharp and colleagues[6] detailed an IMFI model and presented outcomes for the aforementioned 81 patients (age range: 10–230 months) admitted for ARFID manifested as on feeding tube dependence due to inadequate oral intake and chronic food refusal. During admission, patients received 4 therapeutic meals per day, 5 days a week (Monday through Friday), totaling 20 therapeutic meals per week. The average duration of admission was 38 days ± 7 days (range, 11–52 days). The treatment approach combined behavioral intervention as the central method to introduce food, promote oral intake, and expand dietary variety with parent training as the central method to generalize treatment gains from the clinic to the home setting. The approach to behavioral intervention followed a standardized sequence of reinforcement techniques, exposure, and stimulus fading/antecedent manipulation protocols.[21] A team of feeding therapists, working under the supervision of a multidisciplinary team, conducted meals. The progression of treatment followed detailed protocols guided by bite-by-bite data collection.

In addition to behavioral intervention and parent training, the multidisciplinary approach included nutritional counseling, feeding skill assessment and oversight, and medical management to monitor growth and promote a nutritionally complete diet, assess and advance skill deficits, and ensure adequate safeguards to address potential medical concerns that may emerge during the course of therapy (respectively). **Fig. 3** provides additional details regarding the contribution of the multidisciplinary team in this IMFI model. Results suggested positive benefits associated with intervention. Treatment gains included a 70.5% improvement in oral intake; 27 of the 81 patients (33%) completely weaned from tube feeding at discharge. Weight gains were observed, and problem behavior during meals reduced by 68%. Treatment gains continued following discharge, with 72% of patients completely weaned from tube feeding at last follow-up.

### Outcomes for Preterm Infants

Children born premature represent a significant cohort of patients accessing care at IMFI and other specialized feeding programs. In the meta-analysis conducted by Sharp and colleagues,[4] prematurity represented the fourth most documented medical condition, following gastroesophageal reflux, general GI problems, and failure to thrive (respectively). In Sharp and colleagues,[6] preterm birth represented the second most documented medical condition following gastroesophageal reflux, present in 46 of the 81 cases (57%). In a prospective study of 711 tube-dependent children, 378 (53.2%) presented with a history of prematurity; 103 (13%) with a history of prematurity less than 29 weeks.[22] Among this later premature cohort, 86 of the 103 cases (83.5%) presented with no additional medical conditions outside of prematurity and its complications.

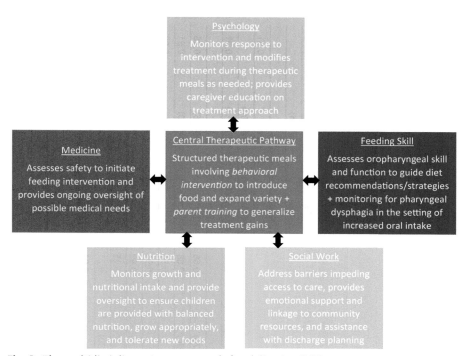

**Fig. 3.** The multidisciplinary team approach for delivering IMFI.

Despite the disproportionate number of children with a history of prematurity being served at IMFI programs, little is known about the experience of this patient population accessing this level of care. The study conducted by Pahsini and colleagues[22] presented outcomes for the 711 children who participated in a feeding program based on the "Graz Model of tube weaning." Graz represents a treatment developed in Austria described as combining tube weaning with psychoanalytically oriented play therapy during meals, nutritional counseling, and oral-motor therapy (eg, tactile stimulation).[4] The analysis included comparing success with tube weaning for preterm infants compared with full-term peers. Findings indicated equivalent outcomes between these 2 groups in terms of success achieving full wean (~87% of the sample). The authors also noted that children with extreme prematurity were more likely to present with a history of consistent feeding tube dependency since birth. This study, however, lacked detail about other feeding-related metrics (eg, weight status, mealtime behaviors, percent oral intake) important when assessing response to feeding intervention.

To extend this line of research, further scrutiny of the 81 patients with feeding tube dependence evaluated by Sharp and colleagues[6] permits closer appraisal of the clinical presentation and treatment outcomes for children with a history of prematurity compared with their full-term peers. This examination also allowed for a subgroup analysis of extremely premature infants, paralleling the work of Pahsini and colleagues.[22] As presented in **Table 1**, few differences were detected between groups in terms of patient characteristics apart from preterm infants being significantly more likely to experience the feeding problem since birth. In addition, children with a history of extreme prematurity were more likely to present with a history of developmental disability and experience more total medical comorbidities compared with other infants born premature.

**Table 1**
**Characteristics of patients entering intensive multidisciplinary feeding intervention by birth status**

| | Full-Term Group (37 wk or greater) N = 35 | Preterm Group (<37 wk) N = 46 | p | Subgroup: Other preterm (28–37 wk) N = 24 | Subgroup: Extreme preterm (<28 wk) N = 22 | p |
|---|---|---|---|---|---|---|
| Age at admission, mo, mean (sd) (range) | 47 (33) (10–118) | 50 (40) (12–230) | 0.35 | 51 (47) (12–230) | 49 (30) (17–117) | 0.43 |
| Sex | | | | | | |
| Female, n (%) | 16 (46) | 19 (41) | 0.86 | 11 (46) | 8 (36) | 0.72 |
| Male, n (%) | 19 (54) | 27 (59) | | 13 (54) | 14 (64) | |
| Ethnicity | | | | | | |
| Hispanic, n (%) | $2^6$ | $1^2$ | 0.81 | $1^4$ | 0 (0) | 0.51 |
| Non-Hispanic, n (%) | 33 (94) | 45 (98) | | 23 (96) | 22 (100) | |
| Total medical comorbidities, mean (sd) | 2.0 (1.2) (0–5) | 2.3 (1.2) (0–5) | 0.11 | 2.0 (1.1) (0–4) | $2.7 (1.1)^{1-5}$ | 0.01 |
| Comorbid medical concern, n (%) | | | | | | |
| Gastroesophageal reflux disease | 25 (71) | 36 (78) | 0.66 | 17 (71) | 19 (86) | 0.36 |
| Developmental disability | 11 (31) | 14 (30) | 0.88 | $3^{13}$ | 11 (50) | 0.01 |
| Autism spectrum disorder | $3^9$ | $7^{15}$ | 0.56 | $3^{13}$ | 4 (32) | 0.90 |
| Failure to thrive | $8^{23}$ | $12^{26}$ | 0.94 | $5^{21}$ | 7 (32) | 0.61 |
| Congenital heart disease with surgery | $6^{17}$ | $9^{19}$ | 0.99 | $5^{21}$ | $4^{18}$ | 0.88 |
| Congenital heart disease without surgery | $2^6$ | $3^7$ | 0.75 | $2^8$ | $1^5$ | 0.94 |
| Pulmonary condition | $6^{17}$ | 14 (30) | 0.27 | $4^{17}$ | 10 (46) | 0.07 |
| Other | $9^{25}$ | $11^{24}$ | 0.94 | 8 (33) | $3^{14}$ | 0.2236 |
| Age of feeding problem onset, mo, mean (sd) (range) | 6.9 (16.8) (0–85) | 6.7 (31.8) (0–211) | | 12.5 (44) (0–211) | 0.59 (2.6) (0–12) | |
| Feeding problem present at birth, n (%) | 17 (49) | 37 (80) | 0.006 | 17 (71) | 20 (91) | 0.18 |
| Previous intervention reported, n (%) | 30 (86) | 40 (87) | 0.87 | 21 (88) | 19 (86) | 0.75 |
| Previous intervention duration, mo, mean (sd) (range) | $14^{12}$ (2.5–84) | $13^{12}$ (.25–60) | 0.25 | $12^9$ 2–29 | $12^{14}$ (.25–60) | 0.44 |

Note: Comparison among groups involved t tests for continuous variables and $\chi^2$ tests for categorical variables.

**Table 2** presents feeding status and anthropometric data at admission to IMFI at admission and at discharge. Results suggest preterm infants experience similar benefits from intervention in terms of weaning from enteral feeding, percent calories met by oral intake, and reduction in inappropriate behavior during meals. Weight gain also occurred across both groups; however, children with a history of prematurity entered treatment with a lower weight z-score by age compared with full-term peers. In addition, children with a history of extreme prematurity entered treatment significantly smaller than other peers with prematurity. The statistical difference between full-term and preterm did not remain at discharge but the difference between children with extreme prematurity and other peers with prematurity did remain.

## DISCUSSION

Preterm infants experience multiple risk factors that contribute to the emergence and maintenance of chronic feeding problems, including underdeveloped systems required to safely and efficiently eat at birth, frequent reliance on enteral feeding to support growth and development, and/or exposure to medical procedures (eg, mechanical ventilation) that may lead to aversive oral experiences. Children with other medical complexities (eg, congenital heart disease) are also at risk for delays or disruptions in oral feeding due to surgical and other lifesaving procedures. When feeding problems persist, PFD is a new diagnosis to capture cases in which a child is either unable to safely eat due to conditions such as aspiration or cardiorespiratory compromise or lack the necessary skills to efficiently consume food due to neurodevelopmental delay and/or lack of exposure and experience with eating.[5] In the United States, PFD has recently been added to the international statistical classification of diseases and related health problems (ICD), defined as a complex and heterogeneous disturbance in oral intake of nutrients associated with dysfunction in multiple domains (medical, nutritional status, feeding skill, psychosocial). ARFID is the corresponding psychiatric diagnosis for case in which the feeding difficulty is associated with avoidance and restriction of food intake, such as behaviorally based food refusal.[18] Both conditions recognize the potential contribution of medical complexities, such as prematurity, in contributing to disordered feeding in infancy and early childhood.

A multidisciplinary team approach is the recommended standard of care for high-risk infants with feeding concerns. Multidisciplinary care often begins in the neonatal intensive care unit (NICU), with a team that may include neonatology, speech pathology, and occupational and physical therapy to provide expertise on the intricacies of feeding issues related to prematurity and the potential interplay of other comorbidities.[13] Therapeutic interventions to promote oral feeding and transition from tube feeds include modifications to feeding position, changes in nipple flow rate, and support for chin, cheek, or jaw.[13,23] For infants who discharge dependent on G-tube feedings, less is known regarding whether access to and/or support from multidisciplinary care continues following hospitalization. This includes important questions about current approaches for managing feeding problems in community settings. Available data indicate speech language pathologists followed by occupational therapists represent the most common disciplines to continue to provide feeding therapy.[24,25] This data, however, are based on nationwide surveys, and there are no well-documented outcome studies or clinical trials involving these providers, raising questions about their effectiveness in improving the feeding status for high-risk infants. It also brings into question the level of expertise and approach to intervention. For example, 70% of respondents in a survey of Australian feeding therapists rated their expertise as limited and average in providing intervention; 58% classified their therapy as somewhat successful.[25]

**Table 2**
Comparison of admission and discharge feeding related metrics by birth status

| | Full Term Group (37 wk or greater) N = 35 | Preterm Group (<37 wk) N = 46 | P | Subgroup: Other preterm (28–37 wk) N = 24 | P | Subgroup: Extreme preterm (<28 wk) N = 22 | p |
|---|---|---|---|---|---|---|---|
| *Admission status* | | | | | | | |
| % Calories met by oral intake, mean (sd) (range) | 2.2 (7.0) (0–38) | 2.1 (6.3) (0–28) | 0.94 | 2.1 (6.9) (0–28) | | 2.2 (5.8) (0–24) | 0.97 |
| Oral feeder, n (%) | 8[23] | 9[20] | 0.76 | 4[17] | | 5[23] | 0.88 |
| % Inappropriate mealtime behavior, mean (sd) (range) | 65.3 (40.0) (0–100) | 57.8 (38.8) (0–100) | 0.39 | 55.8 (41.4) (0–100) | | 59.8 (37.8) (0–100) | 0.73 |
| Anthropometric data, mean (sd) (range) | | | | | | | |
| Weight, kg | 15.4 (6.7) (7.4–36.2) | 15.0 (9.0) (8.6–61.0) | 0.41 | 16.2 (11.5) (8.6–61.0) | | 13.6 (5.2) (9.2–26.3) | 0.17 |
| Weight, percentile for age | 27.2 (26.6) (1–83) | 18.7 (23.2) (1–75.0) | 0.07 | 24.8 (25.7) (1–88.8) | | 12.1 (18.6) (1–67.2) | 0.03 |
| Weight z-score by age | −0.92 (1.03) (−2.98–0.95) | −1.38 (1.17) (−4.01–0.68) | 0.03 | −1.09 (1.24) (−4.01–1.21) | | −1.69 (1.01) (−3.31–0.44) | 0.04 |
| *Discharge status* | | | | | | | |
| *Patients weaned* | | | | | | | |
| Discharge, n (%) | 14 (40) | 13[28] | 0.38 | 7[29] | | 6[27] | 0.85 |
| Follow-up, n (%) | 24 (69) | 34 (74) | 0.77 | 19 (79) | | 15 (68) | 0.61 |
| % Calories met by oral intake, mean (sd) (range) | 72.9 (28.9) (20–100) | 71.6 (24.5) (17–100) | 0.83 | 70.5 (26.8) (17–100) | | 72.7 (22.4) (39–100) | 0.76 |
| % Inappropriate mealtime behavior, mean (sd) (range) | 4.1 (7.8) (0.11–44.85) | 4.83 (5.6) (0–20) | 0.31 | 5.16 (6.3) (0–28.1) | | 3.4 (3.3) (0–14.28) | 0.13 |
| % Treatment goals achieved, mean (sd) (range) | 90.2 (8.4) (71.4–100) | 88.1 (9.0) (71.4–100) | 0.27 | 88.9 (9.1) (71.4–100) | | 87.2 (9.0) (71.0–100) | 0.55 |
| Anthropometric data, mean (sd) (range) | | | | | | | |
| Weight, kg | 15.8 (7.1) (7.9–38.6) | 15.3 (8.9) (8.8–59.1) | 0.39 | 16.7 (11.2) (8.8–59.1) | | 13.9 (5.3) (9.3–26.4) | 0.15 |
| Weight, percentile for age | 27.0 (27.1) (0.2–85.9) | 19.3 (23.4) (0.0–80.1) | 0.08 | 27.2 (26.2) (0.0–80.1) | | 10.7 (16.3) (0.0–70.2) | 0.01 |
| Weight z-score by age | −0.9 (1.1) (−2.97–1.08) | −1.3 (1.12) (−3.77–0.8) | 0.07 | −0.9 (1.2) (−3.8–0.8) | | −1.7 (0.9) (−3.3–−0.5) | 0.01 |
| Weight change | 0.44 (0.77) (−0.6–3.2) | 0.38 (0.71) (−1.9–2.1) | 0.29 | 0.47 (0.77) −1.9–1.5) | | 0.21 (0.64) (−1.2–2.1) | 0.12 |

Note: Comparison between groups involved t tests for continuous variables and $\chi^2$ tests for categorical variables.

Currently, IMFI is the most well-researched and supported treatment of children with chronic and severe feeding difficulties.[4] Children with a history of prematurity and other medical and developmental complexities represent a significant cohort of patients accessing this level of care. Outcomes suggest IMFI holds clear benefit in terms of establishing oral intake, reducing problem behaviors, and improving dietary diversity in pediatric populations, including children with a history of prematurity and longstanding feeding concerns (many since birth). This includes emerging evidence suggesting that children born preterm experience similar improvement with weaning from enteral feeding because their full-term peers, regardless of the severity of prematurity.[22] Of note, patents with prematurity accessing IMFI programs experience a significant, multiyear gap between the onset of the feeding difficulty (often present a birth) and admission to treatment. There are insufficient data to determine what is guiding this delay in accessing care. Possibilities include recent medical clearance to introduce food (eg, passing a swallow study), potential barriers accessing care (eg, insurance coverage), limited recognition of feeding disorders in pediatric settings, and/or lack of a clear referral pathway to IMFI.[26] Ideally, new diagnostic systems (ie, PFD; ARFID) will increase awareness and mitigate previous diagnostic ambiguity that has long plagued the field.[17]

Although IMFI represents the standard of care for complex and longstanding feeding concerns, this level of care is neither available in all communities nor is it likely necessary for all patients. There is a clear need, however, to better understand and evaluate treatments being delivered outside of multidisciplinary clinics. This includes important questions about the timing and intensity of early intervention strategies to reduce the number of patients who develop chronic feeding concerns and require IMFI to establish oral intake.[26] Potential for therapeutic intervention begins in the NICU; however, best practice standards for early oral motor stimulation, initiation, and advancement of oral feeds remain elusive.[13] Increased risk for long-term feeding problems is well known for younger and smaller preterm infants, suggesting one possible avenue may involve closer monitoring and early intervention for this cohort with increased vulnerability.[11] There is also evidence for earlier achievement of feeding milestones for infants fed with breast milk compared with formula, a finding posited to reflect breastmilk's advantage on supporting the infants' immature immune system, promoting GI maturation, and reducing feeding intolerance.[3,27] It is also suggested that the timing of when infants initiate oral feeding may serve as a red flag for inadequate development of feeding skills[3] — providing another potential target for a more focused approach to early intervention.

The long-term effects and health-care costs associated with prematurity continue to expand as infants survive into adulthood.[28] Presence of chronic and severe feeding concerns, such a G-tube dependency, contribute to this cost. A recent economic analysis indicated an 8-year health care utilization and medical expenditure of ∼ US$400,000 per child in cases involve prolonged G-tube use; access to IMFI reduced this cost by half.[29] This suggests clear benefit for investing time, energy, and attention toward developing a comprehensive research agenda that identifies new therapeutic pathways, investigates adjuncts to improve the effectiveness of existing treatments (eg, IMFI), and promotes enhanced detection in pediatric settings to improve earlier access to care.

## SUMMARY

Feeding problems are exceedingly common among children with a history of prematurity, and in many cases, this difficulty is present at birth. Work establishing oral intake is a milestone for this patient cohort that begins in the NICU; a subset of patients will develop a feeding tube dependence and food refusal and seek treatment at a IMFI program. Although available evidence suggest that IMFI holds benefit for patients with prematurity, more research is needed to determine the feeding therapy journey for preterm patients occurring outside these subspecialty programs.

## FUNDING

This work was supported by the Marcus Foundation.

## DISCLOSURE

The author has nothing to disclose.

## ACKNOWLEDGMENTS

I would like to thank the patients, families, and clinicians who participated and/or support this work.

## REFERENCES

1. Pados BF, Hill RR, Yamasaki JT, et al. Prevalence of problematic feeding in young children born prematurely: a meta-analysis. BMC Pediat 2010;21(1):110.
2. Lukens CT, Silverman AH. Systematic review of psychological interventions for pediatric feeding problems. J Pediatr Psychol 2014;38:903–17.
3. Park J, Knafl G, Thoyre S, et al. Factors associated with feeding progression in extremely preterm infants. Nurs Res 2015;64(3):159–67.
4. Sharp WG, Volkert VM, Scahill L, et al. A systematic review and meta-analysis of intensive multidisciplinary intervention for pediatric feeding disorders: how standard is the standard of care? J Pediatr 2017;181:116–24.e4.
5. Goday PG, Huh SY, Silverman A, et al. Pediatric feeding disorder: consensus definition and conceptual framework. J Pediatr Gastroenterol Nutr 2019;68(1):124–9.
6. Sharp WG, Volkert VM, Stubds KH, et al. Intensive multidisciplinary intervention for young children with feeding tube dependency and chronic food refusal: an electronic health record review. J Pediatr 2020;223:73–80.
7. Stoll BJ, Hansen NI, Bell EF, et al. Trend in care practices, morbidity, and mortality of extremely preterm neonates, 1993-2012. JAMA 2016;314(10):1039–51.
8. Kovacic K, Rein LE, Szabo A, et al. Pediatric Feeding disorder: a nationwide prevalence study. J Pediatr 2021;228:126–131 e123.
9. Chapman A, George K, Selassie A, et al. NICU infants who require a feeding gastrostomy for discharge. J Pediatr Surg 2021;56:449–53.
10. Hill R, Tey CS, Jung C, et al. Feeding outcomes after paediatric cardiothoracic surgery: a retrospective review. Cardiol Young 2020;31(4):673–81.
11. Fucile S, Samdup D, MacFarlane V, et al. Risk factors associated with long-term feeding problems in preterm infants: a scoping review. Adv Neonatal Care 2021;22(2):161–9.
12. Jadcherla SR, Khot T, Moore R, et al. Feeding methods at discharge predict long-term feeding and neurodevelopmental outcomes in preterm infants referred for gastrostomy evaluation. J Pediatr 2017;181:125–30.
13. Kamity R, Kapavarapu PK, Chandel A. Feeding problems and long-term outcome sin preterm infants: a systematic approach to evaluation and management. Children 2021;8(12):1158.

14. Piazza CC, Fisher WW, Brown KA, et al. Functional analysis of inappropriate mealtime behaviors. J Appl Behav Anal 2003;36:187–204.
15. Sharp WG, Jaquess DL, Morton JS, et al. Pediatric feeding disorders: a quantitative synthesis of treatment outcomes. Clin Child Fam Psychol Rev 2011;13:348–65.
16. Lindberg L, Bohlin G, Hagekull B. Early feeding problems in a normal population. Int J Eat Disord 1991;10:395–405.
17. Estrem HH, Pados BF, Park J, et al. Feeding problems in infancy and early childhood: evolutionary concept analysis. J Adv Nurs 2017;73:56–70.
18. American Psychiatric Association. Diagnostic and statistical manual of mental disorders (DSM-5). 5th edition. Washington (DC): American Psychiatric Publishing; 2013.
19. Feeding and swallowing disorders in children. American speech-language-hearing association. Available at: https://www.asha.org/public/speech/swallowing/feeding-and-swallowing-disorders-in-children/. Accessed June 1, 2022.
20. Sharp WG, Allen AG, Stubbs KH, et al. Successful pharmacotherapy for the treatment of severe feeding aversion with mechanistic insights from cross-species neuronal remodeling. Transl Psychiatry 2017;7(6):e1157.
21. Sharp WG, Stubbs KH, Adams H, et al. Intensive manual-based intervention for pediatric feeding disorders: results from a randomized pilot trial. J Pediatr Gastroenterol Nutr 2016;62:658–63.
22. Pahsini K, Marinschek S, Khan Z, et al. Tube dependency as a result of prematurity. J Neonatal Perinatal Med 2018;11:311–6.
23. Park J, Pados B, Thoyre SM. Systematic review: what is the evidence for the side-lying position for feeding preterm infants? Adv Neonatal Care 2018;18:285–94.
24. Taylor H, Pennington L, Craig D, et al. Children with neurodisability and feeding difficulties: a UK survey of parent-delivered interventions. BMJ Paediatrics Open 2021;5:e001095.
25. Marshall J, Hill RJ, Dodrill P. A survey of practice for clinicians working with children with autism spectrum disorders and feeding difficulties. Int J Speech Lang Pathol Audiol 2013;15(3):279–85.
26. Noel RJ, Silverman AH. A problem that is difficult to swallow. J Pediatr 2017;181:7–8.
27. Quigley M, McGuire W. Formula versus donor breast milk for feeding preterm or low birth weight infants. Cochrane Database Syst Rev 2014;4:CD002971. https://doi.org/10.1002/14651858.CD002971.pub3.
28. Preterm birth: causes, consequences, and prevention. In: Behrman RE, Butler AS, editors. Institute of medicine (US) committee on understanding premature birth and assuring healthy outcomes. 12, societal costs of preterm birth. Washington (DC): National Academies Press (US); 2007. Available at: http://www.ncbi.nlm.nih.gov/books/NBK11358/. Accessed on 9 June 2022.
29. Serban N, Harati PM, Elizondo JMM, et al. An economic analysis of intensive multidisciplinary interventions for treating Medicaid-insured children with pediatric feeding disorders. Med Decis Making 2020;40(5):596–605.

# Using Telemedicine to Overcome Barriers to Neurodevelopmental Care from the Neonatal Intensive Care Unit to School Entry

Darrah N. Haffner, MD, MHS[a],*, Sarah L. Bauer Huang, MD, PhD[b]

## KEYWORDS

- Neurodevelopment • NICU follow-up • Early intervention • Telemedicine
- Prematurity

## KEY POINTS

- Neonatal Intensive Care Unit follow-up programs are recommended for infants at high risk for neurodevelopmental impairment via a multidisciplinary care clinic, or alternatively by a pediatrician and subspecialist providers.
- Telemedicine may facilitate standardization of evaluations, increased referral rates, and reduced follow-up time, ultimately leading earlier diagnosis and timely access to intervention.
- Although telemedicine can help reduce barriers to care, increasing telemedicine access during the COVID-19 pandemic has shed light on additional obstacles. More attention is needed to address appropriate access to technology and sufficient Internet speed, concerns about data security, and the potential negative impact on the provider–caregiver relationship.

## INTRODUCTION

The American Academy of Pediatrics (AAP) Committee on the Fetus and Newborn recommends referral of all high-risk infants to follow up programs after discharge.[1] High-risk infants include those that are preterm, have special health care needs, or are technology-dependent, at risk because of family issues, or anticipated early death.

Disclosure: The authors have nothing to disclose.
[a] Division of Pediatric Neurology, Department of Pediatrics, Nationwide Children's Hospital and the Ohio State University, 700 Children's Dr, Columbus, OH 43205, USA; [b] Department of Pediatric and Developmental Neurology, Department of Neurology, Washington University in Saint Louis School of Medicine, 660 S. Euclid Avenue, St. Louis, MO 63110, USA
* Corresponding author.
E-mail address: darrah.haffner@nationwidechildrens.org

Clin Perinatol 50 (2023) 253–268
https://doi.org/10.1016/j.clp.2022.10.006
0095-5108/23/© 2022 Elsevier Inc. All rights reserved.

This group also includes other high-risk populations such as children with congenital heart disease, history of extracorporeal membrane oxygenation (ECMO), and hypoxic ischemic encephalopathy (HIE). Preterm infants are at high risk for cognitive impairment, motor disabilities including cerebral palsy (CP), attention-deficit hyperactivity disorder (ADHD), autism spectrum disorder (ASD), and other neurodevelopmental disabilities.[2]

The AAPs statement recognizes that although a multidisciplinary care clinic may be the least cumbersome option for follow-up, additional follow-up can be provided by the pediatrician, medical subspecialist, or additional clinical providers.[1] Although infants receive standard developmental screening during their routine primary care, these screenings may miss subtle findings, especially in cognition and communication.[3] High risk infant follow up (HRIF) programs are in the position to provide detailed assessments leading to timely referral to early intervention (EI) services.[4] HRIF clinics are also designed to optimize the overall health of Neonatal Intensive Care Unit (NICU) graduates, managing common problems including feeding and respiratory issues.

There are many barriers to continued neurodevelopmental follow-up after NICU discharge. For many infants and their families, transporting the child to clinic with equipment needs such as ventilators, supplemental oxygen, feeding equipment, and monitors limits ability to travel for follow-up. Socioeconomic and psychosocial factors also play a large role. Socioeconomic factors include distance from clinic, transportation, and need to work. Psychosocial factors associated with reduced follow-up include parental substance use as well as psychological distress related to the neonatal course.[5–7]

Telemedicine is not a new concept to neonatal care.[8,9] However, until the recent COVID-19 pandemic, telemedicine was not widely used after NICU discharge. The pandemic magnified the need for flexibility in HRIF and to rethink the delivery of developmental care.[10] In a 2021 survey of NICUs in the Vermont Oxford Network, 69% of programs altered their capacity and 65.5% altered the timing, frequency, or content of their assessments during the pandemic.[11] Fourteen percent of programs used telemedicine pre-pandemic and seventy-six percent during the pandemic. Providers reported decreased financial and transportation barriers and increased family-centeredness with a "home-visiting" quality. Sixty-two percent of the programs reported they would continue to offer telemedicine visits after in-person visits could resume.[11]

This review focuses on the major barriers to long-term neurodevelopmental care from discharge to school transition and recent innovations, with an emphasis on telemedicine, designed to ameliorate them (**Fig. 1**).

## NEONATAL INTENSIVE CARE UNIT DISCHARGE
### Identification of Patients

The first barrier to post-NICU neurodevelopmental care occurs before NICU discharge, with the identification and referral to the HRIF. Extensive literature demonstrates disparity in the referral process where infants of Black and Hispanic mothers were less likely to be referred and less likely to follow up.[12–14] In California, due to the disparate referral rates, an initiative to increase referral rates was implemented via a Web-based referral system to match referrals with NICU discharge records. Very low birthweight (VLBW) infants as well as those with moderate to severe HIE and history of ECMO cannulation were included. Although this process increased the referral rates, VLBW infants of African American race were still noted to have lower odds of referral post-implementation. This may be related to differential access to high-quality care.[15]

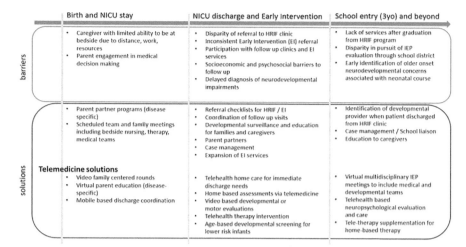

**Fig. 1.** Barriers and telemedicine solutions to neurodevelopmental care from NICU discharge to school transition.

## Transition Plan from Neonatal Intensive Care Unit to Home-Based Care Starts Before Discharge

For those that are referred to an HRIF, a family-focused approach on the transition from the NICU to the outpatient care center has become standard. This transition starts early and many programs use a multidisciplinary approach, including a discharge coordinator, the medical team including the outpatient pediatrician,[16] therapy services,[17] and social work[18–20] (**Fig. 2**). The nurse (bedside and outpatient) helps with supportive and collaborative care at discharge and is the closest with the family to

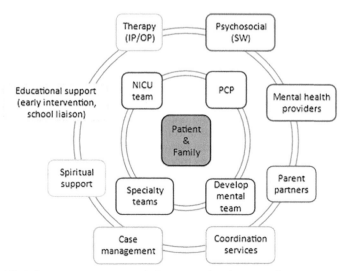

**Fig. 2.** Multidisciplinary support to optimize neurodevelopmental outcomes of high-risk NICU graduates.

reinforce the importance of developmental monitoring for this high-risk group.[21] Psychology and therapy services support the psychosocial and mental health of families, especially given the anxiety surrounding the transition home.[22]

Telemedicine can facilitate the communication and coordination of high-risk infants in the NICU, reducing the need for NICU to hospital transfer before discharge home.[23] In a qualitative study of parents of medically complex NICU graduates, parents supported the use of mobile health technologies in the planning and discharge process, including video chats, health portals, online resources, and a hotline.[24] Parents overall seem accepting of eHealth interventions while still in the NICU and beyond.[25]

### Time to First Follow-Up Appointment

The time frame between discharge and initial follow visit varies widely between programs, ranging from 2 weeks postdischarge, more commonly 3 months, and even up to 12 months corrected age for some infants. Virtual visits post-NICU discharge can help bridge this gap. The use of telehealth-based care for immediate postdischarge care has been used successfully for homecare,[26] lactation support,[27] and feeding.[28] In addition, the standardization of milestone-based telemedicine development screening to allow early diagnosis of developmental concerns may provide an option for families unable to return for multidisciplinary evaluation.

## NEURODEVELOPMENTAL CARE IN THE HRIF
### Diagnosis and Developmental Assessments

Early detection of developmental delays and diagnosis of neurologic conditions such as CP facilitates EI to maximize developmental outcome and prevents associated complications for a wide range of developmental disabilities. CP or "high risk of CP" can reliably be diagnosed before 6 months corrected age.[29] Half of infants with CP have newborn detectable risks,[29,30] many of whom are followed within HRIF. Families report that they prefer earlier diagnosis to facilitate their infants' development, and that early diagnosis fosters acceptance and increased confidence in the medical team.[31,32] Early diagnosis also leads to diagnostic-specific interventions and greater motor and cognitive gains.[29,33,34] These same principles apply to other neurodevelopmental disorders including ASD, cognitive delays, and hearing impairment,[35–37] all of which have increased prevalence in HRIF populations compared with the general public.[2,38,39]

The AAP recommends developmental surveillance at all health supervision settings and the use of standardized screening tests at specific visits through early childhood within the child's medical home.[40] The HRIF provides additional developmental screening and developmental testing for higher risk infants and children. There are, however, many barriers to timely and ongoing care through the HRIF. Telemedicine can provide an important supplement to the services that in-person HRIFs provide. Before the COVID-19 pandemic, most telemedicine visits for NICU follow were related to the infant's medical needs such as monitoring growth, respiratory status, and surgical complications.[41] Multiple studies support that telemedicine visits reduce the need for hospital visits in high-risk infants.[23,42] A group from Boston Children's Hospital took a tiered approach with initial health and developmental history via email to screen those infants at highest risk to triage those that needed in person evaluations.[43]

Within the HRIF community, there has been significant concern for the quality of the assessments performed over telemedicine and subsequent recommendations and referrals.[11] The biggest concerns centered on the inability to obtain adequate assessments and the availability of technology.[11] Maitre and colleagues reported on providers' perspectives on telehealth assessments in a large HRIF. More than 90%

of respondents agreed or strongly agreed that the procedures were valuable and easy to use. There were similar rates of CP and high risk for CP diagnoses in both telehealth and matched cohorts.[44] Providers were positive about ease of use and value.

Examples of assessment tools that have transitioned well to telehealth platforms are the General Movement's Assessment (GMA) and the gross motor assessment tool Alberta Infant Motor Scale (AIMS). The GMA is based on the Prechtl's Method of the Qualitative Assessment of General Movements and estimates the integrity of the infant nervous system by observing the quality of spontaneous movement patterns.[45] General movements evolve at specific time points over the first months of life; aberrant movement patterns are reliable early predictors of subsequent neurodevelopmental impairment (NDI).[46–48] *Baby Moves* is a smartphone application (app), which allows parents to record videos of their infants' movement and securely transmit the clips to trained clinicians for remote GMA performance.[49,50] Although overall quality of uploaded videos was adequate for GMA, lower maternal education, limited English proficiency, and government income support were associated with unscorable videos.[49] Most parents responded positively to the program, but parents of extremely preterm infants were more likely to prefer face-to-face assessments and feel worried while using the app, with increasing concerns of their infant's development. A multi-center Norwegian trial supported the feasibility of parents using the *In-Motion App* to acquire videos for the GMA.[51] Future work is anticipated on using these videos with automated body point software to analyze the GMA. Contrary to the previous work, 90% of families did not become more worried about their child's development while using the *In-Motion app*.[51] Similar parental satisfaction, video quality and reliability have been reported for the *NeuroMotion* app.[52] The AIMS is a norm-referenced tool to assess gross motor performance in infants' ages 0 to 18 months.[53] Although the AIMS does not have a high predictive value for future neurodevelopment in preterm infants,[54,55] it is helpful in identifying infants with current motor concerns.[56] The AIMS has been validated to be applied and scored by video in healthy infants with high parental satisfaction.[57,58]

Not all developmental assessment tools such as the Bayley Scales of Infant Development have been validated for telehealth administration. The ongoing surveillance of behavior and social emotional development is important for the preterm infant, who has high rates of ADHD, ASD, anxiety, and other neurobehavioral problems.[2] Many screening tools are standardized caregiver questionnaires, such as the Infant Toddler Social Emotional Assessment and the Child Behavior Checklist, so can be administered via telehealth or completed independently. There is also a growing body of literature supporting virtual autism evaluations and other more general developmental assessments even pre-pandemic.[59] Although the Autism Diagnostic Observation Scale, the gold standard for ASD diagnosis, has not been validated for telehealth administration, many tools have been adapted or created to be used by telemedicine during the COVID-19 pandemic.[60–64] Most parents were comfortable with the telehealth assessment and appreciated the parent-led format.[65]

Telemedicine provides a unique opportunity for observation of the child in their home environment. During traditional clinic developmental assessments in the clinic, parents report that children are performing skills at home that they do not demonstrate in clinic. In the home environment, the child is likely more comfortable and not encumbered by the clinical environment, including the possible need for personal protective equipment. In telerehabilitation programs, the neurodevelopmental therapist can help parents create a play environment enriched with age-appropriate toys and child-specific advice on home play activities, allowing parents to be more involved in child observation and promoting parenting skills in the home environment.[66,67]

Telemedicine can provide developmental support to poorly resourced areas. Almost 60% of HRIF providers believed that telemedicine increased accessibility to families who might not otherwise be able to participate and reported plans to continue telemedicine after the liberalization of in-person visits.[11] Now that health care has resumed a more normal pace, it will be important to assess how telemedicine continues to be used in HRIF.

### Early Intervention and Therapy Services

EI improves the neurodevelopmental outcomes for high-risk infants, including cognitive outcomes[68] as well as motor outcomes and CP.[29,68,69] The AAP recommends prompt EI referrals for all children at increased risk for developmental delay.[70] Part C EI programs are federally mandated through the Individuals with Disabilities Education Improvement Act to coordinate care and services across the community for children under 3 years of age with developmental delay.[71] Each state establishes the qualifying diagnoses and degree of developmental delay to determine eligibility.[72,73] EI programs have long been shown to improve outcomes across developmental domains including communication, socio-emotional and cognitive skills.[72] There are also considerable psychosocial benefits to the families of children with developmental delays including more comfort in caring for their medically and developmentally complex children, better advocate skills and ability to access other community supports.[72]

There has, however, been a chronic under-enrollment in Part C EI. In one large scale observational cohort (broadly representative of all children in the United States), only 10% of children with developmental delays were receiving EI services at 24 months of age. Infants within the NICU and HRIF setting are already known to the medical system yet continue to be underserved through EI. Less than one-third of low-birth weight infants were enrolled in EI at their first HRIF visit, despite more than 40% of these infants having an automatic qualifying medical diagnosis.[74] The most vulnerable infants (eg, severe developmental delays on standardized testing and longer NICU stays) were more likely to be enrolled.[74]

In general, early intervention/Part C services disproportionately serve white middle and upper-income families.[75] Black children are two to eight times less likely to be referred to services.[71,75–77] Decreased enrollment is also associated with gender, poverty, and lack of health insurance.[71,78] Decreased participation in follow-up is associated with single parenting status, distance to services, and maternal substance use.[6] Compounding these barriers, states with stricter EI requirements have less children receiving services,[78,79] which impact the children with the most severe functional impairments.[79] It is estimated that less than 25% of eligible children may be receiving services.[80]

Given this discrepancy in need and available services, Part C EI programs have long been exploring the use of telehealth to supplement their traditional programs. Telehealth occupational, physical, and speech therapy have all been reported as beneficial and reasonable supplements or alternatives to in-person services.[81,82] Cason reported telehealth EI programs have high parent satisfaction, are cost-effective, and can help compensate for staffing shortages.[83,84] In 2012, nine states used telehealth as part of their Part C early intervention programs.[80] With the COVID-19 pandemic, the use of telerehabilitation services has expanded with benefits including flexibility in scheduling, reduction in time between identification of developmental concern and initiation of services, lowering COVID-19 exposure to high-risk children.[85] A recent systematic review found that telerehabilitation using an applied coaching approach may improve level of functioning in children with disability, including mobility, hand use, and anxiety level.[85]

In infants at high risk for CP, telerehabilitation based on a goal-directed, parent-coaching model has shown clinically significant improvements in GMFM-88 and increase in AIMS percentile by the end of the program.[86] Adherence was high (90%) and costs were low. Caregivers recorded videos for GMA and were guided through the AIMS and portions of the Hammersmith Infant Neurologic Examination and GMFM. Caregivers believed that instructions were easy to understand and replicate the commands; assessors similarly believed that the videos were easy to score.[86] Therapy interventions, such as constraint-induced movement therapy, can be conducted via telehealth for asymmetrical cerebral CP.[87]

Beyond the traditional physical, occupational, and speech therapy, telehealth interventions have been used in a wide array of therapeutic modalities including telehealth ASD-specific therapies. A 2017 and 2020 systematic review demonstrated that telehealth guided parent-mediated intervention training improves social behavior and communication skills.[88,89] The intervention may also improve parent knowledge and increase parent intervention fidelity. Programs targeting parents, via a coaching approach, improved behavioral functioning.[85]

### Neurodevelopmental care post-early intervention

The transition from EI to school-based support at 3 years of age is a time that requires team coordination and oversight to ensure a child does not lose appropriate support. Most EI programs have an individualized transition plan and help guide families through this process. In populations with specific needs, such as those with autism, there is a benefit of a disease-specific school transition plan to improve this transition.[90] Telehealth and digital education could be used to aid in this process, for example, by facilitating medical team involvement in IEP meetings, collaboration with therapy and developmental providers in initiating appropriate therapy and equipment support.[91] School-based therapy support during COVID-19 varied, including telehealth, in person, telephone, send-home assignments or some patients not receiving therapy who previously had. The transition to home-based education, the addition of telehealth-based therapy services was associated with a higher satisfaction of therapy services in general.

In addition to patients with identified neurodevelopmental disability at school entry, early childhood,[92] and elementary school are also times when additional concerns arise in our high-risk populations, including attention, learning differences, and other behavioral concerns.[93,94] Surveillance programs have been recommended for certain at-risk populations, such as congenital heart disease, to ensure reevaluation at these timepoints.[95] The involvement of the multidisciplinary team, including the family, primary medical provider, the school, and the developmental team is essential in identifying these concerns.[96]

## SPECIAL POPULATIONS

Other at-risk neonates that may benefit from expanded neurodevelopment monitoring can be provided by telemedicine/virtual care. For example, moderate and late preterm infants are at an increased risk of developmental delay compared with term-equivalent infants.[97] Telemedicine programming allows for follow-up support for late preterm infants[98] as well as those in a high-risk social situation, including infants with neonatal abstinence syndrome[99] and in utero substance exposure.[100]

Infants with anticipated early death could be supported at home with a combination of face-to-face and telehealth support. Research has been supportive of home-based care in pediatric palliative care, suggesting telemedicine consultations in combination of other multidisciplinary support programs are effective.[101] However, the literature regarding end of life in the care of infants and the use of telemedicine is limited.

## BARRIERS TO TELEMEDICINE ACCESS

Barriers to telemedicine identified before the COVID-19-related expansion included reimbursement and infrastructure barriers.[102] With COVID-19, federal, state, and commercial payer waivers allowed coverage and reimbursement of telehealth services to a degree not seen previously. Some states allowed out-of-state clinicians to provide services to a patient, but this was the minority of states. With the anticipated loss of COVID expansion, there are concerns that interstate telehealth visits will not be reimbursed due to state licensing changes or not reimbursed at the same level as was seen during the public health emergency (PHE) status. Solutions to these concerns include the adoption of multistate licensure agreement and establishing the PHE waivers as permanent.[103]

Additional patient barriers include access to technology, equipment, Internet data or speed necessary to support video-based visits. Ninety percent of low-income parents reported having access to a computer or device, but a significant fraction had too slow connections, frequently exceeded data limits or had services shut off because of difficulty paying bills. Even with access to the appropriate technology, specific considerations are required for a successful telehealth visit.[104] For example, with certain evaluations (such as developmental or behavioral assessment of autistic children), the location, environment, and position of the child is important in the assessment of their interactions.[105]

Although parental satisfaction has been reported regarding the use of telemedicine formats in the care of patients, family-specific concerns regarding the use of telemedicine persist. For example, patients have concerns regarding confidentiality, secure transmission, and data storage.[106–108] There exists perceived increased pressure on caregivers during the telehealth visit, complicated by difficulty accessing Internet, lack of technical support, low ability with the use of e-technologies.[109] Families with limited English proficiency or with hearing impairment require additional communication support.[103] Even without a language barrier, patients also report feeling less involved during the visit with difficulty in speaking up as well as the concern for establishing a therapeutic relationship.[110]

## SUMMARY

This review examines ongoing disparities in the neurodevelopmental support of the high-risk neonate through early childhood and highlights possibility of telemedicine/virtual care to increase access to some children by increasing referrals to HRIF programs, EI programming and facilitating transition to school-based therapy. Telehealth approaches may facilitate early diagnosis and ongoing surveillance of NDI with therapeutic management. Barriers to telehealth care as well as patient-specific concerns regarding virtual visits are reviewed.

## BEST PRACTICES

What is the current practice for the surveillance of NDI for high-risk infants?

NICU follow-up programs are recommended for infants at high risk for NDI, via a multidisciplinary care clinic, or alternatively by a pediatrician, or subspecialist providers.[1]

Before COVID-19, most telemedicine visits for high-risk infants were related to growth monitoring, respiratory, or surgical follow-up.[41]

Early intervention programs have been exploring the use of telehealth to supplement their programs.

Transitions between early intervention and school-based support are coordinated through an IEP evaluation process, which now may include team member participation virtually.[91]

Best Practice/Guideline/Care Path Objective(s):

What changes in current practice are likely to improve outcomes?

Telemedicine may facilitate standardization of evaluations, increased referral rates, and reduced follow-up time.

Standardization of developmental evaluations and motor assessments can lead to diagnosis that benefit from earlier interventions to improve motor and cognitive outcomes.

Increasing surveillance of lower risk infants through telehealth will help identify patients earlier that would benefit from evaluation and intervention.

Pearls/Pitfalls at the Point of Care:

Although telemedicine can help reduce barriers to care, additional obstacles have arisen as increasing telemedicine use during COVID-19, including

1. lack of appropriate technology
2. lack of necessary data/Internet speed
3. concerns about data security
4. impacts on the provider–caregiver relationship
5. state and insurance-based regulatory limitations regarding the requirements for telemedicine

## MAJOR RECOMMENDATIONS

1. Telemedicine can be used predischarge to help facilitate the coordination of high-risk infants before discharge home.[23]
2. For families with financial, transportation barriers, consider use of telemedicine to help reduce barriers to follow up.[11]
3. Supplement in-person developmental assessments with telehealth platforms to allow early diagnosis of neurodevelopmental disorders (eg, CP, ASD) that benefit from early intervention.
4. Telehealth interventions can be used to supplement traditional early intervention services or provide disorder-specific therapies that are not available locally.[88]
5. Facilitate involvement of medical specialist at therapy transition meetings via video conferencing.[91]
6. Consider telehealth surveillance of lower risk infants of NDI who may not qualify for traditional HRIF clinics.

## BIBLIOGRAPHIC SOURCE(S)

1. Hospital discharge of the high-risk neonate. Pediatrics 2008;122:1119-1126.

2. Litt JS, Mercier CE, Edwards EM, Morrow K, Soll R. Follow-through care for high-risk infants during the COVID-19 pandemic: lessons learned from the Vermont Oxford Network. Journal of perinatology: official journal of the California Perinatal Association 2021;41:2625-2630.

3. Gray JE, Safran C, Davis RB, et al. Baby CareLink: using the internet and telemedicine to improve care for high-risk infants. Pediatrics 2000;106:1318-1324.

4. Willard A, Brown E, Masten M, et al. Complex Surgical Infants Benefit From Post-discharge Telemedicine Visits. Adv Neonatal Care 2018;18:22-30.

5. Parsons D, Cordier R, Vaz S, Lee HC. Parent-Mediated Intervention Training Delivered Remotely for Children With Autism Spectrum Disorder Living Outside of Urban Areas: Systematic Review. J Med Internet Res 2017;19:e198.

6. Murphy A, Pinkerton LM, Bruckner E, Risser HJ. The Impact of the Novel Coronavirus Disease 2019 on Therapy Service Delivery for Children with Disabilities. The Journal of pediatrics 2021;231:168-177.e161.

## REFERENCES

1. Hospital discharge of the high-risk neonate. Pediatrics 2008;122:1119–26.

2. Hirschberger RG, Kuban KCK, O'Shea TM, et al. Co-occurrence and Severity of neurodevelopmental Burden (cognitive impairment, cerebral palsy, autism spectrum disorder, and Epilepsy) at age ten Years in children born extremely preterm. Pediatr Neurol 2018;79:45–52.

3. Wong HS, Cowan FM, Modi N. Validity of neurodevelopmental outcomes of children born very preterm assessed during routine clinical follow-up in England. Arch Dis Child - Fetal Neonatal Edition 2018;103:F479.

4. Greene M, Patra K. Part C early intervention utilization in preterm infants: opportunity for referral from a NICU follow-up clinic. Res Dev disabilities 2016;53-54:287–95.

5. Ballantyne M, Stevens B, Guttmann A, et al. Transition to neonatal follow-up programs: is attendance a problem? J Perinat Neonatal Nurs 2012;26:90–8.

6. Ballantyne M, Stevens B, Guttmann A, et al. Maternal and infant predictors of attendance at Neonatal Follow-Up programmes. Child Care Health Dev 2014;40:250–8.

7. Brady JM, Pouppirt N, Bernbaum J, et al. Why do children with severe bronchopulmonary dysplasia not attend neonatal follow-up care? Parental views of barriers. Acta Paediatr (Oslo, Norway : 1992 2018;107:996–1002.

8. Wenger TL, Gerdes J, Taub K, et al. Telemedicine for genetic and neurologic evaluation in the neonatal intensive care unit. J perinatology : official J Calif Perinatal Assoc 2014;34:234–40.

9. Simkin SK, Misra SL, Han JV, et al. Auckland regional telemedicine retinopathy of prematurity screening network: a 10-year review. Clin Exp Ophthalmol 2019;47:1122–30.

10. DeMauro SB, Duncan AF, Hurt H. Telemedicine use in neonatal follow-up programs - what can we do and what we can't - lessons learned from COVID-19. Semin Perinatol 2021;45:151430.

11. Litt JS, Mercier CE, Edwards EM, et al. Follow-through care for high-risk infants during the COVID-19 pandemic: lessons learned from the Vermont Oxford Network. J perinatology : official J Calif Perinatal Assoc 2021;41:2625–30.

12. Litt JS, Edwards EM, Lainwala S, et al. Optimizing high-risk infant follow-up in Nonresearch-based Paradigms: the new England follow-up network. Pediatr Qual Saf 2020;5:e287.

13. Hintz SR, Gould JB, Bennett MV, et al. Referral of very low birth weight infants to high-risk follow-up at neonatal intensive care unit discharge varies widely across California. The J Pediatr 2015;166:289–95.

14. Hintz SR, Gould JB, Bennett MV, et al. Factors associated with successful first high-risk infant clinic visit for very low birth weight infants in California. The J Pediatr 2019;210:91–8, e91.

15. Pai VV, Kan P, Bennett M, et al. Improved referral of very low birthweight infants to high-risk infant follow-up in California. The J Pediatr 2020;216:101–8, e101.
16. Connors J, Havranek T, Campbell D. Discharge of medically complex infants and developmental follow-up. Pediatr Rev 2021;42:316–28.
17. Nwabara O, Rogers C, Inder T, et al. Early therapy services following neonatal intensive care Unit discharge. Phys Occup Ther Pediatr 2017;37:414–24.
18. Hynan MT, Steinberg Z, Baker L, et al. Recommendations for mental health professionals in the NICU. J perinatology : official J Calif Perinatal Assoc 2015; 35(Suppl 1):S14–8.
19. Sharp CG. Use of the chaplaincy in the neonatal intensive care unit. South Med J 1991;84:1482–6.
20. Hummel P, Cronin J. Home care of the high-risk infant. Adv Neonatal Care 2004; 4:354–64.
21. Bondurant PG, Brinkman KS. Developmentally supportive care in the newborn intensive care unit: early intervention in the community. Nurs Clin North Am 2003;38:253–69.
22. Purdy IB, Craig JW, Zeanah P. NICU discharge planning and beyond: recommendations for parent psychosocial support. J perinatology : official J Calif Perinatal Assoc 2015;35(Suppl 1):S24–8.
23. Gray JE, Safran C, Davis RB, et al. Baby CareLink: using the internet and telemedicine to improve care for high-risk infants. Pediatrics 2000;106:1318–24.
24. Lakshmanan A, Kubicek K, Williams R, et al. Viewpoints from families for improving transition from NICU-to-home for infants with medical complexity at a safety net hospital: a qualitative study. BMC Pediatr 2019;19:223.
25. Dol J, Delahunty-Pike A, Anwar Siani S, et al. eHealth interventions for parents in neonatal intensive care units: a systematic review. JBI Database Syst Rev Implement Rep 2017;15:2981–3005.
26. Garne Holm K, Brødsgaard A, Zachariassen G, et al. Parent perspectives of neonatal tele-homecare: a qualitative study. J Telemed Telecare 2019;25:221–9.
27. Demirci J, Kotzias V, Bogen DL, et al. Telelactation via mobile app: perspectives of rural mothers, their care providers, and lactation Consultants. Telemed J E Health 2019;25:853–8.
28. Rasmussen MK, Clemensen J, Zachariassen G, et al. Cost analysis of neonatal tele-homecare for preterm infants compared to hospital-based care. J Telemed Telecare 2020;26:474–81.
29. Novak I, Morgan C, Adde L, et al. Early, Accurate diagnosis and early intervention in cerebral palsy: Advances in diagnosis and Treatment. JAMA Pediatr 2017;171:897–907.
30. McIntyre S, Morgan C, Walker K, et al. Cerebral palsy–don't delay. Dev Disabil Res Rev 2011;17:114–29.
31. Baird G, McConachie H, Scrutton D. Parents' perceptions of disclosure of the diagnosis of cerebral palsy. Arch Dis Child 2000;83:475–80.
32. Rentinck IC, Ketelaar M, Schuengel C, et al. Short-term changes in parents' resolution regarding their young child's diagnosis of cerebral palsy. Child Care Health Dev 2010;36:703–8.
33. Martin JH, Chakrabarty S, Friel KM. Harnessing activity-dependent plasticity to repair the damaged corticospinal tract in an animal model of cerebral palsy. Developmental Med child Neurol 2011;53(Suppl 4):9–13.
34. Eyre J. 2 - corticospinal tract development and activity-dependent plasticity. In: Shepherd RB, editor. Cerebral palsy in infancy. Oxford: Churchill Livingstone; 2014. p. 53–70.

35. Dawson G, Jones EJH, Merkle K, et al. Early behavioral intervention is associated with normalized brain activity in young children with autism. J Am Acad Child Adolesc Psychiatry 2012;51:1150–9.

36. Dawson G, Rogers S, Munson J, et al. Randomized, controlled trial of an intervention for toddlers with autism: the Early Start Denver Model. Pediatrics 2010; 125:e17–23.

37. Spittle AJ, Anderson PJ, Tapawan SJ, et al. Early developmental screening and intervention for high-risk neonates - from research to clinical benefits. Semin Fetal neonatal Med 2021;26:101203.

38. Joseph RM, O'Shea TM, Allred EN, et al. Prevalence and associated features of autism spectrum disorder in extremely low gestational age newborns at age 10 years. Autism Res : official J Int Soc Autism Res 2017;10:224–32.

39. Joseph RM, O'Shea TM, Allred EN, et al. Neurocognitive and Academic outcomes at age 10 Years of extremely preterm newborns. Pediatrics 2016;137.

40. Lipkin PH, Macias MM. Promoting optimal development: identifying infants and young children with developmental disorders through developmental surveillance and screening. Pediatrics 2020;145:e20193449.

41. Willard A, Brown E, Masten M, et al. Complex surgical infants benefit from Post-discharge telemedicine visits. Adv Neonatal Care 2018;18:22–30.

42. Robinson C, Gund A, Sjöqvist BA, et al. Using telemedicine in the care of newborn infants after discharge from a neonatal intensive care unit reduced the need of hospital visits. Acta Paediatr (Oslo, Norway : 1992 2016;105:902–9.

43. Litt JS, Agni M, Jacobi-Polishook T, et al. The acceptability and feasibility of emailed parent questionnaires for medical and developmental surveillance after NICU discharge. J Perinatology 2018;38:392–401.

44. Maitre NL, Benninger KL, Neel ML, et al. Standardized neurodevelopmental surveillance of high-risk infants using telehealth: Implementation study during COVID-19. Pediatr Qual Saf 2021;6.

45. Prechtl HFR, Einspieler C, Cioni G. An early marker of developing neurological handicap after perinatal brain lesions. Lancet (London, England) 1997;339:1361–3.

46. Prechtl HF, Einspieler C, Cioni G, et al. An early marker for neurological deficits after perinatal brain lesions. Lancet (London, England) 1997;349:1361–3.

47. Einspieler C, Marschik PB, Pansy J, et al. The general movement optimality score: a detailed assessment of general movements during preterm and term age. Developmental Med child Neurol 2016;58:361–8.

48. Darsaklis V, Snider LM, Majnemer A, et al. Predictive validity of Prechtl's method on the qualitative assessment of general movements: a systematic review of the evidence. Developmental Med child Neurol 2011;53:896–906.

49. Kwong AK, Eeles AL, Olsen JE, et al. The Baby Moves smartphone app for General Movements Assessment: Engagement amongst extremely preterm and term-born infants in a state-wide geographical study. J Paediatr Child Health 2019;55:548–54.

50. Spittle AJ, Olsen J, Kwong A, et al. The Baby Moves prospective cohort study protocol: using a smartphone application with the General Movements Assessment to predict neurodevelopmental outcomes at age 2 years for extremely preterm or extremely low birthweight infants. BMJ Open 2016;6:e013446.

51. Adde L, Brown A, van den Broeck C, et al. In-Motion-App for remote General Movement Assessment: a multi-site observational study. BMJ Open 2021;11: e042147.

52. Svensson KA, Örtqvist M, Bos AF, et al. Usability and inter-rater reliability of the NeuroMotion app: a tool in general movements assessments. Eur J Paediatric Neurol 2021;33:29–35.

53. Piper MC, Pinnell LE, Darrah J, et al. Construction and validation of the Alberta infant motor scale (AIMS). Can J Public Health 1992;83(Suppl 2):S46–50.

54. Lefebvre F, Gagnon M-M, Luu TM, et al. In extremely preterm infants, do the movement assessment of infants and the Alberta infant motor scale predict 18-month outcomes using the Bayley-III? Early Hum Dev 2016;94:13–7.

55. de Albuquerque PL, Lemos A, Guerra MQ, et al. Accuracy of the Alberta Infant Motor Scale (AIMS) to detect developmental delay of gross motor skills in pre-term infants: a systematic review. Dev Neurorehabil 2015;18:15–21.

56. Darrah J, Piper M, Watt MJ. Assessment of gross motor skills of at-risk infants: predictive validity of the Alberta Infant Motor Scale. Developmental Med child Neurol 1998;40:485–91.

57. Boonzaaijer M, van Dam E, van Haastert IC, et al. Concurrent validity between live and home video observations using the Alberta infant motor scale. Pediatr Phys Ther : official Publ Section Pediatr Am Phys Ther Assoc 2017;29:146–51.

58. Boonzaaijer M, van Wesel F, Nuysink J, et al. A home-video method to assess infant gross motor development: parent perspectives on feasibility. BMC Pediatr 2019;19:392.

59. Juárez AP, Weitlauf AS, Nicholson A, et al. Early identification of ASD through telemedicine: potential value for underserved populations. J autism Dev Disord 2018;48:2601–10.

60. Holtman SJ, Winans KS, Hoch JD. Utility of diagnostic Classification for children 0-5 to assess features of autism: Comparing in-person and COVID-19 telehealth evaluations. J autism Dev Disord 2022;1–12.

61. Stavropoulos KK, Bolourian Y, Blacher J. A scoping review of telehealth diagnosis of autism spectrum disorder. PloS one 2022;17:e0263062.

62. Dow D, Holbrook A, Toolan C, et al. The Brief observation of Symptoms of autism (BOSA): development of a new adapted assessment Measure for remote telehealth administration through COVID-19 and beyond. J autism Dev Disord 2021;52(12):5383–94.

63. Wagner L, Corona LL, Weitlauf AS, et al. Use of the TELE-ASD-PEDS for autism evaluations in Response to COVID-19: Preliminary outcomes and clinician acceptability. J autism Dev Disord 2021;51:3063–72.

64. Talbott MR, Dufek S, Zwaigenbaum L, et al. Brief report: Preliminary feasibility of the TEDI: a Novel parent-administered telehealth assessment for autism spectrum disorder Symptoms in the first Year of life. J autism Dev Disord 2020;50:3432–9.

65. Corona LL, Weitlauf AS, Hine J, et al. Parent perceptions of caregiver-mediated telemedicine tools for assessing autism risk in toddlers. J autism Dev Disord 2021;51:476–86.

66. Caporali C, Pisoni C, Naboni C, et al. Challenges and opportunities for early intervention and neurodevelopmental follow-up in preterm infants during the COVID-19 pandemic. Child Care, Health Development 2021;47:140–1.

67. Vilaseca R, Ferrer F, Rivero M, et al. Early intervention services during the COVID-19 pandemic in Spain: toward a model of family-centered practices. Front Psychol 2021;12:738463.

68. Spittle A, Orton J, Anderson PJ, et al. Early developmental intervention programmes provided post hospital discharge to prevent motor and cognitive

impairment in preterm infants. Cochrane Database Syst Rev 2015;2015: CD005495.

69. Spittle A, Treyvaud K. The role of early developmental intervention to influence neurobehavioral outcomes of children born preterm. Semin Perinatol 2016;40: 542–8.

70. Duby JC. Role of the medical home in family-centered early intervention services. Pediatrics 2007;120:1153–8.

71. Rosenberg SA, Zhang D, Robinson CC. Prevalence of developmental delays and participation in early intervention services for young children. Pediatrics 2008;121:e1503–9.

72. Bailey DB Jr, Hebbeler K, Spiker D, et al. Thirty-six-month outcomes for families of children who have disabilities and participated in early intervention. Pediatrics 2005;116:1346–52.

73. Bailey DB Jr, Nelson L, Hebbeler K, et al. Modeling the impact of formal and informal supports for young children with disabilities and their families. Pediatrics 2007;120:e992–1001.

74. Atkins KL, Duvall SW, Dolata JK, et al. Part C early intervention enrollment in low birth weight infants at-risk for developmental delays. Matern Child Health J 2017;21:290–6.

75. Feinberg E, Silverstein M, Donahue S, et al. The impact of race on participation in part C early intervention services. J Dev Behav Pediatr : JDBP 2011;32: 284–91.

76. Wang CJ, Elliott MN, Rogowski J, et al. Factors influencing the enrollment of eligible extremely-low-birth-weight children in the part C early intervention program. Acad Pediatr 2009;9:283–7.

77. Barfield WD, Clements KM, Lee KG, et al. Using linked data to assess patterns of early intervention (EI) referral among very low birth weight infants. Matern Child Health J 2008;12:24–33.

78. McManus B, McCormick MC, Acevedo-Garcia D, et al. The effect of state early intervention eligibility policy on participation among a cohort of young CSHCN. Pediatrics 2009;124(Suppl 4):S368–74.

79. McManus BM, Magnusson D, Rosenberg S. Restricting state part C eligibility policy is associated with lower early intervention utilization. Matern Child Health J 2014;18:1031–7.

80. Cason J, Behl D, Ringwalt S. Overview of states' Use of telehealth for the delivery of early intervention (IDEA Part C) services. Int J Telerehabil 2012;4:39–46.

81. Heimerl S, Rasch N. Delivering developmental occupational therapy consultation services through telehealth. Developmental Disabilities Spec Interest Section Q 2009;32:1–4.

82. Kelso GL, Fiechtl BJ, Olsen ST, et al. The feasibility of virtual home visits to provide early intervention: a pilot study. Infants Young Child 2009;22:332–40.

83. Cason J. A pilot telerehabilitation program: delivering early intervention services to rural families. Int J Telerehabil 2009;1:29–38.

84. Cason J. Telerehabilitation: an adjunct service delivery model for early intervention services. Int J Telerehabil 2011;3:19–30.

85. Camden C, Pratte G, Fallon F, et al. Diversity of practices in telerehabilitation for children with disabilities and effective intervention characteristics: results from a systematic review. Disabil Rehabil 2020;42:3424–36.

86. Schlichting T, Martins da Silva K, Silva Moreira R, et al. Telehealth program for infants at risk of cerebral palsy during the Covid-19 pandemic: a pre-post feasibility Experimental study. Phys Occup Ther In Pediatr 2022;1–20.

87. Pietruszewski L, Burkhardt S, Yoder PJ, et al. Protocol and feasibility-Randomized trial of telehealth delivery for a Multicomponent upper Extremity intervention in infants with asymmetric cerebral palsy. Child Neurol Open 2020;7. 2329048x20946214.

88. Parsons D, Cordier R, Vaz S, et al. Parent-mediated intervention training delivered remotely for children with autism spectrum disorder Living outside of Urban Areas: systematic review. J Med Internet Res 2017;19:e198.

89. Unholz-Bowden E, McComas JJ, McMaster KL, et al. Caregiver training via telehealth on behavioral procedures: a systematic review. J Behav Education 2020; 29:246–81.

90. Fontil L, Sladeczek IE, Gittens J, et al. From early intervention to elementary school: a survey of transition support practices for children with autism spectrum disorders. Res Dev disabilities 2019;88:30–41.

91. Murphy A, Pinkerton LM, Bruckner E, et al. The impact of the Novel Coronavirus disease 2019 on therapy service delivery for children with disabilities. The J Pediatr 2021;231:168–77, e161.

92. Duncan AF, Matthews MA. Neurodevelopmental outcomes in early childhood. Clin perinatology 2018;45:377–92.

93. Franz AP, GU Bolat, Bolat H, et al. Attention-deficit/hyperactivity disorder and very preterm/very low birth weight: a Meta-analysis. Pediatrics 2018;141.

94. Pritchard VE, Clark CA, Liberty K, et al. Early school-based learning difficulties in children born very preterm. Early Hum Dev 2009;85:215–24.

95. Marino BS, Lipkin PH, Newburger JW, et al. Neurodevelopmental outcomes in children with congenital heart disease: evaluation and management: a scientific statement from the American Heart Association. Circulation 2012;126:1143–72.

96. Spencer T, Noyes E, Biederman J. Telemedicine in the management of ADHD: literature review of telemedicine in ADHD. J Atten Disord 2020;24:3–9.

97. Cheong JL, Doyle LW, Burnett AC, et al. Association between moderate and late preterm birth and neurodevelopment and social-emotional development at age 2 Years. JAMA Pediatr 2017;171:e164805.

98. Das A, Cina L, Mathew A, et al. Telemedicine, a tool for follow-up of infants discharged from the NICU? Experience from a pilot project. J perinatology : official J Calif Perinatal Assoc 2020;40:875–80.

99. MacMillan KDL. Neonatal Abstinence Syndrome: review of Epidemiology, care models, and current understanding of outcomes. Clin perinatology 2019;46: 817–32.

100. Austin AE, Berkoff MC, Shanahan ME. Incidence of Injury, Maltreatment, and developmental disorders among substance exposed infants. Child Maltreat 2021;26:282–90.

101. Bradford N, Armfield NR, Young J, et al. The case for home based telehealth in pediatric palliative care: a systematic review. BMC Palliat Care 2013;12:4.

102. Burke BL Jr, Hall RW. Telemedicine: pediatric applications. Pediatrics 2015;136: e293–308.

103. Curfman A, McSwain SD, Chuo J, et al. Pediatric telehealth in the COVID-19 pandemic Era and beyond. Pediatrics 2021;148.

104. Alkureishi MA, Choo ZY, Rahman A, et al. Digitally Disconnected: qualitative study of patient perspectives on the digital Divide and potential solutions. JMIR Hum Factors 2021;8:e33364.

105. Kryszak EM, Albright CM, Stephenson KG, et al. Preliminary validation and feasibility of the autism detection in early childhood-virtual (ADEC-V) for autism telehealth evaluations in a hospital setting. J autism Dev Disord 2022.

106. Charani E, Castro-Sánchez E, Moore LS, et al. Do smartphone applications in healthcare require a governance and legal framework? It depends on the application. BMC Med 2014;12:1–3.

107. Flaherty JL. Digital diagnosis: Privacy and the regulation of mobile Phone health applications. Am J L Med 2014;40:416–41.

108. Baig MM, GholamHosseini H, Connolly MJ. Mobile healthcare applications: system design review, critical issues and challenges. Australas Phys Eng Sci Med 2015;38:23–38.

109. Ben-Pazi H, Beni-Adani L, Lamdan R. Accelerating telemedicine for cerebral palsy during the COVID-19 pandemic and beyond. Front Neurol 2020;11:746.

110. Gordon HS, Solanki P, Bokhour BG, et al. I'm not feeling like I'm part of the Conversation" patients' perspectives on communicating in clinical video telehealth visits. J Gen Intern Med 2020;35:1751–8.

# Implementation of Early Detection and Intervention for Cerebral Palsy in High-Risk Infant Follow-Up Programs
## U.S. and Global Considerations

Nathalie L. Maitre, MD, PhD[a],*, Diane Damiano[b], Rachel Byrne[c]

## KEYWORDS

- Cerebral palsy • Infant • High risk • Follow-up • Neurodevelopment
- Implementation

## KEY POINTS

- Early detection and intervention for cerebral palsy is best practice for all infants at high-risk for neurodevelopmental delays and impairments.
- Implementation of international guidelines for early detection of Cerebral Palsy is feasible in high-risk infant follow-up programs across the world.
- Parents value the counseling, education and access to supports afforded by early detection of CP.
- Infants at high-risk or with CP benefit from implementation efforts in high-risk infant follow-up programs through access to targeted interventions and research in novel interventions starting earlier in life.

## BACKGROUND

Cerebral palsy (CP) is the most common physical disability across the lifespan, with more than 10,000 new infants being born annually with CP in the US and more than 400,000 in the world.[1,2] While some reports estimate a decreasing incidence of CP among preterm and low birthweight infants,[3–5] it is more likely that the profile of CP is shifting toward the less severe end of a spectrum, making diagnosis potentially challenging. Advances in prenatal (Magnesium sulfate, antenatal steroids)[6,7] and post-

The authors have nothing to disclose.

[a] Department of Pediatrics, Emory University School of Medicine, Children's Healthcare of Atlanta, Atlanta, GA, USA; [b] Rehabilitation Medicine Department, National Institutes of Health; [c] Cerebral Palsy Foundation, New York, NY, USA

* Corresponding author. 1123 Zonolite Rd Suite 22, Atlanta, GA 30306.
*E-mail address:* n.maitre@emory.edu

Clin Perinatol 50 (2023) 269–279
https://doi.org/10.1016/j.clp.2022.11.005
0095-5108/23/© 2022 Elsevier Inc. All rights reserved.

natal care (quality improvement practices to decrease severe intraventricular hemorrhage[8] may account for this change. In support, a large regional study of CP diagnosis with a systematic detection program instituted in 2016 showed rising incidence of CP with GMFCS I-III concomitant with decreasing incidence of GMFCS IV-V patients.[6] In reality, there may not be fewer children with CP, but instead some may be presenting in forms that are more easily confused with mild motor impairments or functional delays. Examples include toe-walking or other gait abnormalities with ankle cord tightness, or persistent balance, fine motor coordination and motor planning problems. These findings have been noted in several large neonatal networks across the world.[9–11] Historically, CP has not been diagnosed in the first year of life. Common misconceptions underlying this practice are that interventions will not change with an earlier diagnosis, and that the only treatments consist of referral to general or perhaps non-specific early intervention services. However, there is growing evidence and multiple reasons why diagnosing CP early is critical to optimizing the long-term trajectories of high-risk infants and families.

First, the consequences of having CP will last a lifetime: the concept of "outgrowing" CP has been disproven,[12,13] while the effects of maturation on CP manifestations have become more evident, especially at developmental stages when hormonal surges typically drive rapid bone and muscle growth.[13] For example, a toddler with CP and a fully functional and symmetric ambulation pattern can become a teenager with dysfunctional gait if scoliosis or leg length discrepancies manifest. Equally important, parents want information with honest conversations surrounding the diagnosis.[14] They favorably view early dialogue about risks of CP, even when certainty is lacking. Conversely, parental dissatisfaction, mistrust and anger with healthcare providers grows with the time elapsed between their suspicions and a physician directly addressing the concept of CP.[15] Research has also shown that parents have positive ways of coping with early diagnoses while they are more likely to experience adverse mental health issues when diagnosis is delayed.[15]

Finally, delaying CP diagnoses can result in missed opportunities for targeted, safe and effective interventions. A recent systematic review and international practice statement demonstrated a range of CP-specific interventions and other less specific interventions addressing co-morbidities of CP, all before the age of two.[16] Neuroplasticity and potential for recovery of function may be greatest in the first two to three years,[17,18] making early diagnosis central to the start of interventions when they have the highest likelihood of being successful and the greatest downstream effects.

While early diagnosis of CP might appear challenging due to the sometimes uncertain etiology or heterogeneity of clinical presentations,[19] medical decisions are facilitated by examining a comprehensive dataset of objective clinical variables.[20–22] This dataset includes a clinical history suspicious for disrupted neural development, neuroimaging findings consistent with perinatal lesions,[23] a comprehensive neurological exam, an assessment of motor function, biomarkers such as abnormal patterns on the General Movements Assessment (GMA)[24] or Hammersmith Infant Neurological Examination (HINE) scores below cut-offs for age,[25] and increasingly, genetic evaluation results. The diagnosis optimally occurs in a team where physicians assessing neurophysiology partner with therapists evaluating function, parents reporting on a child's abilities in daily life, and psychosocial health professionals assessing the family environments while supporting their emotional adjustment.[26] The role of the provider is then to synthesize and summarize diagnosis, parent goals and potential approaches to achieving an optimal developmental trajectory.

New systematic reviews and international guidelines provide a framework for early detection of CP,[27] summarizing the evidence into risk factors and tools for standardized assessments. Particularly relevant to high-risk infant follow-up programs, a class of "newborn attributable risks" such as prematurity, encephalopathy, neurological factors (intrauterine growth retardation, birth defects, stroke) and – most recently – intrauterine drug exposure,[28] are known to neonatology teams while infants are still hospitalized. These patients can then be directed toward surveillance pathways that may include some or all elements of best evidence evaluations for early CP detection.

Most follow-up programs see a spectrum of children, either due to state mandates, perinatal regionalization or due to the nature of their referring NICUs.[29] Patients meeting criteria for follow-up are the same as those transferred to Level 3 or level 4 NICUs, with the goal being easy access to high-level specialty care and improved perinatal outcomes. For more on this, an article in this issue addresses the types of patients and outcomes in follow-up programs. Currently, certification for NICU levels of care does not include follow-up,[29] but this is changing in 2023 with new checklists for certifying examiners, who will record the characteristics of follow-up referrals from NICUs during certification.[30]

Reflecting the complex and heterogeneous etiologies of CP, NICU graduates, whether they are born preterm, have congenital heart defects, intrauterine substance exposure or neural insults originating in the perinatal period, are all at increased risk for CP compared to the general population.[31] Premature birth, especially before 28 weeks of gestation, is the leading risk factor for the development of CP.[32] The birth prevalence of CP can reach up to 15% among preterm neonates who were born between 24 and 27 weeks of gestation.[33] The odds of having CP for these groups ranges from 4.7 times the general population for those with non-cerebral congenital defects, to 3.4 times in late preterm infants who are small for gestational age,[34] to a rough approximation of 17.3 times in those with intrauterine drug exposure[28] or 57.6 in moderate to severe neonatal encephalopathy treated with hypothermia.[35,36]

Traditionally, these infants are followed in high-risk infant follow-up programs, with a variety of schedules, assessments, personnel and models.[37] Some programs provide primarily research endpoints while others systematically follow all high-risk children from 0 to school-age, as standard care. Because no mandates from pediatric academic organizations have specified the exact nature or timing of service, this variability persists, with multiple specialties involved in often-disjointed care. High-risk NICU graduates, when not part of research studies, may be seen in primary care and only referred to specialists such as in neurologists or developmental pediatricians when an area of concern is identified.

Often, NICU follow-up is perceived by neonatologists and follow-up personnel alike as a type of safety net, to address issues that may have originated during the NICU stay, but with a longitudinal requirement compared to time-limited intensive care needs. Care coordination between numerous specialties, screening for psychological and social determinants of health, and feeding, growth and nutrition checks and nutrition all fall within these categories,[38] though not all clinics offer all medical services. Other issues that lend themselves to coordinated care between the NICU and outpatient settings include neurodevelopmental concerns and interventions promoting an empowered transition to home for parents and children.[39] For all these follow-up clinic functions and opportunities to develop health care models to better serve these children, articles in the current issue provide excellent points of reference. Overall, high-risk infant follow-up clinics provide an ideal setting for a transitional specialty system, maintaining rapid communication with the NICU and necessarily close ties to community pediatric providers. Follow-up clinics identify those children at highest risk for CP to diagnose them early and to intervene through multidisciplinary partnerships.

## IMPLEMENTATION OF EARLY DETECTION FOR CP IN CLINICAL PRACTICE

While multiple implementation science frameworks are available, with overlap between them and with quality improvement models, one of the easiest to understand is the active implementation framework.[40] Four main steps graduate from planning to installation to early implementation to full implementation. Scale up efforts across networks or countries can also follow local sustaining efforts. Tools and metrics used for implementation are variable, ranging from surveys and standardized questionnaires to Institute for Healthcare Research methodology (eg, Key Driver Diagrams, Plan-Do-Study-Act cycles, Run/Control Charts); and for those transforming systems, business and manufacturing principles such as Six Sigma (eg. Process Flow, Value Added, SIPOC analyses).[41,42]

### Phase 1: Planning/Preparation

Multiple examples of planning/preparation phases have been published. Many are focused on preparation of regional or field research in the field of CP, but a few notable exceptions are entirely focused on implementation science and the high-risk follow-up clinic setting. The planning phase of the first documented clinical implementation of the early detection of CP guidelines occurred in Columbus, Ohio,[21] where Strengths, Weaknesses, Opportunities and Threats (SWOT) analyses were conducted to form an action plan. The follow-up clinic there had ~4500 annual visits, a catchment area of 200 square miles in a state with ~12 million inhabitants. Notable weaknesses included staffing utilization, lack of standardized assessments, high no-show rates, limited research experience, lack of knowledge base in early CP assessments and effective interventions, and inconsistent use of clinic documentation in the EMR. Threats included sustainability/return on investment and home-based program offerings at other institutions. Recently, Williams and colleagues conducted a year-long planning phase study in New Zealand during which they assessed enablers and barriers to implementation of the early detection guidelines.[43] Among the 159 surveyed participants, while the vast majority were aware that tools existed often-cited, systems barriers to utilization ranged from time, workload and staffing concerns, to lack or inconsistent referral pathways. Funding for education was also cited as a barrier along with confidence in using tools and lack of clinical pathways. Interestingly, in the 54 diagnosing providers, MRI was used as a tool for diagnosis more frequently in the under 1 year than lower resource tools such as the GMA and HINE (MRI: 46% and 59% vs. 25% for GMA and 15% for HINE).

### Phase 2: Installation

Installation usually includes training to build capacity in a system; in the case of early detection of CP, this includes high-evidence assessments. Two concrete examples of this phase across the world include new use of the GMA in India and Bangladesh[44] and development of a standardized HINE workshop followed by routine use in a large high-risk infant follow-up clinic in the US.[22]

Prechtl's GMA relies on observation of spontaneous movement patterns which originate in fetal life and evolve into characteristic patterns in periods termed writhing (near-term equivalent age) and fidgety (at 12–16 weeks post term age). Prechtl's GMA has 97% sensitivity and 89% specificity at fidgety age and has 93% sensitivity and 59% specificity at writhing age for later CP in select high risk populations.[45] In more mixed follow-up clinic settings (as opposed to primarily research settings), the GMA appears somewhat less specific.[46] Implementation into practice of Prechtl's GMA can be challenging due to a limited number of Prechtl's Trust trainers in the world, the high resource demands of the training, the need for regular practice and recalibration with advanced trained Prechtl's Trust trainers to maintain accuracy over time.[47] Exporting video recording of infants can prove challenging depending on HIPAA and other privacy concerns, hospital information technology safeguards; storing these videos into EMRs can require additional protected cloud storage. Nonetheless, the GMA remains a rapid, non-invasive bedside assessment. Based on this, an Australian team led by Dr. Benfer [44] was able to train providers to use this as an early CP screen and use it to enroll patients in an RCT of 142 infants. Others have developed phone apps to allow remote recording of GMAs to be read by a central reader with the main difference being the use of HIPAA compliant Redcap apps in the US, and cloud-based apps in Australia.[48] Ultimately, the challenges inherent in using human visual recognition for four-dimensional patterns will be overcome through various artificial intelligence solutions; currently though, these machine-based tools are still imprecise and have yet to become widely feasible.

In the case of the HINE, an installation challenge was the lack of any standardized training programs to achieve reliability with a neurologic exam used in many research publications. Development of a clinical workshop for a follow-up team that included theory, video demonstration, hands on practice and testing of fidelity was published in 2016.[49] It was refined with input from some of the neurologists trained by Dr. Dubowitz, the initial developer of the examination.[50–52] Finally, a train-the-trainer program and reliability check process were developed to allow capacity building with this critical tool for high-risk infant follow-up.

### Phase 3: Early Implementation

In 2018, the Monash Children's Hospital in Australia leveraged their Early Neurodevelopment Clinic to implement evidence-based guidelines for the early diagnosis of CP in high-risk infants.[53] This clinic showed for the first time in Australia that it was feasible to implement the early CP diagnosis guidelines into a high-risk infant follow-up clinic, and in one year, 9 children were diagnosed with CP and 11 classified as having high-risk for CP, using best evidence tools. It was unclear if the implementation was effective in decreasing the age at CP diagnosis, previously reported at 19 months in Australia, as no baseline or post-intervention age at diagnosis were presented. However, decreased age at diagnosis is likely since the age at visits for reported patients was on average 13 months. In the single clinic example reported above for Phase 1,[21] process metrics such as 3 to -4 month visits with HINE and GMA increased and age at CP diagnosis for new patients in the clinic pathway decreased from 18 to 13 months on average. In this case, those patients already in the clinic may have also benefitted from the initiative, as mean age at CP diagnosis for all patients decreased from 28 to 16 months. While others have reported recent implementation initiatives, none were in traditional high-risk infant follow up programs after the NICU.

### Phase 4: Full Implementation

In the case of the first clinical program to implement the CP early detection guidelines in their entirety, full implementation occurred after an initial phase of verification, troubleshooting and development of a support program and process for those providers who may initially have difficulties with diagnostic conversations. The high-risk infant follow-up clinic's initial success was followed by outreach to community primary care providers, with dissemination of tools to help with CP referral pathways and training of regional early intervention therapists in the HINE.[54] Following this, referrals from the community increased and resulted in addition of patients with newborn attributable risks. The HRIF clinic diagnosed ~100 new cases annually, or ~1/3 of the state's new cases.[21,49]

In a CP clinical in New South Wales, Australia, Velde and colleagues described the single-center implementation of early detection guidelines.[55] Parent and referrer acceptability of the clinic was high, supporting access to CP-specific early interventions when they are likely to be most effective.

Across a US Early Detection and Implementation (EDI) Network of high-risk follow-up programs, examination of drivers decreasing the age at CP diagnosis revealed the importance of a 3–4-month visit completion, with basic elements at least the HINE, GMA, a medical history, and a motor function assessment. This visit itself constituted a process metric that drove the success of the project, especially since 90% of sites did not have such a visit prior to implementation, and none had it with all elements consistently. As important as the data obtained from the standardized elements may appear, the opportunity a the 3-4-month visit provided was in starting conversations about risk of CP and engaging caregivers in critical diagnostic planning and execution. As the number of these visits tripled over full implementation, the age at diagnosis decreased from a weighted average of 19.5 to 9.5 months corrected age.[22]

### Phase 5: Scale-up and Sustainability

Currently, only one example of sustainability across an HRIF network can be found, due to the recent nature of most implementation efforts. The previously mentioned CP Early Detection Implementation (EDI) Network, has been in existence for 5 years, allowing the examination of various sustainability data. In particular, the Network faced the challenges of sustaining their primary aim, an average age of diagnosis of 12 months through the challenges of the COVID pandemic. High-risk infant follow-up at this time had highly variable responses to the shut-down and resumption of outpatient visits, from telehealth, to in person to hybrid models.[56] To address this challenge, the lead site quickly developed a standardized telehealth version of their basic detection elements, and ensured their integration in clinical processes through a value-added-analysis.[57] Sites then quickly rolled these out and improved the telehealth tools, with the result that early CP diagnosis was maintained throughout the network, even with the addition of 3 new sites and subtraction of 2 original sites (**Fig. 1** A). A new metric, the "High-Risk for CP designation", was adopted across

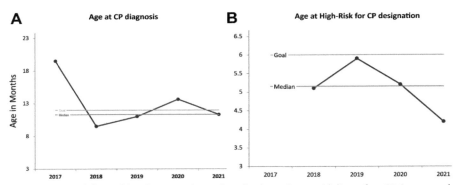

**Fig. 1.** Sustainability of implementation of early detection guidelines for CP in an early detection network. Green lines indicate goal age while red lines indicate the median for the 5-year period. (A) (left): Weighted-mean age at CP diagnosis; (B) (right): Weighted-mean age at "High risk for CP" designation (note that no designation was available at baseline before guidelines were implemented.

---

**Box 1**
**"High-Risk for Cerebral Palsy" clinical designation**

Basic elements of diagnosis include: clinical history consistent with etiology of CP, neurological exam with qualitatively documented impairments, quantitative decreases in motor function on standardized assessments, positive CP biomarkers (genetic test positive for conditions associated with CP and not progressive disorders, HINE scores below threshold for age or general movements pattern (cramped synchronized or absent fidgety)

| *Situation 1* | *Situation 2* |
| At the time of evaluation, A basic element is missing/an assessment was not performed or OR An basic element had a negative result for predicting later CP but others are positive | A clinician is evaluating the child for the first time well before the age of 2 years and no previous evaluations have demonstrated clear concerns. |

---

the network. Despite an increase at the age at which this designation was given during the height of the pandemic, sites steadily returned to a baseline near their goal of 12 months CA (**Fig. 1**B).

The importance of the designation prompted the EDI Network to circulate a consensus statement for this clinical concept, aimed to develop a common language across providers and start shared decision-making with parents, beyond the purpose of varied definitions used in research studies or systematic reviews (**Box 1**). In 2022, more than 150 clinicians and patient-oriented researchers across the US, Canada and Europe endorsed the consensus.[58] The majority were part of follow-up programs, supporting a new paradigm for care models in these settings.

## CONCLUSION AND FUTURE DIRECTIONS

Early efforts across implementation phases and sustainability of early CP diagnosis have now paved the way for international scale-up efforts. Some have started through knowledge translation and dissemination efforts, for example, at research and implementation conferences.[54,59] Others have partnered with international organizations to expand and adapt implementation to developed and low middle income countries (LMIC). Examples include the new partnership between the Cerebral Palsy Foundation (CPF), the US EDI Network and INFANT -the Irish Center for Maternal and Child Health Research,[60] to implement early detection of CP in the Irish Network of high-risk infant follow-up programs. Another example is a partnership between the CPF, Emory University, and United Nations Children's Fund (UNICEF) to detect CP and intervene early in LMIC, this time leveraging previous work in the US and adapting the best evidence in CP interventions to in-country and provider types within follow-up clinics as well as community-based environments.[61] This last example allows us to conclude with a return to the purpose of early detection of CP in high-risk follow-up clinics: ultimately, the goal is to improve the outcomes of infants who have perinatal insults or disorders contributing to their CP presentation. By implementing early detection of CP in these programs, children and their families should have access to safe, specific, efficacious and effective interventions that can change their developmental trajectories. By providing the best care for those at high risk for CP, high-risk follow-up clinics fulfill not only surveillance missions but also those of actively improving developmental outcomes.

## DISCLOSURE

NLM has equity in Thrive Neuromedical and a patent licensed to Enlighten Mobility. No conflict of interest is present with the review above.

## REFERENCES

1. CDC. CP data 2021. 2021. Available at: https://www.cdc.gov/ncbddd/cp/data.html. Accessed 01 25, 2022.
2. UNICEF Child Demo. 2021. Available at: https://data.unicef.org/resources/dataset/the-state-of-the-worlds-children-2021-statistical-tables/. Accessed January 25, 2022.
3. Sellier E, Platt MJ, Andersen GL, et al. Decreasing prevalence in cerebral palsy: a multi-site European population-based study, 1980 to 2003. Dev Med Child Neurol 2016;58(1):85–92.
4. Durkin MS, Benedict RE, Christensen D, et al. Prevalence of cerebral palsy among 8-year-Old children in 2010 and Preliminary evidence of trends in its Relationship to low birthweight. Paediatr Perinat Epidemiol 2016;30(5):496–510.
5. Galea C, McIntyre S, Smithers-Sheedy H, et al. Cerebral palsy trends in Australia (1995-2009): a population-based observational study. Dev Med Child Neurol 2019;61(2):186–93.
6. Stetson BT, Buhimschi CS, Kellert BA, et al. Comparison of cerebral palsy severity between 2 Eras of antenatal Magnesium Use. JAMA Pediatr 2019; 173(2):188–90.
7. Linsell L, Malouf R, Morris J, et al. Prognostic factors for cerebral palsy and motor impairment in children born very preterm or very low birthweight: a systematic review. Dev Med Child Neurol 2016;58(6):554–69.
8. Kramer KP, Minot K, Butler C, et al. Reduction of severe intraventricular hemorrhage in preterm infants: a quality improvement project. Pediatrics 2022;149(3). e2021050652.
9. Adams-Chapman I, Heyne RJ, DeMauro SB, et al. Neurodevelopmental impairment among extremely preterm infants in the neonatal research network. Pediatrics 2018;141(5). e20173091.
10. Taylor GL, O'Shea TM. Extreme prematurity: risk and resiliency. Curr Probl Pediatr Adolesc Health Care 2022;52(2):101132.
11. Charkaluk ML, Truffert P, Fily A, et al. Neurodevelopment of children born very preterm and free of severe disabilities: the Nord-Pas de Calais Epipage cohort study. Acta Paediatr 2010;99(5):684–9.
12. Haak P, Lenski M, Hidecker MJ, et al. Cerebral palsy and aging. Dev Med Child Neurol 2009;51(Suppl 4):16–23.
13. Yi YG, Jung SH, Bang MS. Emerging issues in cerebral palsy associated with aging: a Physiatrist Perspective. Ann Rehabil Med 2019;43(3):241–9.
14. Byrne R, Duncan A, Pickar T, et al. Comparing parent and provider priorities in discussions of early detection and intervention for infants with and at risk of cerebral palsy. Child Care Health Dev 2019;45(6):799–807.
15. Baird G, McConachie H, Scrutton D. Parents' perceptions of disclosure of the diagnosis of cerebral palsy. Arch Dis Child 2000;83(6):475–80.
16. Morgan C, Fetters L, Adde L, et al. Early intervention for children aged 0 to 2 Years with or at high risk of cerebral palsy: international clinical practice guideline based on systematic reviews. JAMA Pediatr 2021;175(8):846–58.
17. Johnston MV. Plasticity in the developing brain: implications for rehabilitation. Dev Disabil Res Rev 2009;15(2):94–101.
18. Maitre NL, Jeanvoine A, Yoder PJ, et al. Kinematic and Somatosensory Gains in infants with cerebral palsy after a multi-Component Upper-Extremity intervention: a Randomized controlled trial. Brain Topogr 2020;33(6):751–66.

19. Badawi N, Watson L, Petterson B, et al. What constitutes cerebral palsy? Dev Med Child Neurol 1998;40(8):520–7.
20. Rosenbaum P, Paneth N, Leviton A, et al. A report: the definition and classification of cerebral palsy April 2006. Dev Med Child Neurol Suppl 2007;109:8–14.
21. Byrne R, Noritz G, Maitre NL, et al. Implementation of early diagnosis and intervention guidelines for cerebral palsy in a high-risk infant follow-up clinic. Pediatr Neurol 2017;76:66–71.
22. Maitre NL, Burton VJ, Duncan AF, et al. Network implementation of guideline for early detection decreases age at cerebral palsy diagnosis. Pediatrics 2020; 145(5).
23. Krageloh-Mann I, Helber A, Mader I, et al. Bilateral lesions of thalamus and basal ganglia: origin and outcome. Dev Med Child Neurol 2002;44(7):477–84.
24. Maitre N. Skepticism, cerebral palsy, and the general movements assessment. Dev Med Child Neurol 2018;60(5):438.
25. Romeo DM, Ricci D, Brogna C, et al. Use of the Hammersmith Infant Neurological Examination in infants with cerebral palsy: a critical review of the literature. Dev Med Child Neurol 2016;58(3):240–5.
26. Damiano DL, Longo E, Carolina de Campos A, et al. Systematic review of clinical guidelines related to care of Individuals with cerebral palsy as part of the world health organization efforts to develop a Global Package of interventions for rehabilitation. Arch Phys Med Rehabil 2021;102(9):1764–74.
27. Novak I, Morgan C, Adde L, et al. Early, accurate diagnosis and early intervention in cerebral palsy: Advances in diagnosis and treatment. JAMA Pediatr 2017; 171(9):897–907.
28. Benninger KL, Purnell J, Conroy S, et al. Intrauterine drug exposure as a risk factor for cerebral palsy. Dev Med Child Neurol 2022;64(4):453–61.
29. Handley SC, Lorch SA. Regionalization of neonatal care: benefits, barriers, and beyond. J Perinatol 2022;42(6):835–8.
30. Pediatrics AAo. 2022. Available at: https://www.aap.org/en/patient-care/neonatal-care/nicu-verification-program-process-and-fees/. Accessed 10 24, 2022.
31. Beaino G, Khoshnood B, Kaminski M, et al. Predictors of cerebral palsy in very preterm infants: the EPIPAGE prospective population-based cohort study. Dev Med Child Neurol 2010;52(6):e119–25.
32. O'Shea TM, Allred EN, Dammann O, et al. The ELGAN study of the brain and related disorders in extremely low gestational age newborns. Early Hum Dev 2009;85(11):719–25.
33. Himpens E, Van den Broeck C, Oostra A, et al. Prevalence, type, distribution, and severity of cerebral palsy in relation to gestational age: a meta-analytic review. Dev Med Child Neurol 2008;50(5):334–40.
34. Zhao M, Dai H, Deng Y, et al. SGA as a risk factor for cerebral palsy in moderate to late preterm infants: a system review and meta-analysis. Sci Rep 2016;6: 38853.
35. Blair E, Al Asedy F, Badawi N, et al. Is cerebral palsy associated with birth defects other than cerebral defects? Dev Med Child Neurol 2007;49(4):252–8.
36. Zhang S, Li B, Zhang X, et al. Birth Asphyxia is associated with increased risk of cerebral palsy: a meta-analysis. Front Neurol 2020;11:704.
37. Kuppala VS, Tabangin M, Haberman B, et al. Current state of high-risk infant follow-up care in the United States: results of a national survey of academic follow-up programs. J Perinatol 2012;32(4):293–8.
38. Bockli K, Andrews B, Pellerite M, et al. Trends and challenges in United States neonatal intensive care units follow-up clinics. J Perinatol 2014;34(1):71–4.

39. Phillips RM, Goldstein M, Hougland K, et al. Multidisciplinary guidelines for the care of late preterm infants. J Perinatol 2013;33(Suppl 2):S5–22.

40. Blanchard C, Livet M, Ward C, et al. The active implementation frameworks: a roadmap for advancing implementation of comprehensive Medication Management in primary care. Res Social Adm Pharm 2017;13(5):922–9.

41. Ogrinc GSHL, Barton AJ, Dolansky MA, et al. Fundamentals of health care improvement: a Guide to improving Your patients' care. 4th ed. Joint Commission Resources and Institute for Healthcare Improvement; 2022.

42. Rathi R, Vakharia A, Shadab M. Lean six sigma in the healthcare sector: a systematic literature review. Mater Today Proc 2022;50:773–81.

43. Williams SA, Mackey A, Sorhage A, et al. Clinical practice of health professionals working in early detection for infants with or at risk of cerebral palsy across New Zealand. J Paediatr Child Health 2021;57(4):541–7.

44. Benfer KA, Novak I, Morgan C, et al. Community-based parent-delivered early detection and intervention programme for infants at high risk of cerebral palsy in a low-resource country (Learning through Everyday Activities with Parents (LEAP-CP): protocol for a randomised controlled trial. BMJ Open 2018;8(6): e021186.

45. Kwong AKL, Fitzgerald TL, Doyle LW, et al. Predictive validity of spontaneous early infant movement for later cerebral palsy: a systematic review. Dev Med Child Neurol 2018;60(5):480–9.

46. Stoen R, Boswell L, de Regnier RA, et al. The Predictive accuracy of the general movement assessment for cerebral palsy: a prospective, observational study of high-risk infants in a clinical follow-up setting. J Clin Med 2019;8(11):1790–801.

47. Peyton C, Pascal A, Boswell L, et al. Inter-observer reliability using the General Movement Assessment is influenced by rater experience. Early Hum Dev 2021; 161:105436.

48. Spittle AJ, Olsen J, Kwong A, et al. The Baby Moves prospective cohort study protocol: using a smartphone application with the General Movements Assessment to predict neurodevelopmental outcomes at age 2 years for extremely preterm or extremely low birthweight infants. BMJ Open 2016;6(10):e013446.

49. Maitre NL, Chorna O, Romeo DM, et al. Implementation of the Hammersmith infant neurological examination in a high-risk infant follow-up program. Pediatr Neurol 2016;65:31–8.

50. Haataja L, Cowan F, Mercuri E, et al. Application of a scorable neurologic examination in healthy term infants aged 3 to 8 months. J Pediatr 2003;143(4):546.

51. Haataja L, Mercuri E, Regev R, et al. Optimality score for the neurologic examination of the infant at 12 and 18 months of age. J Pediatr 1999;135(2 Pt 1):153–61.

52. Dubowitz L, Mercuri E, Dubowitz V. An optimality score for the neurologic examination of the term newborn. J Pediatr 1998;133(3):406–16.

53. King AR, Machipisa C, Finlayson F, et al. Early detection of cerebral palsy in high-risk infants: translation of evidence into practice in an Australian hospital. J Paediatr Child Health 2021;57(2):246–50.

54. Foundation CP. Implementation of early detection & intervention for cerebral palsy conference. 2022. Available at: https://cpearlydetection.org. Accessed 10 20, 2022.

55. Te Velde A, Tantsis E, Novak I, et al. Age of diagnosis, fidelity and acceptability of an early diagnosis clinic for cerebral palsy: a single site implementation study. Brain Sci 2021;11(8):1074–87.

56. Panda S, Somu R, Maitre N, et al. Impact of the Coronavirus pandemic on high-risk infant follow-up (HRIF) programs: a survey of academic programs. Children (Basel) 2021;8(10):889–99.

57. Maitre NL, Benninger KL, Neel ML, et al. Standardized neurodevelopmental surveillance of high-risk infants using telehealth: implementation study during COVID-19. Pediatr Qual Saf 2021;6(4):e439.

58. Maitre NL, Byrne R, Duncan A, et al. High-risk for cerebral palsy" designation: a clinical consensus statement. J Pediatr Rehabil Med 2022;15(1):165–74.

59. Queensland Uo. LEAP-CP Symposium 2019. 2019. Available at: https://qcprrc. centre.uq.edu.au/article/2019/12/LEAPCPsymposium2019. Accessed 20 10, 2022.

60. University C. Infant center. Available at: https://www.infantcentre.ie/. Accessed 10 20, 2022.

61. Damiano DL, Forssberg H. International initiatives to improve the lives of children with developmental disabilities. Dev Med Child Neurol 2019;61(10):1121.

# The Future of High-Risk Infant Follow-Up

Nathalie L. Maitre, MD, PhD[a,b,]*, Andrea F. Duncan, MD, MS[c,d]

## KEYWORDS

- High-risk • Follow-up • Infant • High-risk infant follow-up programs

## KEY POINTS

- High-risk infant follow-up has evolved from primarily documentation of outcomes to developing novel models of care, including new high-risk populations and psychosocial factors, and incorporating targeted interventions to improve outcomes.
- Technology, systems, and scientific research and humanism can combine to build a far different future for our patients and their families.
- Environmental factors and social determinants of health are our responsibility to address and within our capacity to change.

As this issue of Clinics in Perinatology illustrates, a profound shift has occurred in the driving purpose of high-risk infant follow-up (HRIF) over the past 5 years. As a result, HRIF has evolved from primarily providing an ethical compass, concerned surveillance and documentation of outcomes. It is now understood that developing novel models of care, considering new high-risk populations, settings, and psychosocial factors, and incorporating active, targeted interventions to improve outcomes (**Fig. 1**) are critical components of exemplary HRIF care. High-risk infant follow-up programs are less concerned about providing "prognostic" information for families of hospitalized infants, recognizing that parents do not care as much about abstract or general concepts, but instead prefer specific, goal-oriented conversations about the future. Instead, HRIF programs focus on standardized surveillance, continuous improvements in care through quality improvement or implementation science, and partnerships with researchers that allow the testing of new interventions to change developmental outcomes, whether at the transition to home or in the outpatient setting. After decades of documenting poor outcomes, the focus is shifting to

[a] Department of Pediatrics, Emory University School of Medicine, Atlanta, GA, USA; [b] Children's Healthcare of Atlanta, Atlanta, GA, USA; [c] Division of Neonatology, Department of Pediatrics, Children's Hospital of Philadelphia, 3401 Civic Center Boulevard, 2nd Floor Main, Neonatology, Philadelphia, PA 19104, USA; [d] Department of Pediatrics, University of Pennsylvania Perelman School of Medicine, Philadelphia, PA, USA
* Corresponding author. Baby Brain Optimization Project at Emory, 1123 Zonolite Road Suite 22, Atlanta, GA 30306.
*E-mail address:* nmaitre@emory.edu

Clin Perinatol 50 (2023) 281–283
https://doi.org/10.1016/j.clp.2022.11.006
0095-5108/23/© 2022 Elsevier Inc. All rights reserved.

perinatology.theclinics.com

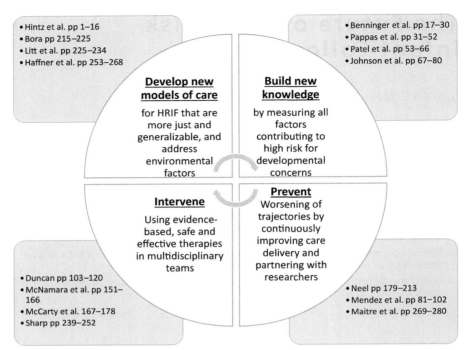

**Fig. 1.** Framework for improving high-risk infant outcomes via follow-up programs and corresponding *clinics* articles.

performing interventions, resilience, and understanding those children who have better than expected outcomes. What can these children, their families, and their providers teach us? How can we aspire, in the funny yet prescient words of Garrison Keillor, for all our children to be above average?[1]

Every one of the articles in this issue recommends an avenue for future improvement or research. We are finally at a phase of HRIF history where technology, systems, scientific research, and humanism can combine to build a far different future for our patients and their families. We are fortunate that interdisciplinary clinicians, advocates, and researchers currently work toward a common goal across social, medical, and geographical settings. However, there are still two pressing issues that may slow us down. First, we cannot accept the status quo that environmental factors and social determinants of health are neither our responsibility to address nor within our capacity to change. Although these problems may seem too enormous for HRIF programs to tackle alone, they can certainly partner together, with community partners, state institutions, and stakeholder foundations to intervene early, when the return on investment for disadvantaged populations is greatest.[2] Secondly, we must, as for the first point, work in synergy across disciplines and continents. With the globalization of Internet-based platforms and advances in telecommunications, there is no longer any reason why an outpatient therapist and a neonatologist cannot work as research partners, or a social worker/community health worker and clinic-based developmental pediatrician cannot collaborate on new care model development. Similarly, through continued communication with national and international stakeholders, successful practices implemented in other environments may be adapted for new geographic, institutional, or community areas without having to start the creative process from scratch. The reasons that propel providers to care for those who are most vulnerable should make it easy for us to successfully work as teams across variable environments and resource strata; the selflessness, caring, and passion that push us to give all of ourselves to these patients and their families despite challenges that are far greater than those of controlled hospital settings should help us break artificial, self-imposed barriers. If we cannot do it completely for ourselves, we should at least learn from this issue and its articles; we can empower our families and our trainees to learn and advocate for change, because they are the true future of HRIF.

## DISCLOSURE

Dr Maitre is co-founder and has equity in SmallTalk. Dr Maitre is funded by the National Institutes of Health (R01HD081120;R01HD093706) and a Cerebral Palsy Foundation Network Award. There are no conflicts to report regarding this submission.

## REFERENCES

1. Maxwell NL, Lopus JS. The lake wobegon effect in student self-reported data. Am Econ Rev 1994;84(2):201–5.
2. Heckman JJ. Skill formation and the economics of investing in disadvantaged children. Science 2006;312(5782):1900–2.

# Moving?

## Make sure your subscription moves with you!

To notify us of your new address, find your **Clinics Account Number** (located on your mailing label above your name), and contact customer service at:

**Email: journalscustomerservice-usa@elsevier.com**

**800-654-2452** (subscribers in the U.S. & Canada)
**314-447-8871** (subscribers outside of the U.S. & Canada)

**Fax number: 314-447-8029**

**Elsevier Health Sciences Division**
**Subscription Customer Service**
**3251 Riverport Lane**
**Maryland Heights, MO 63043**

*To ensure uninterrupted delivery of your subscription, please notify us at least 4 weeks in advance of move.